AIDS

AIDS

The Making of a Chronic Disease

Edited by
Elizabeth Fee and
Daniel M. Fox

UNIVERSITY OF CALIFORNIA PRESS
Berkeley · *Los Angeles* · *Oxford*

University of California Press
Berkeley and Los Angeles, California

University of California Press, Ltd.
Oxford, England

© 1992 by
The Regents of the University of California

Library of Congress Cataloging-in-Publication Data

AIDS : the making of a chronic disease / edited by Elizabeth Fee and
  Daniel M. Fox.
    p. cm.
  Includes bibliographical references and index.
  ISBN 0-520-07569-2 (cloth : alk. paper)
  ISBN 0-520-07778-4 (paper : alk. paper)
  1. AIDS (Disease)—History. I. Fee, Elizabeth. II. Fox, Daniel M.
  [DNLM: 1. Acquired Immunodeficiency Syndrome—epidemiology.
  2. Acquired Immunodeficiency Syndrome—history. 3. Acquired
  Immunodeficiency Syndrome—legislation. 4. Ethics, Medical.
  5. Health Policy. WD 308 A288544]
  RA644.A25A3769   1992
  614.5'993—dc20
  DNLM/DLC
  for Library of Congress   91-731
                                                                CIP

Printed in the United States of America

9 8 7 6 5 4 3 2 1

Contents

Introduction:
The Contemporary
Historiography of AIDS

Elizabeth Fee and Daniel M. Fox

AIDS "has stimulated more interest in history than any other disease of modern times," as we wrote in the introduction to *AIDS: The Burdens of History* in 1988.[1] This interest led many commentators to employ history, and sometimes even historians, to explain what this epidemic has in common with devastating infections in the past. Now, a decade after AIDS was first recognized, there is increasing evidence that analogies to the past can be misleading, as they usually are in the history of war or economies or anything else. In this essay we summarize and criticize the brief historiography of the epidemic and suggest research questions and methods that may lead to more valid and useful historical writing. We then introduce the essays in this volume, essays that lead us in the directions we have proposed as both necessary and useful.

The history of AIDS is a problem in contemporary history. The problem the epidemic raises for historians and for others who use historical methods is to understand the intricacies of the relationships among people and the institutions they have created in the closing decades of the twentieth century.

In the early 1980s most accounts presented AIDS as a radical break from the historical trends of the twentieth century, at least in the industrialized nations: a sudden, unexpected, and disastrous return to a vanished world of epidemic disease. Historians and most other people who paid attention to AIDS addressed it as a startling discontinuity with the past. The new epidemic seemed to bear little relationship to the diseases that absorbed the most attention and resources—the chronic diseases of an aging population. Epidemic disease belonged to history, a history that most had comfortably forgotten. But faced with the new threat of AIDS, people felt a need to reach back into history to discover how previous epidemics had been handled: how had societies dealt with plague, cholera, and polio? We searched for analogues in the past.

We found some apparently significant parallels and some similar themes in past epidemics: themes that seemed useful. Most of the essays in *AIDS: The Burdens of History* followed this pattern, as did a set of conference papers published in *Social Research*.[2] The editor of the latter collection made explicit the analogy to past epidemics by choosing the title "In Time of Plague." Media accounts of the epidemic increasingly made use of historians' references to past plagues, and Susan Sontag drew on the work of historians for her influential *AIDS and Its Metaphors*.[3] Sontag, however, inverted the historians' argument that diseases must be understood in their social and cultural context; she wanted to strip disease of its social and cultural meanings, or metaphors, leaving behind only what she regarded as pure biology. Barbara Rosenkrantz's note of warning has largely gone unheeded: "The ordinary vices that tempt us to make simple sense of history are, not surprisingly, embedded in our culture. They offer the same temptations that we face in mounting resistance to the uncertainties of epidemic disease: the vice of 'whiggery' through which we celebrate linear progress and reassuringly demonstrate how evil is overwhelmed by good, and the vice of relativism, which separates the event from its context so we may conclude that nothing has really changed."[4]

Several aspects of the early years of the AIDS epidemic had made analogies with past epidemics seem relevant. AIDS was an infectious disease that defied cure and, for a few years, even the implication of a causal organism. More important, AIDS seemed to resonate to great historical themes—notably the victimizing and stigmatizing of helpless members of minority groups and the indifference of public officials callous to human suffering. The disease attacked gay men just a few years after they had, for the first time in modern history, been freed from the most overt oppression and, at least in major cities, had asserted a visible political presence. The disease allowed some journalists and politicians a ready opportunity to express—more accurately, to resurrect—fear and resentment toward newly visible and assertive gay communities. Moreover, the disease struck at the time when containing health costs had become a major objective of governments in the United States and Western Europe, and these governments were reluctant to recognize, let alone deal with, the potentially devastating costs of coping with a new epidemic. The battle between a beleaguered gay community and a government apparently indifferent to the epidemic provided the dramatic point and counterpoint for Randy Shilts's *And the Band Played On*.[5] Indeed, many of the themes of early AIDS historiography dealt with the insensitivity of governments, socially and morally repressive attitudes to sexual behavior, the tendency of those in power to blame the poor or other disenfranchised groups for harboring dread diseases, and the potential threat of quarantines or other attacks on individual rights—all themes that were complaints or fears of a gay community facing an unsympathetic, indeed hostile, administration in Washington (and, by some accounts, in the capital cities of Europe).

Debates about how to respond to the epidemic reinforced the belief that AIDS was discontinuous with the recent past. Oversimply, these were arguments between alarmists on the one hand and advocates of equanimity on the other. The alarmists found analogies to the present in the great epidemics of infectious disease—notably bubonic plague, cholera, yellow fever, influenza, and polio. They urged adoption of what had become the classic repertoire of public health responses to epidemics: enhanced surveillance, mobilization of medical resources, and increased research. Advocates of equanimity used different historical parallels. They recalled times in the past when exaggeration of the severity of an outbreak of infectious disease had led to the deflection of resources from areas of greater need, the exchange of individual rights for an illusory collective good, and diminished repute for the enterprise of public health. These advocates needed to go no further back than the flu nonepidemic of 1976, although historians soon supplied them with many earlier examples.

Both the alarmists and the advocates of equanimity agreed that AIDS was a contemporary plague. They shared the belief that history was pertinent to understanding the epidemic and that the events in the past that were most pertinent were those surrounding sudden, time-limited outbreaks of infection. This agreement was the result of the shock of discontinuity in the early 1980s. Many people were unwilling to believe that a disease that had emerged (it seemed) so suddenly, and appeared to be invariably fatal, was either deeply rooted in the past or likely to become part of the human condition for the foreseeable future.

Because the history of visitations of plagues was the only history that appeared relevant to the new epidemic, most people ignored the alternative historical models that were available. For example, most of those who used historical analogies avoided the most pertinent aspects of the histories of venereal disease and tuberculosis, emphasizing issues of surveillance and personal control policy and ignoring the problems of housing, long-term care, public education, and the financing of palliative care for people suffering from chronic infections. Tuberculosis and venereal disease had been, for many years, both endemic and intractable. For individuals, they were chronic, debilitating conditions; lifetime burdens. For the people who provided and paid for health services, these diseases were characterized by a few acute episodes and long periods when patients required no care or only supportive care. For public health officials, venereal disease and tuberculosis raised difficult problems about surveillance, public education, and the long-term control of noncompliant patients. Yet in the early years of the AIDS epidemic, people who sought historical analogies explored venereal disease and tuberculosis mainly for what they could learn about screening, contact tracing, and the restraint of patients who were dangerous to others. The history of the two leading chronic infectious diseases of modern times, that is, was used to understand a very different situation, a polity threatened by devastating plague.[6]

At the end of the first decade of what is now called the epidemic of HIV infection, the initial sense of discontinuity with the past seems ironic. For some people, especially those with the infection or close to people who have it, the psychological alternative to discontinuity is devastating. The alternative to discontinuity is admitting that the threat of disease is not transient, not a matter of a bad season or a terrible year; not, that is, like the Black Death or cholera or yellow fever. For public officials, health industry leaders, and physicians, the idea that AIDS would become another killer chronic disease, like heart disease, cancer, and stroke, has been unpalatable because it adds to the already overwhelming financial and organizational problems of health policy. Yet for all these people it is becoming increasingly plain that AIDS, like tuberculosis during most of the nineteenth century, may be, for particular populations, an endemic life-threatening condition.

By the mid-1980s concerned physicians, public officials, and gay leaders no longer had to demand attention to an unrecognized life-threatening epidemic. AIDS was institutionalized within academic medicine and the medical care establishment. The patterns of research, services, and financing of care in the 1990s have more to do with long-term strategies for responding to diseases such as cancer than with the epidemic diseases of the past. It may well be horrifying to realize that

AIDS is fitting our patterns of dealing with chronic disease, since it puts the problem into a long-term perspective. But if we assume that the rate of HIV infection will continue for the 1990s much as it did for the 1980s; if we assume that, as with cancer, most treatments will prolong life rather than cure the disease; if we assume that scientific research will continue to expand our knowledge rather than soon provide a means of prevention or cure; and if we assume that we will continue to respond to AIDS through the provision of specialized hospital units, long-term care, and other institutional services, we must also conclude that we are dealing not with a brief, time-limited epidemic but with a long, slow process more analogous to cancer than to cholera.

When, separately and together, we presented an earlier version of this argument in March 1989, it generated considerable distress and skepticism. Three months later, by June 1989, the idea that AIDS should be regarded as a chronic illness was widely accepted; in a speech at the final plenary session of the international AIDS meeting in Montreal, Samuel Broder, head of the National Cancer Institute, publicly declared that AIDS is a chronic disease and cancer the appropriate analogue for therapy.[7] Such rapid shifts in public perception illustrate how quickly things change in the world of AIDS. As contemporary perceptions of AIDS change, so too does its history; historical accounts that at one time seemed most relevant to understanding the epidemic need to be replaced by new interpretations. Such shifts in the relevance of historical texts are, of course, familiar—but in the case of AIDS, they can be especially rapid.

As a result of huge increases in funding for AIDS research and services, AIDS has now entered mainstream medicine in the United States and Western Europe. AIDS services are being financed by the existing system of private medical insurance and government programs. The costs of AIDS are being met by shifting around budgets. Today the problem of health policy is not so much to provoke a more generous official response to AIDS as to make sure that other health programs are not sacrificed to feed the swelling budgets appropriated for AIDS research and services.

Today, moreover, there is relatively little talk about quarantine, isolation, and mass testing for the disease. The immediate panicked reactions to the disease have been replaced by medical management; even if we can do little more to treat the disease than we could five years ago, we know that responsibility for its management has now passed into the hands of those who organize and control our medical care system.

The lessons of contemporary history, when they are assessed, will be different from those drawn from the epidemic diseases of the past.

The analogy between AIDS and past plagues—the argument that this epidemic constitutes a sharp break with recent history and can best be understood in relation to more distant events—is itself data for contemporary history. The insistence on discontinuity was useful, politically as well as psychologically, in the early years of the epidemic. Discontinuity was a story that many people used to comprehend dangerous, distracting, and depressing events. It was also a theme that could be used to leverage additional resources for surveillance, research, and treatment of the disease.

Professional historians were not casual bystanders in the making of a history of the AIDS epidemic as discontinuous with the recent past and best understood by examining past plagues. Many historians, including ourselves, found analogies to AIDS in time-limited visitations of infectious disease in the past. It became fashionable to make references to AIDS at the beginning and the end of historical articles and monographs ostensibly dealing with other subjects in the history of medicine or sexual behavior.[8]

Historians should not be faulted for making AIDS a minor industry or for sharing an interpretation of the past that made sense to most other people who talked and wrote about the epidemic. It is pleasant to find one's work suddenly regarded as relevant, or to have it disseminated, even if in caricature, by the media. Historians of medicine have, in general, been consulted about recent events less often than, say, our colleagues who study war and foreign affairs.

Most historians have no special knowledge about contemporary events. Their hard-won, archive-based knowledge about the past events in which they specialize may easily seduce them into arguing by analogy to their own times. Moreover, knowledge that is derived from the close reading of archival (that is, unpublished manuscript) sources is both the strength and the weakness of professional history. It is a strength because it helps to sustain scholars' resistance to reading the present backward into the past, and it provides a strong basis for dismissing stories (or models or theories) about human behavior that have no empirical basis. It is a weakness because it creates a fondness for the particular, which, carried to extremes, becomes a mindless antiquarianism that relishes facts and artifacts at the expense of explanation.

The historians who properly claim special knowledge about contemporary events may have troubled relations both with other historians and with colleagues in adjacent disciplines. Although contemporary history flourishes, with journals, grant awards, and numerous professorial appointments, its practitioners are often on the defensive. During most of the century and a half in which some people have earned their living as historians making claims to knowledge on a scientific basis, contemporary studies have been in professional disrepute. Until the early twentieth century, studies of ancient history or of the origins of modern nation-states earned scholars more prestige from their peers. Moreover, because the analysis of archival sources properly has been the basis of historians' claims to valid and reliable knowledge, contemporary history, for which many pertinent archives are closed, has been suspect. In dealing with the distant past, historians have only the dead and each other with whom to contest their interpretations; in dealing with the recent past and the present, they must confront the living—who have memories of their experience, and who may also have powerful and perhaps partisan explanations of the same events. The political and ideological struggles over interpretations of the present are usually waged with a special intensity rarely displayed in arguments over the more distant past.

Contemporary historians have, especially in the past several decades, had equivocal relationships with colleagues in adjacent disciplines—notably political science, economics, sociology, epidemiology, anthropology, and moral philosophy. Similarly, they have had equivocal relationships with professionals, such as physicians, lawyers, managers, and policy analysts, who are often paid to make informed judgments about the recent past. *Equivocal* may be too polite a word: the methods of historical inquiry have ceased to matter to many scholars and professionals in fields in which, earlier in this century, formal historical study would have been required. This is not the place to explain this circumstance, which has complicated causes. The essential point for our argument—and the basis for this book—is that practitioners of these fields are contributing to the historiography of the epidemic of HIV infection, that they will continue to do so, and that they would benefit from alliance with contemporary historians.

People in several disciplines and professions have been notable contributors to the contemporary history of this epidemic. The most thorough analysis of the responses of public health officials and gay community leaders has been written by a political scientist.[9] Other political scientists have written about the responses of the media.[10] An economist is the principal author of the only history to date of the effectiveness of educational measures.[11] Two policy analysts (one a professional historian) and an economist have analyzed the history of perceptions of the cost of treatment for AIDS.[12] Sociologists have synthesized the history of the responses of philanthropic foundations[13] and the history of outreach to intravenous drug users.[14] Epidemiologists have told us the most about the origins and spread of infection;[15] physicians, about treating patients;[16] ethicists, about moral dilemmas.[17] A sociolinguist has written extensively about the history of women and HIV infection.[18] Lawyers have contributed important histories of measures to control the behavior of persons perceived as dangerous to others, discrimination, and the problems of public health statutes governing the classification of disease and surveillance.[19] And policy analysts have written the only systematic comparative history of AIDS policies in Western countries.[20]

This rapidly accumulating body of secondary sources in contemporary history has had an important, but as yet unacknowledged, impact on the historiography of the epidemic. The cumulative weight of these publications has made history by analogy obsolete and, implicitly, has challenged the assumptions about discontinuity and the pertinence of the classic plague model on which it was based. These rich secondary sources make plain the continuity between the HIV epidemic and the recent past, and they demonstrate the linkage between events during the epidemic and such matters as how we have thought about disease, minority groups, women, drug users, public health law, and the organization and financing of health services.

Most of the people who have written these histories have little interest in historiography. They did not write history to test hypotheses about the past, much less to examine the validity of a discontinuity model. They wrote because they were concerned about their own disciplinary or professional agendas or about certain areas of policy or advocacy. Insofar as they are conscious of other disciplines that contribute to their practice of a social science or a policy profession, they would, typically, credit statistics or economics.

Although the displacement of history as a fundamental discipline of the social and policy sciences accounts for the relative lack of interest in historiography, it does not justify resignation among contemporary historians. Historians of our own times may find an even more receptive audience among social scientists or the policy professionals than they do among colleagues who study the more distant past. Such a potential community of scholars, like all communities, would be based on reciprocity. Contemporary historians now appreciate and use the theories and methods of adjacent disciplines. The problem for contemporary historians is to convince their colleagues who do history, but only incidentally, that they could do it better with the help of historians.

The HIV epidemic provides an opportunity to demonstrate the potential reciprocity of contemporary history and studies in other disciplines and the policy professions. The problem in achieving reciprocity is that historians must make a convincing case that their theories, methods, and ways of asking questions will help other people comprehend contemporary events more profoundly and with greater practical effect.

Although contemporary historians may disagree about what stance to take on particular theoretical issues, most would, we believe, urge their colleagues in other disciplines to pay more attention to three issues. Most historians would argue that having a considered position on each of these issues would improve the ability of scholars in any discipline or profession to make claims with reasonable objectivity. The first issue is social construction: the claim that historical reality does not exist as a truth waiting to be discovered but, rather, is created by people. Some social constructionists include the data of the biological sciences in their analysis. Others, rejecting this radical relativism, would maintain that biology or at least some forms of scientific knowledge have a validity independent of the social context in which they have been produced. For contemporary history, social constructionism means an emphasis on the complex processes by which disease is negotiated, the ways in which our concepts of pathology are defined and redefined, and the ways in which these conceptions of disease in turn govern our changing social and medical responses to illness.

AIDS is a particularly good example of the social construction of disease. In the process of defining both the disease and the persons infected, politics and social perceptions have been embedded in scientific and policy constructions of their reality and meaning. Human beings make disease in the context of biological and social conditions.

A second issue for historians is skepticism about the idea of progress. Skeptical historians worry about pseudo-causal statements that substitute metaphors for data-driven analysis of why events occurred and in what direction history (reified) is tending. Pseudo-causal statements are often driven by organic metaphors ("evolve," "develop," "unfold," "mature"). Skeptics also try to look behind polite synonyms for social or medical progress ("advance" is the most common of these synonyms) and to examine instead who did what to, for, or with whom, with what documentable results. The AIDS epidemic, or epidemic of HIV and related diseases, makes plain the danger of naive ideas about progress. At a meeting of the American Academy of Arts and Sciences in early 1988, Nobel laureate David Baltimore stated that AIDS is a medical problem; the only issue is when we will solve it. Many of the debates and much of the anger between gay activists and scientists have revolved around the idea of scientific progress or the lack of it: the accusation on the part of many activists that scientists have not lived up to the promises of progress, and the defensive reaction from scientists that an enormous amount has been learned about the disease in the time available.

A third theoretical issue is wariness about presentism; that is, distorting the past by seeing it only (or even mainly) from the point of view of our own time. Among contemporary historians presentism is often a result of using analogies from current events to interpret earlier events that are comprehended only superficially. It is the reverse of the use of analogies discussed earlier, when historians who have research-based knowledge about the past use that knowledge to project simple moral statements or conclusions about events in the present. The desire for "lessons from history," while generally welcome, must be treated with caution and laced with an awareness of the problems of extrapolating from one historical context to another.

The boundary between theory and method is somewhat artificial, since a scholar's theoretical stance often accounts for his or her choices among methods. Nonetheless, there are several methodological concerns that contemporary historians can commend to their colleagues. The most important of these is comprehensiveness, the necessity of basing a historical account on the greatest possible variety of data—on, if possible, manuscript sources, artifacts, memoirs (oral and written), printed primary sources, and a critical analysis of the theory and methods of earlier accounts of the same events. The sociologist who allegedly complained to a historian colleague that "you people read too much" either got or missed the point, depending on the level of self-irony he intended.

In particular, contemporary historians are aware that they must be skeptical of data from interviews (or, more formally, oral history) even though, in the absence of manuscript sources, they often must rely heavily on such data. The historical literature contains considerable evidence that spoken history is an account of what respondents find memorable and choose to present, using the conventions of contemporary storytelling. Such memories are notoriously fallible and often self-serving, although they may also provide insights and information not otherwise available. Whereas journalists seek corroborating interviews (double-sourcing), historians are more comfortable checking oral accounts against documentary evidence. Journalists and contemporary historians, however, may often share the same problem when oral sources are the only ones available. Like journalists, historians may then check one person's memory against another's, with due regard for the specific context and interests of their sources. Historians usually do have more time to explore information and hypotheses in depth, being less subject to immediate deadlines; they may also be under less pressure to tailor their accounts to the views and interests of their editors. Nevertheless, there is considerable similarity between contemporary historians and investigative reporters, and both have a proper disdain for armchair commentators.

The final area in which contemporary historians can contribute to their colleagues who write historically is in helping to set the questions. Among people who write about contemporary events, historians are almost alone in asking what has been left out. Scholars in other social sciences and in the policy and advocacy professions usually write history because they already have a question to answer; they look to the past for evidence, not as a source of questions. Journalists must respond to definitions of newsworthiness that they often do not set. Historians, by contrast, have been trained to think about what is and is not known about the past, even the recent past. In the HIV epidemic it is obvious that a great deal more study could be given to the history of research on the virus, the development and testing of drugs, sexual behavior, and the behavior of particular government and private organizations.

Historians should apply their skills and training to constructing a more adequate and complete history of AIDS than can be created by the press, by activists, or by physicians and scientists. This task requires an understanding of contemporary health politics and the methods of contemporary history. Moreover, a great deal of this history should be comparative; much more, for example, is known about events in the United States than in the countries of Western Europe or Africa. The politics, policies, and practices of responding to the AIDS epidemic within different cultures and national boundaries influence not only the internal affairs of other countries but also the future shape of national and international politics. As in the United States, AIDS in the countries of the Third World must be examined as an issue of contemporary history and politics.

Historians, who usually have to deal with the scattered and often inadequate sources left by past events, have an opportunity in the AIDS epidemic to help gather more complete records of contemporary events. Historians and their archivist colleagues should be developing principles for collecting materials that will allow us to explore as fully as possible the many dimensions of this disease and our social, political, and cultural responses to its progression. Collaborators and informants—on the streets, in the clinics, and in executive boardrooms—have perspectives on the epidemic that must be documented.

Perhaps most important, the proliferation of events since the epidemic was first identified suggests that the contemporary history of science, medicine, and public health, like that of war, must be studied prospectively. Just as combat historians are identified during a conflict and follow their assigned units, so historians of fast-breaking events in health affairs could benefit from such privileged access. Prospective research on contemporary history has resulted in several superb histories of space and defense initiatives and, in Britain during World War II, of social policy.[21] There are obvious problems with giving historians privileged access to primary sources, notably those involving objectivity and potential censorship. But there is a rich literature about these problems and the ways in which people in other fields have addressed them.

The history of the epidemic of HIV infection and related diseases is now rapidly being transformed. As the contemporary history of the epidemic is being written, many people have recognized that in important aspects AIDS is continuous with the recent past and that its history is linked to our patterns of behavior, both personal and institutional. The new historiography of the epidemic creates an opportunity for reciprocity between professional contemporary historians and their colleagues in other fields, for whom history is useful but not central.

This book attempts to encourage such reciprocity. The contributors belong to what could be called, with apologies for sounding imperialistic, the Greater Historical Profession. That is, each of them uses historiography—the theory and methodology of historical studies—to explain contemporary events. As the Notes on Contributors make plain, our colleagues who are the authors of the essays in this volume have formal training and vast experience in a variety of disciplines. They represent diverse fields and professions, including epidemiology, history, law, medicine, political science, communications, sociology, social psychology, sociolinguistics, and virology. Some of the contributors use their historical accounts as the basis for advocating particular changes in contemporary policies and practices.

The essays in Part One, "The Virus and Its Publics," explore scientific and public efforts to present and represent HIV and AIDS. Stephen S. Morse, for example, is a virologist who brings an unusually broad historical perspective to his field. Here he discusses HIV in the context of the evolutionary relationship of viral species to their human and animal hosts. He suggests that the process of viral emergence involves two major steps. In the first step, a new agent or, more commonly, an existing virus, is introduced into the human species. In the second step, the virus is disseminated in the human population. Morse develops the concepts of "viral traffic" between species and of "traffic laws" governing transmission. He provides examples of viral emergence and urges the establishment of much more systematic methods for detecting viral species. He suggests that a broader concept of environmental planning should be instituted to take into consideration the possible effects of human social behavior on viral transmission, thus enabling us to predict, and possibly prevent, the emergence of new epidemics.

Gerald M. Oppenheimer here expands his earlier study of the role of epidemiology in the social and scientific construction of AIDS.[22] Like Morse, he extends his view beyond the biological aspects of disease. He discusses the social impact of the early epidemiological characterization of AIDS by the life-style hypothesis, the definition of high-risk groups, and the analogy with hepatitis B; he then shows how the isolation of HIV led to reconceptualizing the disease in terms of a virus. He explores the continuing role of epidemiology and social science research in the process of redefining the disease and outlines the conflicts between different professional groups in the definition and management of the epidemic. The history of the epidemic, he concludes, demonstrates a dynamic process in which "different scientific specialties negotiated definitions that . . . reflected their relative power."

David C. Colby and Timothy E. Cook explore the social construction of AIDS, this time as a public problem presented through the mediation of the television nightly news. They trace the cycles of attention and inattention, of alarm and reassurance, that have been part of the logic of media attention in framing and responding to the disease. They thus explain the changing messages about AIDS that have been transmitted to the general public and show the ways in which these messages have unintentionally helped generate fearful public responses. Their essay provides an interesting parallel to the epidemiological construction of AIDS and helps explain some aspects of the public response to AIDS as they have been at least partially determined by the internal logic of the mass media.

The essays in Part Two address the political, legal, and ethical aspects of contemporary AIDS policies. Daniel M. Fox emphasizes the problems of financing patient care for persons with infection and disease. The heaviest financial burden continues to be borne by state and local government. This burden is increasing as HIV infection, which is now perceived as a chronic disease of lengthening duration, becomes a disease of the disadvantaged, especially of poor blacks and Hispanics. Moreover, the problems of financing health services for persons with HIV infection are inextricable from the larger policy and political issues of health care financing in the United States. Since prospects for general health care reform are modest in the political and economic climate of the early 1990s, Fox finds reason to conclude that social generosity toward persons with HIV infection will decrease.

Larry Gostin writes history as both an analyst and an advocate. His detailed synthesis of 149 legal cases of discrimination since the epidemic was recognized is solid legal history. These cases provide the only systematic data that have been collected about past, current, and potential future patterns of discrimination in education, employment, housing, and health services. Gostin also sketches the current state of antidiscrimination law, including the likely impact of the Americans with Disabilities Act, which became law in 1990 and was first enforced in 1991. But Gostin is also an advocate who detests discrimination in all its forms; his essay places historical evidence and methods in the service of legal advocacy.

Harvey M. Sapolsky and Stephen L. Boswell analyze the impact of the HIV epidemic on blood services in the United States, taking issue with conventional accounts in the medical and social science literature and in the media. Their new interpretation concurs with standard accounts in many particulars. Thus, they describe how transfusion recipients and health care personnel became subject to new risks of infection as a result of the epidemic. Though these risks are relatively small, fear of AIDS became so intense that high priority was given to efforts to reduce risk, forcing long-needed changes in medical practice and in the policies of blood collection and banking agencies. Sapolsky and Boswell differ from most other experts, however, in presenting evidence that most of the "significant improvements in the overall quality of American blood services . . . could have been achieved without the existence of this new health menace." They also provide an explanation, grounded in historical research, of why blood services failed to make these improvements before the HIV epidemic.

David J. Rothman and Harold Edgar compare the standards used by the federal government to judge the safety and efficacy of drugs against cancer and HIV. They undertook their inquiry in order to test the hypothesis that a chronic disease model of disease had different implications for policy than did a plague model. They conclude that, in this instance at least, the choice of a specific historical model had important policy implications. Had AZT been a drug for people with advanced cancer, the Food and Drug Administration would most likely have given much earlier approval for its use outside experimental situations. Using a plague, or infectious disease, model, however, federal scientific and regulatory officials believed that they were obligated to base their decisions exclusively on data from placebo-based, randomized clinical trials.

Ronald Bayer argues that privacy was the central political and ethical issue of the HIV epidemic in the United States in the 1980s, but that it has now been "joined, although not displaced, by the question of equity." By equity he means providing resources for "care and counseling—especially to the poor, among whom intravenous drug use plays a critical role in HIV transmission." Bayer says that he is now less pessimistic about the generosity of public policy in the United States than he was in 1988, the publication date of his important book *Private Acts, Social Consequences.*[23] In his view, there is evidence that the "culture of responsibility" may govern the United States response to the epidemic in the 1990s. By examining different kinds of evidence, Bayer thus comes to very different conclusions from those reached by Daniel Fox about the likely future of AIDS politics and policy.

The essays in Part Three deal with some of the groups most directly affected by AIDS. This section begins with a selection of photographs of women with AIDS by Ann Meredith. These are from an exhibition shown, and favorably reviewed, in cities around the United States and Europe. The photographs are accompanied by comments from the women who were interviewed about their lives and experiences.

Robert A. Padgug, a historian of sexuality turned health policy analyst, and Gerald M. Oppenheimer, a historian-epidemiologist, have previously collaborated on studies of AIDS financing; here they provide a sensitive account of the complex relationships of the gay community to

AIDS. They place AIDS in the historical context of sexual politics and practices and the construction of gay identity, as the gay community came to "own" the AIDS epidemic, at least in its early stages. In the process of taking responsibility for AIDS services and organizing around AIDS policies, the gay community and its organizations were themselves transformed. Padgug and Oppenheimer trace the political shifts of the 1980s and speculate what may happen when gay communities move beyond the stage of being consumed and defined by the AIDS crisis.

Don C. Des Jarlais and his colleagues Samuel R. Friedman and Jo L. Sotheran write about events with which they have been deeply involved: the history of the epidemic of HIV infection among intravenous drug users in New York. Des Jarlais and his colleagues have been doing research on the epidemic among intravenous drug users in New York City since 1981. Their methods have been widely emulated, and their findings have had a wide international audience. In this essay they look back on their experience and propose a "staging system," or model, of the history of the epidemic among intravenous drug users. This model is, they argue, useful for cities in which HIV infection among intravenous drug users began later than in New York or has not been as extensive. They note that, in the more recent stages of the epidemic among drug users in New York and other cities, HIV seroprevalence has stabilized.

The fourth and final section provides a sampling of perspectives on the social and scientific construction of AIDS in other nations. Virginia Berridge and Philip Strong first analyze the development of AIDS policies in the United Kingdom. They suggest three stages of AIDS policy development in their country: the first, a period of slow growth and bottom-up organizing, which developed a "policy community"; the second, a period when AIDS was treated as a national emergency; and the third, a period of normalization. They highlight the early leadership of the Department of Health, the strategy of gay groups to emphasize the possibility of heterosexual transmission, and the energetic public education campaign that followed. They stress the themes of continuity versus change in AIDS policies, provide a basis for comparing AIDS politics in the United Kingdom and other countries, and list some areas for further research.

James W. Dearing examines health policy development in Japan, a country with a small number of cases and a very distinct epidemiological profile. He thus shows how a very different society and economy responded to the epidemic. At first Japan reacted to the problem of AIDS as it was defined by the American media—namely, a disease of homosexuals and intravenous drug users. However, since the first two persons with AIDS identified in Japan were prostitutes, national fears of heterosexual transmission were raised. But AIDS in Japan, at least in the 1980s, was largely a disease of hemophiliacs, spread by the use of imported blood products. Dearing show how a foreign curiosity thus became a domestic problem, as public-interest groups in Japan struggled to redefine the issue. The major policy issues became the regulation, importation, and use of blood products and the compensation of those who had suffered as a consequence of Japanese industrial practices. Dearing thus implicitly makes the case that AIDS is a very distinct problem in different cultural contexts.

Randall M. Packard and Paul Epstein provide a critical view of the work of epidemiologists, social scientists, and medical researchers dealing with AIDS in Africa. They draw on earlier historical studies to show how diseases in Africa, particularly tuberculosis and endemic syphilis, have been viewed through the lens of Western cultural assumptions about Africa and Africans. On the question of heterosexual transmission of HIV, they note that social scientists had a very limited role in framing the research questions and were limited to exploring behavioral assumptions about sexual promiscuity. Here they suggest the need for a broader analysis, with much more attention paid to the role of malnutrition, background infections, and other immunosuppressant conditions with respect to susceptibility to infection, and to the role of injections and transfusions in HIV transmission.

Paula A. Treichler critically deconstructs First World discourses about AIDS in the Third World. She is less interested in arriving at a single "truth about AIDS" than in examining the process and consequences of particular forms of narrative construction of disease. These narratives, she suggests, may also serve, and mask, relations of power. Treichler calls into question many accounts of AIDS in Third World countries, from the eyewitness reports of traveling experts to the compilations of statistical data that may seem better to represent hard fact. She tries to show how language works in culture, "how narratives perform as well as inform, how information constructs reality." By doing so, she hopes to help Western commentators become more self-reflective about their forms of knowledge and belief.

We thus begin and end this book with unconventional accounts of the international problem of AIDS and HIV-related diseases. We have gone from the ecology of viral transmission to the cultural environment of the scientific power to name, and from the mutation of disease agents to the mutation of cultural meanings. In the process, we have included many different voices, all of them helping to define the contemporary history of AIDS. At this stage in the process of coming to terms with AIDS, no one collection of essays can pretend to cover all aspects of the problem, but we have tried to provide a rich sampling of what we consider the most interesting current work in the field.

NOTES

An earlier version of this essay, "The Contemporary Historiography of AIDS," is reprinted with permission from *Journal of Social History* 23 (1989): 303–14.

1. Elizabeth Fee and Daniel M. Fox, "Introduction: AIDS, Public Policy, and Historical Inquiry," in *AIDS: The Burdens of History*, ed. Fee and Fox (Berkeley: University of California Press, 1988), p. 1.
2. Arien Mack, ed., "In Time of Plague: The History and Social Consequences of Lethal Epidemic Disease," *Social Research* 55 (1988): special issue.
3. Susan Sontag, *AIDS and Its Metaphors* (New York: Farrar, Straus and Giroux, 1988).
4. Barbara Gutman Rosenkrantz, "Case Histories—An Introduction," *Social Research* 55 (1988): 399.
5. Randy Shilts, *And the Band Played On: Politics, People, and the AIDS Epidemic* (New York: St. Martin's Press, 1987).
6. Most of the references to Allan Brandt's *No Magic Bullet* (New York: Oxford University Press, 1985, 1988) have addressed the analogies with plagues, what we call discontinuities, not the chronic disease aspects of venereal disease.
7. Cited in Lawrence K. Altman, "A New Therapy Approach: Cancer as a Model for AIDS," *New York Times*, June 13, 1989.
8. Those studying past epidemics began to claim special relevance for their work in the age of AIDS. See, for example, the ending of the study by Richard Evans, *Death in Hamburg: Society and Politics in the Cholera Years, 1830–1910* (Oxford: Oxford University Press, 1987), p. 568.
9. Ronald Bayer, *Private Acts, Social Consequences* (New York: Free Press, 1988). See also Dennis Altman, "Legitimation through Disaster: AIDS and the Gay Movement," in *AIDS: The Burdens of History*, ed. Fee and Fox, pp. 301–15.
10. David Colby, Timothy Cook, and Timothy Murray, "Social Movements and Sickness on the Air: Agenda Control and Television News on AIDS," paper presented at the annual meeting of the American Political Science Association, Chicago, September 1987.
11. Jane E. Sisk, Maria Hewitt, and Kelly L. Metcalf, "The Effectiveness of AIDS Education," *Health Affairs* 7 (Winter 1988): 37–51.

12. Daniel M. Fox and Emily H. Thomas, "AIDS Cost Analysis and Social Policy," *Law, Medicine and Health Care* 15 (1987–88): 186–211; Anne A. Scitovsky, "The Economic Impact of AIDS," *Health Affairs* 7 (Fall 1988): 32–45.

13. James A. Wells, Andrea Zuercher, and John Clinton, "Foundation Giving for AIDS Education," *Health Affairs* 7 (Winter 1988): 146–68.

14. For an interview with Don C. Des Jarlais that summarizes his research, see William Booth, "AIDS and Drug Abuse: No Quick Fix," *Science* 239 (February 12, 1988): 717–19. See also in this volume Don C. Des Jarlais, Samuel R. Friedman, and Jo L. Sotheran, "The First City: The Spread of HIV among Intravenous Drug Users and the Treatment Program Response in New York City."

15. For example, Gerald M. Oppenheimer, "In the Eye of the Storm: The Epidemiological Construction of AIDS," in *AIDS: The Burdens of History*, ed. Fee and Fox, pp. 267–300.

16. Deborah J. Cotton, "The Impact of AIDS on the Medical Care System," *Journal of the American Medical Association* 260 (July 22, 1988): 519–23; Gerald Friedland, "Clinical Care in the AIDS Epidemic," *Daedalus* 118, no. 2 (Spring 1989): 59–84.

17. Many pertinent articles have appeared in the *Hastings Center Report;* an influential article by a group sponsored by Hastings is Ronald Bayer, Carol Levine, and Susan M. Wolf, "HIV Antibody Screening: An Ethical Framework for Evaluating Proposed Programs," *Journal of the American Medical Association* 256 (October 3, 1986): 1768–74.

18. Paula A. Treichler, "AIDS, Gender, and Biomedical Discourse: Current Contests for Meaning," in *AIDS: The Burdens of History*, ed. Fee and Fox, pp. 190–266.

19. See, for example, Lawrence Gostin, William J. Curran, and M. Clark, "The Case against Compulsory Case Finding in Controlling AIDS," *American Journal of Law and Medicine* 12 (1987): 7–53.

20. Daniel M. Fox, Patricia Day, and Rudolf Klein, "The Power of Professionalism: AIDS in Britain, Sweden and the United States," *Daedalus* 118, no. 2 (Spring 1989): 93–112. An exception to our generalizations in this paragraph is M. Grmek, *Histoire du SIDA* (Paris: Payot, 1989), an excellent work of contemporary history by a historian.

21. The modern classic in military history is Samuel Eliot Morison's multi-volume history of the United States Navy in World War II. Morison was even made an admiral in order to facilitate prospective research. The classic in social policy history is Richard Titmuss, *Problems of Social Policy* (London: Her Majesty's Stationery Office, 1950). Titmuss's book was commissioned during the war as part of the larger wartime history project.

22. Oppenheimer, "In the Eye of the Storm."

23. Bayer, *Private Acts, Social Consequences*.

PART I

The Virus and Its Publics

AIDS and Beyond: Defining the Rules for Viral Traffic

Stephen S. Morse

The lesson of AIDS demonstrates that infectious diseases are not a vestige of our premodern past; instead, like disease in general, they are the price we pay for living in the organic world. AIDS came at a time of increasing complacency about infectious diseases. The striking successes achieved with antibiotics, together with widespread application of vaccines for many previously feared viral diseases, made many physicians and the public believe that infectious diseases were retreating and would in time be fully conquered. Although this view was disputed by virologists and many specialists in infectious diseases, it had become a commonplace to suggest that infectious diseases were about to become a thing of the past and that chronic, noninfectious diseases should be our major priorities.[1] Rudely jolted back into an awareness of infectious diseases by AIDS, we now find ourselves in a period of great uncertainty, poised for the AIDS of the future. We cannot help but wonder what other catastrophes are waiting to pounce on us. In this essay I consider what we now know about the "AIDS of the future." In particular, I discuss the origins of "new" viruses and the question of whether their emergence can be anticipated and prevented.[2]

I argue that AIDS and HIV are novel but that biological antecedents and parallels can be found in nature. The novelty of AIDS therefore probably reflects our imperfect knowledge of the natural world rather than a diabolical new development in viral evolution. It is of note, though, that the conditions favoring rapid dissemination of the virus were comparatively recent social developments of great importance. In essence, they served as highways to expedite "viral traffic," from animal sources to humans and from small or isolated human populations to larger groups. This "viral traffic," as I call it, is central to the origin of most epidemics of viral disease. Most "new" or "emerging" viruses are the result of changes in traffic patterns, which give viruses new highways. Perhaps most important, human actions often precipitate viral emergence. Apart from such obvious human factors as the role of behavior in HIV transmission, many episodes of emergence have been the result of agricultural or environmental changes brought about by human intervention. We therefore bear greater responsibility for emergence, and may have greater ability to influence it, than has been supposed.

The emphasis placed by scientists and the public on the diversity of viruses—of which the stress on the novelty of HIV is one example— may have made us oblivious to these recurrent patterns and common features shared by many emerging viruses. Most "new" viruses are of zoonotic (animal) origin and are not really new; instead, they are existing viruses that have been given new opportunities or new settings.[3] Viral evolution, while a fascinating phenomenon to scientists, has generally been less important per se as a mechanism of viral emergence than this transfer of existing or slightly modified viruses to new hosts. The optimistic message is that the possibly unpredictable path of viral evolution need not necessarily be fully charted before we can anticipate new diseases like AIDS. The central problem concerns the changing relationships between viruses and human society, reflecting changes in relationships between humans and their environment.

In this regard, focusing on the uniqueness of AIDS has tended to obscure the many features that this virus shares with other viruses.[4] AIDS is unquestionably unusual, and its viral cause, human immunodeficiency virus (HIV), has many novel features. Nothing in our knowledge of viral disease prepared us for the unique features of AIDS. Much was known about interactions of viruses with the immune system, but a virus that caused human disease by depleting the cells responsible for specific immunity was unprecedented. AIDS was also one of the few documented examples of what appears to be a truly new virus entering the human population to cause a previously unknown disease (but see below). Most notably among its unusual properties, HIV has a predilection for T lymphocytes (and other cells) bearing the surface protein called CD4 (or T4). Various types of T lymphocytes are responsible for orchestrating and regulating all immune responses, as well as for carrying out certain types of immune functions known collectively as cell-mediated. Their roles are determined by specific proteins on the cell surface, which serve as recognition markers. T lymphocytes bearing the CD4 protein, colloquially known as "T4 cells," are generally responsible for turning on and amplifying immune responses. Without these CD4$^+$ T cells, the body is unable to mobilize an immune response, so that the host becomes vulnerable to the opportunistic infections that are the hallmark of AIDS.

As was shown several years ago, the predilection of HIV for CD4$^+$ T cells is due to the fact that the CD4 protein is a receptor for the virus.[5] That is, the virus enters T cells by attaching specifically to CD4 on the cell surface. Other viruses have specific receptors; what made HIV tragically unique was that its receptor was CD4 rather than some other protein on the cell surface. This allowed HIV access to the CD4$^+$ T cell that is so crucial in the immune response. However, for reasons to be discussed, it seemed improbable that the property of infecting and killing CD4$^+$ cells would be found in only one virus and not in any of its relatives.[6] Thus, the discovery of this mechanism led to a search, ultimately successful, for other examples of viruses that infect or kill CD4 T cells. HIV belongs to the Lentivirus subfamily of retroviruses. One might expect that relatives of HIV among other lentiviruses would behave similarly; indeed, Luc Montagnier has pointed out that most, if not all, primate lentiviruses have a predilection for CD4$^+$ lymphocytes of their hosts.[7] In addition to these, some lentiviruses of other species, such as the bovine and feline immunodeficiency viruses, also appear to attack similar targets in their respective species.[8]

But the ability to infect and kill CD4$^+$ T lymphocytes may not even be unique to retroviruses. Herpesviruses are DNA-containing viruses unrelated to HIV. In my laboratory we have found that a mouse herpesvirus, mouse thymic virus (MTLV; murid herpesvirus 3), can specifically kill CD4$^+$ T lymphocytes developing in the thymus of young mice.[9] T cells not possessing CD4 are not affected. Recent reports suggest that the recently described human herpesvirus 6 (HHV-6; also called HBLV) is probably T lymphotropic as well.[10] In cell culture at least, HHV-6 can infect and kill cells bearing CD4.[11] Despite these worrisome properties, these viruses have never been associated with AIDS-like disease and are probably not responsible for any serious illnesses in mice or humans, although HHV-6 has been suggested as a possible cofactor for AIDS.[12] The mouse virus does not appear to cause overt disease, even though individuals remain infected for life and chronically secrete virus, probably from T lymphocytes.[13] The human virus seems to cause roseola, a mild childhood disease, and may be one of the commonest of all human viruses.[14] I shall say more about HHV-6 later. We do not know why, unlike HIV, these apparently T lymphotropic infections rarely if ever cause severe disease and do not appear to result in AIDS-like syndromes. Although they might someday become the cause of new AIDS-like diseases, that is unlikely; in distinction to HIV, these viruses were probably in their respective host species for many generations and appear well adapted to their hosts.

The lesson from such findings is that infectious agents do not develop in a vacuum but are the result of an ongoing evolutionary process. Most life forms existing today evolved from organisms already in existence, and viruses appear to be no exception. Appearance of viruses *de novo* seems extremely rare, for the same reasons that other species rarely arise *de novo*. Thus, "new" viruses are likely to come from existing viruses, and, in general, viruses of today have antecedents and relatives. In a sense, viruses have "parents" just as we do. As Luc Montagnier put it, "We're boarding a train that's already in motion. New species aren't being created. We're seeing the old ones evolve."[15] It has taken us a long time to assimilate this lesson, and I am not sure that even now we fully grasp its implications. In the words of Joshua Lederberg, "the historiography of epidemic disease is one of the last refuges of the concept of special creationism."[16] We still tend to think of each infectious agent as if it arose in a vacuum, and not as the result of an ongoing evolutionary process.

Viruses show great variety, and in addition many of the viruses of greatest concern mutate rapidly and unpredictably.[17] Because previously unrecognized viruses are involved, mechanisms of viral emergence must mirror the unpredictability of these mutations in the genotype. It was usually assumed that most emerging viruses had to arise through the evolution of a new variant, and the emphasis on variation in the viral genome may have engendered a widespread feeling that the significance of viral evolution is to generate unpredictable or unexpected new variants. As we cannot foretell the future, and thus cannot predict the future evolution of any organism, the problem of emerging viruses has always appeared insoluble because it seemed to require predicting the course of viral evolution—an impossible task.

The valuable implication of evolutionary theory for viral origins is that if "new" viruses must arise from closely related preexisting viruses, it is not really essential to answer the question in those terms. While variability has undoubtedly contributed to the success of many of the most troublesome viruses, including influenza, HIV, and many others, the more germane question is how an existing virus that normally infects one host species would be able to cross over into humans to become a human disease problem.[18] When restated this way, the seemingly insoluble problem of viral origins thus reduces to a more manageable (although not trivial) question of viral traffic, and attacking the problem includes better understanding and appreciating the viruses that already exist in nature, including some viruses not yet discovered. Even more usefully, however, by focusing attention on viral traffic, especially between species, this concept shifts attention to more approachable questions concerning conditions, or the "rules of the road" for viral traffic. What conditions, for example, on the part of the virus or of the host or in the environment, will permit a virus to infect people? Novelty will evolve—even new mechanisms of pathogenesis, as was the case with AIDS. But we may have some advance warning in nature if we know where to look (see also note 6). On the other hand, the factors leading a virus, perhaps as yet unseen in nature, toward emergence can be more more readily predicted and studied. In addition, some emerging viruses may already be in a human population, but they may be geographically isolated.

This explanation allows us to consider viral emergence as a process in two major steps. The first step is the advent of what may at first seem to be (or, rarely, actually is) a "new" agent and its initial introduction into the human population. Depending on the virus, this step could have occurred recently or long ago, or it may even have occurred repeatedly before a successful infection. I have made this one step rather than two, because, for the reasons discussed above, a "new" agent is just as likely to be an "old" agent of another species. The virus may perhaps sometimes be slightly altered, although that is usually not necessary. The second step, dissemination in the human population, occurs once a virus infects its first human being. This model, then, presumes that emergence is simply a matter of a virus's getting into the human population and then spreading within the population. Many viruses may never achieve this second step. Although this simplification covers a multitude of sins, it provides a conceptual framework with which to begin. One consequence of this model is that—without requiring detailed advance knowledge of the virus—it permits us to analyze emergence by considering what contributes to each of these steps and what conditions could affect each step, the "traffic laws."

For the first step, even apparently new viruses, such as HIV, have usually left tracks; often we have just failed to spot them in time. The conceptual problem of viral evolution is also in the first step. But because the requirements of evolution constrain novelty somewhat, there are only a few ways a "new" virus can arise. It can be a truly new virus, a major evolutionary variant, arising by genetic processes such as (for example) mutation or recombination; it can be an existing virus of another species, introduced virtually unchanged or with minor variations into humans from the other species; or it may be an existing human virus of limited scope. The "truly" new virus or major variant is possible but, for the reasons discussed above, is likely to be a rare event. While it is unlikely that we can predict its occurrence, we fortunately will not often be required to do so.[19]

Several different factors can influence this first step profoundly. Many of the important changes responsible for new viral traffic are made by humans. Just as with other kinds of traffic, viral "traffic" has its traffic indicators, stop-and-go signals, and rules of the road. For example, certain types of environmental changes may be "go" signals for viral traffic. They act by increasing chances or frequency of introduction, or by favoring spread of a natural host or carrier (vector) for a virus. Deforestation and agricultural practices are among the factors most often responsible. To illustrate, I will sketch several instances of viral emergence. Although the examples may appear exotic at first, they will eventually come closer to home.[20]

Argentine hemorrhagic fever is caused by Junin virus. It emerged from obscurity to cause about 400–600 cases annually over an area of 100,000 square kilometers (up from the original 16,000 square kilometers of 1958). The emergence of Argentine hemorrhagic fever was precipitated by agricultural changes as people cleared the pampas for agriculture and began to plant maize. A natural host for this virus is a mouse, *Calomys musculinus;* infected individuals of this species chronically shed virus in their urine. Although this rodent was always in the Argentine pampas, it began to flourish when natural grassland was cleared and maize was planted, so that ultimately it outnumbered the other rodents. Studies show an enormous difference in numbers of this mouse in cornfields, as opposed to natural grasslands,[21] and the first recognition of Argentine hemorrhagic fever (1953) corresponds to increased corn planting in the region. Additional data corroborate the association. The rodent population fluctuates in a three- to five-year cycle, as does the incidence of Argentine hemorrhagic fever cases, and percentage of infected mice is higher in areas with many human Argentine hemorrhagic fever cases. Bolivian hemorrhagic fever is caused by a related virus (Machupo virus) with a similar story; here the rodent is *Calomys callosus*. For various economic reasons, agriculture, primarily cattle raising, increased in the affected areas of Bolivia over the past thirty years. *Calomys callosus* adapted well to the new conditions, with the result that more people came in contact with the virus carried by this rodent. Increasing agriculture caused increasing cases. In the 1960s about 1,000 cases were reported, with 20 percent mortality. A program of rodent control, trapping and killing infected mice, has been very effective; as a result, there have been no new cases since 1974. This decrease further indicates that the putative association of rodent and disease was correct. An Old World relative of these two viruses, the notorious Lassa fever of Africa, follows an almost identical pattern.[22] The major natural host of this virus is another mouse, *Mastomys natalensis,* which adapts readily to humans, thriving on the food people leave and sharing human habitation. It unwittingly sheds Lassa fever virus, and humans become infected by contact.

The unrelated Korean hemorrhagic fever (Hantaan) falls into the same pattern. The natural host is *Apodemus,* basically a field rodent, and people come in contact with infected animals during rice harvesting. Increased rice planting has provided food for *Apodemus* as well as for people, and prevalence of Korean hemorrhagic fever has increased accordingly.

Not all of these viruses originate in rodents, although a remarkable number do. A number of important disease-causing viruses are also transmitted by arthropod vectors, such as insects or ticks. Most of these are viruses that can infect both mammals and the arthropod vector, a rather rigorous requirement that bespeaks evolutionary intimacy, on the part of the virus, with both invertebrates and vertebrates. They cause diseases that usually have long histories, and the arthropod vectors (really, arthropod hosts) serve primarily to disseminate a virus or to transport it into new individuals from a natural zoonotic (animal) source. Factors encouraging the arthropod vector can be important in disease emergence, as is demonstrated by several arthropod-transmitted diseases that have emerged recently. Rift Valley fever, found in Africa, caused serious outbreaks in Egypt in 1977 and more recently in Mauritania; the infection is characterized by a fever, usually with hemorrhaging; is naturally transmitted by various mosquitoes; and normally infects ungulates, such as sheep. Because the larvae of most mosquitoes involved in virus transmission develop in water, the addition of large open sources of water often increases the mosquito population and has a major impact on transmission. In Egypt, although it is not known for certain why the virus emerged, the Aswan high dam was a possible factor precipitating emergence. The factors were more clearly defined in the Mauritanian Rift Valley fever outbreaks. Here the human cases occurred near areas along the Senegal River where large dams (for hydroelectric power) had recently been constructed. Similarly, sporadic outbreaks in other parts of Africa were usually associated with unexpectedly heavy rains.

There have been several incidents of Oropouche fever, first seen in Trinidad around 1957, in the Amazon region of Brazil. Appearance of the disease coincided with the introduction of cacao as a cash crop to the Amazon region. The vector, a biting *Culicoides* midge, breeds well in empty cacao hulls discarded after harvesting. The virus is also widespread in Panama, where a number of cases have been reported since 1989, and in Venezuela, where a notable outbreak occurred in early 1990. I will have a few words shortly about Lyme disease, not viral but also arthropod borne.

In all these cases, expanding agriculture, often accompanied by deforestation, played a major role in precipitating emergence—that is, in introducing a zoonotic (animal) virus into a new population. The role of agriculture seems logical on consideration. After all, if many "new" viruses are zoonotic, how would people come in contact with animal species bearing unfamiliar zoonotic viruses? Agricultural practices, as well as increased human habitation, may change the ecology of an area to allow a previously minor species to proliferate, as in the cases above. Expanding human habitation in a region, which may include or be the result of clearing land for agriculture, may also put people in direct contact with new animal species (and thus their viruses), as in the example of monkeypox. Monkeypox is an African virus that is related to smallpox but causes a milder form of illness upon infecting humans. It has often been named as a possible successor to smallpox following the recent eradication of the human virus. Monkeypox is so called because it was first identified in infected monkeys, but it is actually a virus of rodents, especially squirrels. People become infected when they develop settlements at the edge of the rainforest and, encroaching on the forest, come in contact with infected rodents inhabiting the forest.[23]

More remarkably, the same principles also often apply to viruses whose emergence can clearly be ascribed to viral evolution. Influenza A virus is one of the few known examples (aside from some arguable cases, such as HIV, it may be the only example) of such a virus. Every twenty years or so, influenza A undergoes a major antigenic shift in one key protein, known as the hemagglutinin (H) protein, and a pandemic results.[24] Although most changes in influenza virus H proteins occur by so-called antigenic drift, involving the accumulation of random mutations (this drift can lead to the smaller influenza epidemics seen every few years), new pandemic influenza viruses arise by a different route, that of major antigenic shifts. These invariably involve a reassortment of viral genes carried by different influenza strains. Thus, the important event in generating new pandemic influenza strains has, oddly, been not mutational evolution but a reshuffling of existing genes. Where do the genes come from? It has recently been found that most influenza genes are maintained in wildfowl; every known subtype of the H protein can be found in waterfowl. A number of virologists believe that pigs are an important "mixing vessel," allowing influenza virus to make a transition from birds to humans.[25] Every major flu epidemic known has originated in south China, which has also long practiced a traditional and unique form of integrated pig-duck farming.[26] Agriculture may play the leading role in emergence of this virus as well. Here, too, viral traffic— reassortant viruses from the mixing of animal influenza strains and the transmission of the resulting virus to humans—is more important than viral evolution for human disease.

Human immunodeficiency virus is a more difficult case. Where did HIV come from? We do not know the origin of HIV, but a probable primate origin is often suggested and appears highly plausible, at least for HIV-2. The origin of HIV-1 is more problematic. The existence of animal lentiviruses with a predilection for CD4$^+$ T lymphocytes strongly suggests the possibility of a zoonotic origin for HIV at some time in the past. What is currently unknown is how and when the virus was first introduced into humans.[27]

The principles involved in these examples apply to all types of infectious diseases in all parts of the world. For example, it is hard to imagine a part of the world more heavily populated and thoroughly explored than the northeastern United States, but Lyme disease, the media's star disease of the 1989 and 1990 summer seasons, follows the same principles. Although bacterial rather than viral, Lyme disease is also zoonotic, being naturally found in several other mammals and probably originating in wild mice, and is transmitted by a tick. It is not clear why Lyme disease has recently emerged, but conditions favoring increased contact of people and infected tick vectors are likely to be principal reasons. These conditions appear to include changes in forestland around

houses. Malaria, a major cause of death worldwide, is caused by a pro-
tozoan parasite and not a virus. It is so widespread that one can hardly
consider it emerging. But the recent completion of a new highway (SR
364) through the Amazonian rainforest of Brazil resulted in a massive
increase in malaria cases in the region.[28]

The second step, dissemination within the human population, is obviously crucial. Not only for newly introduced viruses, but also for many
viruses long established in humans, emergence is the result of increased
or accelerated dissemination. For this step, there is a vast epidemiological literature, which it is beyond the scope of this essay to review. Instead, I will mention a few recent developments, extending the metaphor of viral traffic by adding traffic in the more familiar sense. Modern
transportation offers rich possibilities for rapid dissemination of new
or exotic viruses. Recently a man who contracted Lassa fever while
visiting Africa became sick after returning to the United States.[29] As
another example, HIV undoubtedly traveled along the Mombasa-Kin-
shasa highway and came to the United States presumably through travel.[30]
I have already mentioned malaria and the Brazilian highway. Of course,
this is hardly a new phenomenon in infectious diseases, as witness the
classic example of bubonic plague. In this vein, the dissemination of
dengue and yellow fever, both transmitted by the same species of mosquito, is a particularly instructive example. The viruses and the mosquitoes were both probably spread by the African slave trade. It has
been suggested that the mosquitoes that spread these diseases were inadvertently carried to the New World in the large open water containers on slave vessels. The mosquitoes lay their eggs in water, where the
larvae hatch and develop; availability of water is therefore a major factor in population growth for many mosquito species. *Plus ça change:* A
new, and more aggressive, mosquito, *Aedes albopictus* (the Asian tiger
mosquito), was recently found in the United States and is now established in seventeen states. An effective vector for dengue and several
other mosquito-borne viruses, the mosquito was introduced into the
United States in 1985 in containers of used tires imported into Houston,
Texas, from Asia. Wet tires are known as excellent breeding grounds
for several species of mosquitoes, and have been shown to harbor many
more tiger mosquito larvae than dry tires. Thus, carriers of disease are
still themselves carried, however inadvertently, in commerce.

Human population movements are of obvious importance for dis-
seminating viruses. Migration to cities from remote areas may pose a
particular challenge. People in a remote area may come in contact with

an isolated virus, as in the examples of monkeypox and Lassa fever. If they move to a city, an increasingly common event, they bring their diseases with them. The population growth strains the city's infrastructure and can cause serious problems, as shown by the impressive expansion of dengue virus (a mosquito-borne infection). In many tropical cities open water storage is used increasingly as the city enlarges; as a result, additional breeding grounds are provided for mosquito vectors. At the same time, the high density of these urban areas places infected people and susceptible people in close contact, so that a cycle of infection is established.

Public health measures—such as mosquito control programs, health certification of travelers, and health inspection of imported livestock—have traditionally been directed to combating this stage, which has generally been the most vulnerable to attack. These programs have been instrumental in containing many potential threats, but they also have several drawbacks. Their success with the targeted diseases depends on vigilance and assiduity. Sadly, even when adequate weapons to combat disease are available, we may fail to use them effectively. As a case in point, the recent resurgence of measles in some U.S. cities seems largely due to the failure to ensure that all children are adequately immunized early in life. Efforts may fall victim to their own success, being prematurely relaxed or abandoned, usually to save money; as a result, the conditions that precipitated the program in the first place may reestablish themselves. Many mosquito control programs have met with this fate after initial partial success. These programs are reactive and can generally succeed only with known diseases, although some programs may confer broader benefits. Most of these programs also cannot contain viruses that can spread efficiently from person to person, such as influenza. Present strategy with influenza is to attempt to track emerging new strains and to immunize when feasible.

The modern world also offers additional gateways for viral traffic. For example, as has tragically been demonstrated with HIV, such medical procedures as blood transfusion and tissue transplantation offer the donor's viruses direct access to new hosts. Since many viruses, including HIV, are not able to spread efficiently from person to person, these procedures circumvent the lack of effective means of transmission. As these lifesaving procedures become more widely used, and as the scarcity of donors forces medical centers to look farther afield, it is reasonable to expect more instances. Agriculture again provides an interesting analogy. Viroids, small pieces of genetic information that lack the protein coat normally needed by viruses to infect host cells, are spread, as far as we know, entirely by mechanical transmission on agricultural implements such as pruning knives and harvesters. It is speculation, but the evolution of viroids could very likely have been shaped, unbeknownst to its human agents, by these human activities.

How do we assess the nature of a viral threat? Before we address this question, let us put aside one class of emerging viruses that occasionally make the news (and rightfully so) but that probably would not represent a major threat. These are viruses that have only recently been identified because of advances in diagnostic technology, but have probably been with us a long time. Two recent examples are non-A, non-B hepatitis and human herpesvirus 6, both viruses that have been discovered within the last three years. In the case of non-A, non-B hepatitis, there is considerable evidence that the virus had been a major cause of posttransfusion hepatitis for years, but the virus itself remained elusive. The application of molecular technology, using DNA cloning, finally made it possible to identify the virus.[31] I have already mentioned human herpesvirus 6 (HHV-6).[32] HHV-6 was originally reported from Robert Gallo's laboratory under the name "human B lymphotropic virus" (HBLV); it was discovered fortuitously when it interfered with the growth of HIV isolates in tissue culture. At first thought rare, HHV-6 was later associated with the very common childhood disease called roseola. Since roseola has been known for many years,[33] it is likely that HHV-6 has been a ubiquitous virus for decades, probably centuries. Many known diseases in search of causes can be placed in this category. There are likely to be many surprises here, but few threats, because the viruses are already widely disseminated. On the other hand, the importance of technological advances in making these discoveries cannot be overemphasized. These viruses became apparent because the means were developed to demonstrate their existence.[34] It is conceivable that a change in some critical condition could cause one of these already widespread viruses to become a threat, but such an occurrence appears unlikely.

Predicting the greatest threats is a more difficult task, made more difficult by significant gaps in our knowledge. Of course, we cannot foretell the future. Many would say that the only sure bet is that the next threat will be one not on any list today, as was the case with AIDS. That is why I think it is much more important and useful to emphasize the general principles underlying viral emergence, rather than to attempt to compile a list. However, since I am flinging about a plethora of virus names as examples, I list here some of the viruses that might be perceived as future threats. Several have already been discussed. Most lists would probably include the following: influenza; the hantaviruses (Hantaan, Seoul, and related viruses); Rift Valley fever; yellow fever; dengue fever; Junin (Argentine hemorrhagic fever); Lassa fever; Marburg and Ebola viruses (members of the family Filoviridae); and various encephalitides, all arthropod borne, such as Japanese encephalitis, Venezuelan equine encephalitis, and Eastern equine encephalitis.

Influenza, of course, is familiar. The hantaviruses—Hantaan, Seoul, and related viruses—cause hemorrhagic fevers with renal syndrome (that is, fevers accompanied by severe bleeding and kidney involvement); these viruses, found in Asia, Europe, and the United States, are naturally occurring viruses of rodents (in the case of Hantaan, a rodent called *Apodemus agrarius*). Seoul virus is found in rats, including urban rats in Korea as well as in Baltimore and other American cities. James Le Duc has recently found a possible association between this virus and chronic renal disease in people living in inner-city Baltimore.[35]

Yellow fever, a mosquito-borne disease characterized by fever and jaundice, originated in Africa and is now widespread in Africa and South America; it probably originated as a virus of monkeys. Dengue fever, a virus in the same family that is also transmitted by the same mosquitoes as yellow fever, probably also originated in the Old World but is now in tropical areas worldwide (Africa, Asia, the south Pacific, South America, and the Caribbean). Other viruses, classified by virologists as members of the Arenavirus family, cause hemorrhagic fevers and are natural infections of rodents. These include Junin (Argentine hemorrhagic fever) and Machupo (Bolivian hemorrhagic fever), and the once infamous (because of its high mortality rate in Western medical missionaries who first came in contact with the virus in the early 1970s) Lassa fever of West Africa, which originated in the rodent *Mastomys natalensis*, all of which viruses were discussed above. Among viruses believed to have originated in monkeys or apes are two related African viruses, Marburg and Ebola, which cause fever with hemorrhage; the unrelated HIV also can be placed in this category. The various equine encephalitides are mosquito borne but tend to have natural animal hosts as well.

Of the viruses listed, I think that influenza, dengue, and the hantaviruses are of greatest potential importance to North America; the recent outbreaks of Oropouche in the Caribbean and Central America are also notable. All these viruses either are widening their scope (dengue, hantaviruses, and recently Oropouche) or still cause recurrent pandemics (influenza). Because of its proximity, dengue might be a special concern. It is widespread in Asia and is also spreading over the Caribbean basin. A dengue outbreak in Cuba in 1981 involved over 300,000 cases. Under certain circumstances an individual who was previously infected with one variety (technically, subtype) of dengue virus can develop a severe form known as dengue hemorrhagic fever upon later infection with a different subtype. The frequency of dengue hemorrhagic fever is increasing as several subtypes of dengue virus extend their range. Aside from the viruses I have listed, there is also always a likelihood that other, as yet undescribed or presently obscure, zoonotic viruses may emerge, as did HIV and Lassa fever. That is why I have emphasized the principles and used these viruses only as examples.

Although the framework offered here identifies the essential conditions for viral emergence, there is still a great deal to learn. Consider influenza. With all the possibilities for recombination, and many human infections annually (perhaps 100,000,000), pandemic influenza strains appear only once every twenty years or so. Why? To put the question in more technical terms, what restrains the emergence of new viruses? Comparatively little is known about this fascinating question, although some patterns are beginning to appear. We also only vaguely understand what factors are required for efficient transmission of viruses in humans. Apart from influenza, many of the other viruses discussed here—such as Junin (Argentine hemorrhagic fever), Marburg, Hantaan, and Lassa fever—fortunately have limited ability to spread from person to person. They would have been devastating if they had that ability or if they were to acquire it. We also need to know more about the mechanisms and determinants of interspecies transfer of viruses. This is a complex matter involving both viral and host factors, but some information is already available and the question is susceptible to further scientific attack. Equally little is known about constraints on viral evolution. In particular, the role of natural selection in shaping or restraining viral evolution has been little explored. Certainly, constraints operate at the level of the virus—host interaction and the maintenance of the virus in nature. In order to survive, viruses must be maintained in nature in some living host. This requirement alone must impose strong selective pressures on a virus.

Even with these gaps in knowledge, we now possess, at least embryonically, the necessary intellectual foundation and tools for attacking these questions, and are faced with the challenge of dealing with the problem of disease emergence. We are not outside the problem; we are learning that emerging viruses do not come as a malevolent rain from above. Human actions have influenced many of these calamities, including HIV. This is, perhaps, both the good news and the bad: We are not completely helpless; but before we can begin to do something, this issue must become a social and economic priority. In many ways, this may prove to be a harder problem than the virological one. However, the essential conclusion is that we must learn to be aware of the consequences of our own actions.

Despite its limitations, the historical record provides clues to traffic patterns. As McNeill has noted, new diseases tend to emerge when populations cross disease boundaries.[36] Recurrent patterns, and near recurrences, abound in history. As pointed out by Elizabeth Fee and Daniel Fox in their Introduction to this volume, such recurrences can be misleading when they are used as analogies. However, they can also be instructive when viewed as manifestations of similar biological processes and traffic patterns that have continued throughout history. The historic association of bubonic plague with rats, and its entry at seaports, is well known.[37] Hence the concern when a virus resembling Hantaan was found only a few years ago in rats living around Baltimore harbor. Although an imperfect analogy, the discovery should remind us that the historic association of rodents, ports, and disease dissemination is not an antiquarian oddity.

More recently the epidemiology of AIDS itself—although, tragically, not its effects—could have been inferred from what was known about hepatitis B, which had a remarkably similar epidemiology. Long before the viral etiology of AIDS was defined, epidemiologists had demonstrated the similarity of transmission patterns for AIDS and for hepatitis B, with identical high-risk practices and risk groups.[38] This information began pointing the way toward suitable precautions to limit spread.

If we had a science of traffic patterns, part biology and part social science, we might have made these inferences more readily, with many lives saved. Perhaps such a field may be struggling to emerge, and among those in the forefront might be mentioned Joshua Lederberg, Baruch Blumberg, Frank Fenner, Edwin Kilbourne, Karl M. Johnson, Thomas Monath, Christoph Scholtissek, Luc Montagnier, D. A. Henderson, Mirko Grmek, William McNeill, the late Fernand Braudel, and Daniel Fox.

Enthusiasm, of course, must be tempered by reality. Even if such a science were developed, and even if there were universal agreement on an agenda, it will probably never be possible to anticipate or prevent every episode of disease emergence. Aside from human factors, our knowledge and ability to act will always be imperfect: not every consequence can be anticipated, the world is too complex, and the generation of new pathogens by viral evolution, however constrained and rare it may be, is still possible. At the moment perhaps the most we can hope for realistically is to begin making inroads into the problem.

Why has it taken so long to develop such thinking? For one thing, we may have been misled by our own preconceptions. Virologists and microbiologists have been concerned with the properties of the disease agents—physical and molecular—and of the diseases they cause, and have tended to concentrate on the particular, possibly to the detriment of defining features in common. Until very recently there were many examples of viral traffic and some examples of mutations, but we had not critically evaluated the contributions of each mechanism to viral emergence. It also seemed too daunting a problem. But, as the examples discussed here should demonstrate, the variations in the agents themselves may be less crucial than the traffic laws, the conditions that allow introduction and dissemination in the human population. While this idea is possibly a logical extension of the Darwinian emphasis on natural selection in the environment, it is nevertheless rarely considered. An appropriate global emphasis on conditions, as in historical thinking, would therefore be valuable in combination with the powerful molecular tools now available for virus detection.

Biological scientists may also find it difficult to believe that people themselves bear much of the responsibility for what may seem at first to be natural processes. Historians and social scientists are more accustomed than virologists and microbiologists to think in terms of the consequences of human actions, and of conditions that cause or permit certain developments, and try to infer these predisposing conditions from the results. This perspective is valuable and complements the kind of analytic and causal thinking in which biological scientists are trained. As the historian Marc Bloch put it, "The virus [sic] of the Black Death was the prime cause of the depopulation of Europe. But the epidemic spread so rapidly only by virture of certain social—and, therefore, in their underlying nature, mental—conditions."[39]

Like every other kind of traffic, viral traffic is increasing. What we are now learning about viral emergence shifts the burden to society at large, to all of us. The conditions I have described are really manmade. Consequently, we need to develop greater sensitivity to our environment and the complex ecological relationships that have evolved. In many cases viral emergence follows deforestation and is another unanticipated consequence of despoiling the environment. As deforestation progresses worldwide, as human activities continue to alter the environment, as population influx into Third World cities continues unabated, as every part of the world becomes more accessible, one would expect disease emergence to accelerate. Our first line of defense is to recognize that these and similar human activities can have serious health consequences, and to anticipate these consequences. We need effective strategies to deal proactively, before their spread becomes critical, with viruses as yet unrecognized and with those that disseminate efficiently. To put it simply, if we are often the engineers of viral traffic, we need better traffic engineering. We need viral traffic studies and road maps of disease. I mean this not only literally, in the sense of medical geography, but also metaphorically. When agricultural development is desirable, it would also be wise to consider and plan for disease emergence as a possible side effect. Environmental impact surveys, conducted thoroughly and systematically, should also include consideration of the microbial and viral fauna in the region.

How might such studies be done? Until a more systematic approach can be defined, we have only the rudiments of an answer, but some generalizations can be made. Certain activities, notably the sorts of environmental changes I have discussed, should be recognized as potentially hazardous, especially in tropical regions. Surveys can test for a known virus when there is a proposed expansion of conditions favorable to viral transmission in areas where this virus is endemic. For example, in view of the history of Argentine hemorrhagic fever, plans to clear new areas of the pampas could trigger field surveys to test for the presence of Junin virus in local rodents. Plans for dam building in certain parts of Africa should bring Rift Valley fever to mind, with appropriate field surveys for this virus.

Unknown viruses will present more of a challenge. One can work from analogy with known examples, and search for viral relatives in similar environments. We do not know what other viruses exist in nature, but using the biotechnological tools now available (such as PCR, discussed in note 34) for broad and rapid testing, we can make more systematic efforts to find out. Fenner has noted that our knowledge of arbo (arthropod-borne) viruses increased dramatically in the 1950s and 1960s largely because the Rockefeller Foundation funded a program to screen for arboviruses in the field by the methods then available.[40] This screening was done mostly by simple biological assays in which samples of ground-up mosquitoes were injected into mice in order to detect viruses pathogenic for mammals that might be present in the mosquitoes. Crude as this sort of screening was, it yielded many new viruses. However, such screening has many disadvantages and is not cost-effective. It is also difficult to evaluate the actual human or animal disease potential of the viruses discovered in this way. Present technology makes it much easier to identify families of viruses in human, primate, rodent, or arthropod populations by broad-based PCR and serological techniques.

Industrialized nations must learn to assist the Third World in financing the needed planning and protective measures to accompany development projects. In many cases relatively simple measures could help greatly, if they are chosen well and if there is sufficient global resolve to implement them. For example, rebuilding water systems in tropical cities to reduce or eliminate open water sources could have a real impact on dengue. Perhaps such projects could someday become priorities before their need reaches the crisis stage. In the intellectual arena our best strategy may be to encourage expanded attempts to find answers to the scientific questions mentioned above, and to forge stronger alliances between molecular virology and such organism-based approaches as field biology, evolutionary biology, and pathogenesis (mechanisms of disease and host-virus interactions). Several scientists have expressed concern that field virologists will soon be in critically short supply; with a paucity of training programs and trainees, the outlook for the future is bleak. In the Third World, for example, there are few well-staffed and thoroughly equipped field laboratories, and their number is decreasing.

The tragedy of AIDS has spurred us on to a consideration of these issues, but it is an unfortunate comment on human nature that such adversity is required before these issues are considered at all. Even with AIDS, the virological problems were largely secondary to a social problem: the failure to recognize the threat and mobilize responses in a timely way.[41] The "moral equivalent" of war, as many leaders have learned to their chagrin, is a poor substitute for the actual thing. It is hard to sustain fervor without a visible adversary. There are also insufficient economic incentives to mobilize concerted action in advance of a crisis. One can only hope that the value of doing so will be appreciated before we are in the throes of another crisis. Ironically, the costs are likely to be small in comparison with major military projects. As Henderson has pointed out, the eradication of smallpox, a landmark in infectious disease control, was accomplished at a total cost of about $300 million.[42]

It is unlikely that infectious diseases will ever be totally eliminated. Our desire to believe that they can be eliminated may reflect the irrational feelings of terror and loss of control that thoughts of these diseases inspire.[43] We have no recourse but to confront these feelings and to deal constructively with them. Even in this highly technological age, we cannot control our biological milieu. At the same time, we must recognize the role that we ourselves play in shaping this milieu. We are part of a complex, interlinked world that we can alter but do not fully control, and science is the study of this complexity. The periodic appearance of "new" infectious diseases serves to remind us of this reality.

NOTES

I thank Dr. Richard L. Landau, editor, and the University of Chicago Press for their permission to reprint this essay, which appeared in modified form in the journal *Perspectives in Biology and Medicine* (34 [Spring 1991]: 387–409, © 1991, The University of Chicago) under the title "Emerging Viruses: Defining the Rules for Viral Traffic."

I also thank Dr. Daniel M. Fox for many helpful comments on this essay, especially on viral traffic and its implications. Many of the examples presented here were drawn from examples discussed at the conference "Emerging Viruses: The Evolution of Viruses and Viral Diseases" (see note 2 below). Special thanks to Dr. John R. La Montagne, Director, Division of Microbiology and Infectious Diseases, and Dr. Ann Schluederberg, Virology Program Director, National Institute of Allergy and Infectious Diseases of the National Institutes of Health; to Drs. Frank Fenner (Australian National University), Dennis M. Stark (The Rockefeller University), S. Gaylen Bradley (Medical College of Virginia), Paul J. Edelson (Cornell University Medical College), and Pravin Bhatt (Yale University School of Medicine); and to the speakers and members of the organizing committee of the conference on emerging viruses for their enthusiastic and generous response, including their sharing of unpublished data. I am grateful to historians Marilyn Gewirtz, Daniel J. Abrams, Daniel M. Fox, Mirko D. Grmek, and Edward Tenner for helpful discussions on historical approaches. Research in my laboratory is supported by grant RR 03121 from the National Institutes of Health, DHHS.

1. Donald A. Henderson, M.D., Dean Emeritus, School of Public Health, Johns Hopkins University (personal communication, 1989) recalls a speech at Johns Hopkins University in 1969 in which the surgeon general of the United States Public Health Service, expressing the optimism typical of this period, assured his audience that infectious diseases were now of marginal interest in the United States and that we should thus shift our focus of attention to the chronic diseases.

2. Emerging viruses and viral evolution were the subject of a conference that I chaired in May 1989 ("Emerging Viruses: The Evolution of Viruses and

Viral Diseases"), the first ever held on this subject. One purpose of the conference, which was sponsored by the National Institutes of Health with The Rockefeller University, was to unite historical, epidemiological, and molecular approaches. I am editing a book containing contributions by the participants. Several popular summaries of this conference have recently appeared; see, for example, Julie Ann Miller, "Diseases for Our Future," *BioScience* 39 (1989): 509–17. For a more technical summary, see Stephen S. Morse and Ann Schluederberg, "Emerging Viruses: The Evolution of Viruses and Viral Diseases," *Journal of Infectious Diseases* 162 (1990): 1–7.

3. This point has also been discussed in a very readable essay by Edwin D. Kilbourne, "Are New Diseases Really New?" *Natural History* 92 (December 1983): 28–32.

4. See Howard M. Temin, "Is HIV Unique or Merely Different?" *Journal of Acquired Immune Deficiency Syndromes* 2 (1989): 1–9.

5. Angus G. Dalgleish et al., "The CD4 (T4) Antigen Is an Essential Component of the Receptor for the AIDS Retrovirus," *Nature* 312 (1984): 763–67; David Klatzmann et al., "T-Lymphocyte T4 Molecule Behaves as the Receptor for Human Retrovirus LAV," *Nature* 312 (1984): 767–70; P. J. Maddon et al., "The T4 Gene Encodes the AIDS Virus Receptor and Is Expressed in the Immune System and the Brain," *Cell* 47 (1986): 333–48.

6. It is hypothetically possible that a particular virus could be the only surviving member of an extinct group possessing a distinctive characteristic (in which case one might be forced to conclude that the characteristic would not have been of much survival value to the virus); however, the tendency in nature is usually the opposite: vestigial characteristics are often retained long past any apparent utility. Virtually nothing is known about viral "extinction," or even whether it occurs, except for the intentional case of smallpox. On the other hand, it is also possible, and actually not improbable, that a new characteristic could arise as a small change by mutation from an existing virus. Thus, CD4 tropism of HIV could have arisen by a fortuitous mutation in the *env* (viral envelope) protein required for attachment to the appropriate cell receptor for virus entry; such a mutation would enable the protein to attach to CD4 on cells. This was the view originally held by many people, including many virologists. Although HIV itself did not arise this way, for the very reasons discussed, one would suppose that an ancestor of HIV could have arisen in this fashion. Howard M. Temin has discussed the role of mutation; see "Is HIV Unique or Merely Different?" (referred to in note 4) and "Evolution of Cancer Genes as a Mutation-Driven Process," *Cancer Research* 48 (1988): 1697–1701. Alternatively, the virus could conceivably have acquired the capability for CD4 binding by picking up a host cellular gene for this property; retroviruses are well known for their propensity to exchange genetic information with host cells. It is hard to make any predictions about how important mutation is as a way of generating new viruses. My personal feeling is that, for statistical reasons, it is less important in human disease. Ours is only one of many mammalian species, and many other species are more numerous; if there is a finite probability of the critical step's happening in any particular species, the numerical chance of its happening first in humans is therefore comparatively small. However, such an

event could someday happen, although perhaps at a lower frequency than would suit our own anthropocentrism.

7. Luc Montagnier, "Origin and Evolution of HIVs and Their Role in AIDS Pathogenesis," *Journal of Acquired Immune Deficiency Syndromes* 1 (1988): 517–20.

8. Matthew A. Gonda et al., "Characterization and Molecular Cloning of a Bovine Lentivirus Related to Human Immunodeficiency Virus," *Nature* 330 (1987): 388–91; Niels C. Pedersen et al., "Isolation of a T-Lymphotropic Virus from Domestic Cats with an Immunodeficiency-Like Syndrome," *Science* 235 (1987): 790–93. These viruses were all characterized after the discovery of the CD4 tropism of HIV as researchers became alerted to the possibility that related viruses with this property might exist. The example of mouse thymic virus, discussed below, was the first case of an *unrelated* virus shown to cause a similar effect.

9. Stephen S. Morse and Jay E. Valinsky, "Mouse Thymic Virus (MTLV): A Mammalian Herpesvirus Cytolytic for DC4$^+$ (L3T4$^+$) T Lymphocytes," *Journal of Experimental Medicine* 169 (1989): 591–96. The virus has been known since 1961. Rather than suggesting a common evolutionary relationship with HIV, which seems unlikely, this similarity probably indicates that unrelated organisms can evolve similar ways to go about a particular process. This apparent convergence is likely due to such limitations of the viral life-style as dependence on host cells.

10. Dharam V. Ablashi et al., "HBLV (or HHV-6) in Human Cell Lines," *Nature* 329 (1987): 207; Carlos Lopez et al., "Characteristics of Human Herpesvirus-6," *Journal of Infectious Diseases* 157 (1988): 1271–73. HHV-6, although cytolytic for CD4$^+$ T cells, probably does not enter the cell via a CD4 receptor.

11. Ablashi et al., "HBLV (or HHV-6) in Human Cell Lines."

12. S. Z. Salahuddin et al., "Isolation of a New Virus, HBLV, in Patients with Lymphoproliferative Disorders," *Science* 234 (1986): 596–600.

13. Wallace P. Rowe and Worth I. Capps, "A New Mouse Virus Causing Necrosis of the Thymus in Newborn Mice," *Journal of Experimental Medicine* 113 (1961): 831–44; Sue S. Cross et al., "Biology of Mouse Thymic Virus, a Herpesvirus of Mice, and the Antigenic Relationship to Mouse Cytomegalovirus," *Infection and Immunity* 26 (1979): 1186–95; Stephen S. Morse, "Mouse Thymic Necrosis Virus: A Novel Murine Lymphotropic Agent," *Laboratory Animal Science* 37 (1987): 717–25, and "Mouse Thymic Virus (MTLV; Murid Herpesvirus 3) Infection in Athymic Nude Mice: Evidence for a T Lymphocyte Requirement," *Virology* 163 (1988): 255–58. This does not rule out more subtle effects; we have recently found an association with autoimmune disease.

14. K. Yamanishi et al., "Identification of Human Herpesvirus-6 as a Causal Agent for Exanthem Subitum," *Lancet* 1 (1988): 1065–67; Lopez et al., "Characteristics of Human Herpesvirus-6."

15. Interview with Thomas Bass, *Omni* 11 (1988): 102–6, 128–34; remark quoted, p. 130.

16. Personal communication; see also note 2 above. For other comments by

Lederberg on this subject, see Joshua Lederberg, "Medical Science, Infectious Disease, and the Unity of Humankind," *Journal of the American Medical Association* 260 (August 5, 1988): 684–85.

17. Esteban Domingo and John J. Holland, "High Error Rates, Population Equilibrium and Evolution of RNA Replication Systems," and Manfred Eigen and C. K. Biebricher, "Sequence Space and Quasispecies Distribution," both in *RNA Genetics*, ed. E. Domingo, J. J. Holland, and P. Ahlquist (Boca Raton, Fla.: CRC Press, 1988), 3: 3–36, 211–45; David Steinhauer and John J. Holland, "Rapid Evolution of RNA Viruses," *Annual Reviews of Microbiology* 41 (1987): 409–33. As these reviews show, HIV is highly variable but is not unique in this respect.

18. This essay deals with emergence of human disease, but the principles apply equally to other species.

19. Howard Temin provides evidence that a number of neutral mutations can accumulate and lead in time to a virus possessing drastically different properties from its "parents." Therefore, he argues, it is impossible to predict what new variants will emerge. For an exposition of this argument, see his papers cited in note 6. On the other hand, other factors, such as the limited number of routes by which a virus can enter the body, impose certain constraints. It appears likely that the rules I have described here for the first step are the most important factors in the short run; on a longer time scale, over hundreds or thousands of years, genuine evolutionary change might occasionally be significant.

20. Because of their number, I have not provided specific references for most of the examples mentioned. For some references, see also Morse and Schluederberg, "Emerging Viruses." Many examples were discussed at the May 1989 conference on emerging viruses, and a forthcoming volume (see note 2) on emerging viruses will describe many of them in greater detail. I am grateful to Karl M. Johnson for providing much of the information on the hemorrhagic fever viruses; to Drs. Robert G. Webster, Peter Palese, and Edwin D. Kilbourne for information on influenza; and to Dr. Thomas P. Monath for information on the arthropod-borne viruses. For the reader desiring additional detailed scientific information, at a more advanced level, and references, the following can be recommended: For background on viruses, viral diseases, and immunology, a general textbook of medical microbiology, such as Bernard D. Davis et al., *Microbiology*, 4th ed. (New York: Lippincott, 1990), can be consulted. For a general treatment of infectious organisms and their hosts and of viruses as the causes of disease (principles of pathogenesis), see Cedric A. Mims, *The Pathogenesis of Infectious Diseases*, 3rd ed. (New York and London: Academic Press, 1987); see also Sir Macfarlane Burnet and David O. White, *Natural History of Infectious Disease*, 4th ed. (London and New York: Cambridge University Press, 1972), which has become a classic. Finally, for specific viruses, the most detailed reference is Bernard Fields, ed., *Virology*, 2nd ed. (New York: Raven Press, 1990).

21. Gloria de Villafañe et al., "Dinámica de las comunidades de roedores en agro-ecosistemas pampásicos," *Medicina (Buenos Aires)*, 37, Suppl. 3 (1977): 128–40.

22. The recognition of Lassa fever, and its astonishing mortality, was the

subject of a popular book about fifteen years ago, *Fever! The Hunt for a New Killer Virus*, by John Fuller (New York: Reader's Digest Press, 1974). A recent incident was reported in the press (Lawrence K. Altman, "When an Exotic Virus Strikes: A Deadly Case of Lassa Fever," *New York Times*, February 28, 1989, p. C3).

23. Z. Jezek and Frank Fenner, *Human Monkeypox*, Monographs in Virology, vol. 17 (Basel: S. Karger, 1988). Fortunately, monkeypox has only a limited ability to spread from person to person and therefore is probably not a major threat, at least in its present form. Frank Fenner considers human monkeypox a transient phenomenon in areas undergoing transition from forest to cleared land. He points out that risk of exposure to monkeypox increases as people begin to encroach on the forest but that the risk decreases considerably after deforestation is largely complete in an area.

24. Robert G. Webster and R. Rott, "Influenza Virus A Pathogenicity: The Pivotal Role of Hemagglutinin," *Cell* 50 (1987): 665–66. Robert Webster (personal communication) calls influenza the oldest emerging virus that is still emerging.

25. H. Kida, K. F. Shortridge, and R. G. Webster, "Origin of the Hemagglutinin Gene of H3N2 Influenza Viruses from Pigs in China," *Virology* 162 (1988): 160–66. In contrast, Chinese scientists believe that the pig is the recipient (getting virus from people) rather than the donor; see Zhu Ji-ming, "Human Virus Diseases in China: Research and Control," *Impact of Science on Society* 150 (1988): 137–47.

26. Christoph Scholtissek and Ernest Naylor, "Fish Farming and Influenza Pandemics," *Nature* 331 (1988): 215. For further information on the traditional Chinese pig-duck agriculture systems, see K. Ruddle and G. Zhong, *Integrated Agriculture-Aquaculture in South China: The Dike-Pond System of the Zhujiang Delta* (New York: Cambridge University Press, 1988). I thank Wallace Parham, U.S. Congress Office of Technology Assessment, for valuable information on this subject.

27. It is also unknown how many times the virus may have been previously (but unsuccessfully) introduced to humans. A great deal has been written on the origins of HIV. For an excellent discussion of several aspects of this question, see Mirko D. Grmek, *Histoire du SIDA* (Paris: Payot, 1989; English trans., *History of AIDS* [Princeton, N.J.: Princeton University Press, 1990]). A chapter by Gerald Myers in my forthcoming volume on emerging viruses (note 2) will consider the origin and spread of HIV. For an earlier discussion of these views, see T. F. Smith et al., "The Phylogenetic History of Immunodeficiency Viruses," *Nature* 333 (1988): 573–75 (and accompanying "News and Views" commentary by David Penney, "Origins of the AIDS Virus," 494–95). See also S. Conner and S. Kingman, *The Search for the Virus* (London: Penguin Books, 1988); and Montagnier, "Origin and Evolution of HIVs." An alternative hypothesis, that HIV-1 is an ancient virus in humans, has been suggested, notably by Montagnier.

28. Thomas Lovejoy, personal communication, May 1989; Richard House, "Malaria Spreads in Brazil as Development Opens Up the Amazon," *Washington Post*, July 18, 1989, p. 5.

29. Altman, "When an Exotic Virus Strikes." This example demonstrates how comparatively easy it is for a disease to be spread rapidly by travel.

30. I thank Gerald Myers for this example. See also Conner and Kingman, *The Search for the Virus*, pp. 212ff, and Peter Piot et al., "AIDS: An International Perspective," *Science* 239 (1988): 573–79.

31. Qui-Lim Choo et al., "Isolation of a cDNA Clone Derived from a Blood-Borne Non-A, Non-B Viral Hepatitis Genome," *Science* 244 (1989): 359–62.

32. Another T lymphotropic human herpesvirus, dubbed "human herpesvirus 7" (HHV-7), has recently been described (N. Frenkel et al., "Isolation of a New Herpesvirus from Human CD4$^+$ T Cells," *Proceedings of the National Academy of Sciences (USA)* 87 (1990): 748–52).

33. J. Zahorsky, "Roseola Infantilis," *Pediatrics* 22 (1910): 60.

34. A few words on the importance of technology in disease recognition may be appropriate here. The recognition of HIV was dependent on the previous development of methods for growing T lymphocytes in culture, including key methods that were developed in Gallo's laboratory. For an excellent discussion of the history of HIV and of the role of technology in the discovery of HIV, see Grmek, *Histoire du SIDA*. In a more general sense, the introduction of tissue culture methods, in the 1940s, was a major breakthrough in the study and characterization of viruses. The identification of non-A, non-B hepatitis virus (now called hepatitis C virus), described above, is another example of the successful application of technology. It can be expected that new tools for detection will uncover new viruses. In particular, many new avenues are opened by the recent development of an exceptionally sensitive technique—the polymerase chain reaction, or PCR (Randall K. Saiki et al., "Primer-Directed Enzymatic Amplification of DNA with a Thermostable DNA Polymerase," *Science* 239 (1988): 487–91; Chin-Yih Ou et al., "DNA Amplification for Direct Detection of HIV-1 in DNA of Peripheral Blood Mononuclear Cells," *Science* 239 (1988): 295–97). PCR is capable of detecting one HIV-infected cell in a hundred thousand (Richard A. Gibbs and Jeffrey S. Chamberlain, "The Polymerase Chain Reaction: A Meeting Report," *Genes and Development* 3 (1989): 1095–98). Because PCR can detect and amplify DNA in minuscule amounts of sample, and is comparatively undemanding, it is rapidly finding favor in many applications. PCR has great potential for disease archaeology and the study of evolution. One difficulty with conventional virological methods is that they often require a sample that has been carefully handled. It is often difficult to detect viable virus, for example, in fixed tissues or in samples that have been stored carelessly or for long periods. By PCR many otherwise intractable samples can now be tested, even mummified human bodies 7,000 years old (Svante Pääbo, "Ancient DNA: Extraction, Characterization, Molecular Cloning, and Enzymatic Amplification," *Proceedings of the National Academy of Sciences (USA)* 86 (1989): 1937; S. Pääbo, R. G. Higuchi, and Allan C. Wilson, "Ancient DNA and the Polymerase Chain Reaction: The Emerging Field of Molecular Archaeology," *Journal of Biological Chemistry* 264 (1989): 9709). This technique also has possibilities for detecting viral genetic information in ancient samples. There have been many speculations about the antiquity of HIV and AIDS. Mirko Grmek (personal communication, Paris, July 1989) has suggested using PCR to

test for HIV or HIV-like viruses in century-old tissues preserved in pathological museums, and this would be quite a feasible way to determine whether HIV infection might have existed then. Even older samples can be tested for specific viruses. PCR techniques are available now for detecting entire families of viruses based on limited genetic resemblances and offer powerful tools for studying viral "paleontology" and evolution (see, for example, David H. Mack and John J. Sninsky, "A Sensitive Method for the Identification of Uncharacterized Viruses Related to Known Virus Groups: Hepadnavirus Model System," *Proceedings of the National Academy of Sciences (USA)* 85 (1988): 6977–81; Andy Shih, Ravi Misra, and Mark G. Rush, "Detection of Multiple, Novel Reverse Transcriptase Coding Sequences in Human Nucleic Acids: Relation to Primate Retroviruses," *Journal of Virology* 63 (1989): 64–75. As a result, one can now "go fishing" for viral ancestors and relatives in formerly untestable samples. PCR makes multiple copies of the specific piece of DNA it detects, and the resulting product can be analyzed and compared with known viruses. This capability is a boon for the study of viral evolution over long periods of time. Such study was previously impossible because, as has often been remarked by viral evolutionists, "viruses have left no fossil footprints" (quote from Darryl C. Reanney, "Evolutionary Virology: A Molecular Overview," in *The Human Herpesviruses,* ed. André J. Nahmias, W. R. Dowdle, and Raymond R. Schinazi (New York: Elsevier, 1981), p. 519; for a more recent review of molecular evolutionary studies of viruses, see Adrian Gibbs, "Molecular Evolution of Viruses: 'Trees,' 'Clocks' and 'Modules,' " *Journal of Cell Science* Supp. 7 (1987): 319–37, and earlier forms could only be inferred from vestigial genetic information in existing viruses.

35. James LeDuc, personal communication, May 1989.

36. William H. McNeill, *Plagues and Peoples* (Garden City, N.Y.: Doubleday, 1976). His recent essay "Control and Catastrophe in Human Affairs," *Daedalus* 118 (Winter 1989): 1–12, giving his views on human attempts to control catastrophic events, may also be of interest.

37. Philip Zeigler, *The Black Death* (New York: Harper and Row, 1969); Robert S. Gottfried, *The Black Death* (New York: Free Press, 1983). As a non-historian, I have sometimes idly wondered whether the history of Europe would have been different if the people of this period had known sooner about this association and if the simple metal rat-catcher that prevents rats from leaving ships had been available in the Middle Ages.

38. W. Thomas London and Baruch S. Blumberg, "Comments on the Role of Epidemiology in the Investigation of Hepatitis B Virus," *Epidemiologic Reviews* 7 (1985): 59–79.

39. Marc Bloch, *The Historian's Craft,* trans. Peter Putnam (New York: Knopf, 1953), chap. 5, quoted sentences, p. 194.

40. Frank Fenner, "Keynote Address," in *Viral and Mycoplasmal Infections of Laboratory Rodents,* ed. Pravin N. Bhatt et al. (Orlando, Fla.: Academic Press, 1986), p. 21; amplified in personal communication, November 1989.

41. Randy Shilts, *And the Band Played On: Politics, People, and the AIDS Epidemic* (New York: St. Martin's Press, 1987), describes many of these failures and their disastrous consequences.

42. Donald Henderson, personal communication May 1989, February 1991; and D. A. Henderson, in F. Fenner et al., *Smallpox and Its Eradication* (Geneva: World Health Organization, 1988). Dr. Henderson directed the world smallpox eradication program.

43. The subject of much literature, from antiquity to now. Susan Sontag, *AIDS and Its Metaphors* (New York: Farrar, Straus and Giroux, 1988), demonstrates the power of these images even now.

Causes, Cases, and Cohorts: The Role of Epidemiology in the Historical Construction of AIDS

Gerald M. Oppenheimer

In his history of the HIV (human immunodeficiency virus) epidemic, Mirko Grmek reports that the term *acquired immune deficiency syndrome,* the first generally accepted name for this new disorder, was coined at a 1982 meeting held at the Centers for Disease Control (CDC) in Atlanta. Thereafter, the CDC epidemiologists spread and legitimated the neologism by using it extensively in official publications.[1] By attributing to the CDC the power to control the name of the disease, Grmek indirectly demonstrates how prominent a part that agency and its epidemiologists played in defining this new "medical mystery."

In this essay I examine the role of epidemiologists, in the CDC and elsewhere, in characterizing HIV infection. Faced with a new disease of unknown origin, epidemiologists and their collaborators constructed, over time, hypothetical models to explain the disorder in order to contain it. Prior to the isolation of a causal virus, epidemiologists played a central role in defining the new syndrome, developing first a "life-style" model and later a model based on hepatitis B. Though subsequently supplanted from their special position by virologists and other "bench" scientists working in laboratories (who named the virus and thereby redesignated the disease), epidemiologists have continued to define important dimensions of the disorder and to raise disquieting questions. Specifically, they were concerned with discovering risk factors for HIV infection, its modes of transmission, the natural history of the disease, the extent to which it had spread within population groups, and the projection of future prevalence and incidence rates.

Although epidemiologists have increasingly lost to biomedical scientists the power to construct the meaning of the HIV infection, epidemiologists in the CDC retain an important prerogative: they continue to frame the population-based definition of AIDS. Because the CDC has responsibility for monitoring infection in the United States, it has formulated, over time, the surveillance definitions of AIDS. Recently this population-based definition, as well as the reporting system itself, has been found deficient by demographers and quantitative social scientists. Their critiques raise the possibility that the power of epidemiologists to frame the disorder, already limited by biomedical scientists, may be further eroded by social scientists newly attracted to the study of AIDS. Nonetheless, since 1981 epidemiology has had a profound effect on the characterization of HIV infection in the United States. To a large degree, that characterization reflects something of the nature and concerns of American epidemiology itself.

Epidemiology, unlike virology, has a strong social dimension in that it explicitly incorporates perceptions of a population's social relations, behavioral patterns, and experiences into its explanations of disease processes. Given their training, epidemiologists fairly consistently defined HIV infection as a biological process occurring within a determinant social matrix. That the infection was first identified among young male homosexuals and intravenous drug users certainly reinforced that professional proclivity.

The results of this exercise in epidemiological imagination were complex and equivocal. On the one hand, the epidemiologists' approach may have skewed the choice of models and hypotheses, determined which data were excluded from consideration until later in the epidemic, and offered scientific justification for popular prejudice, particularly against gay men. On the other hand, the epidemiological approach gave the new disease a human face. By defining the behaviors and the multiple social experiences of groups as risk factors for the disease, epidemiology countered attempts to reduce the etiology of HIV infection to a virus alone. In addition, epidemiology offered the possibility of primary prevention in the form of health education and follow-up, particularly important in the absence of a vaccine or a successful therapy.

The various characterizations of HIV infection examined in this essay will span the period from early 1981, when physicians first encountered anomalous medical facts, to mid-1990, when epidemiologists had attempted to define the distribution of the HIV across subpopulations; to project future rates of HIV infection and illness for the population as a whole; and to establish wih some specificity the natural history of the new disease. This essay draws almost entirely on the medical literature of the period.

EPIDEMIOLOGY AND PUBLIC HEALTH

Epidemiology played a key role in the AIDS epidemic for at least two reasons—one institutional, the other scientific. The institutional link was the Centers for Disease Control (CDC) in Atlanta. Part of the Public Health Service, which falls under the jurisdiction of the U.S. Department of Health and Human Services, the CDC is responsible for monitoring morbidity and mortality trends in the United States and for responding to acute outbreaks of disease—infectious disease in particular. To fulfill its mission, the CDC depends heavily on case reports, surveillance, and epidemiological investigations.

Epidemiology is particularly well suited to explore, portray, and explain new medical phenomena. It seeks to measure and analyze the occurrence and distribution of diseases and other health-related conditions in human populations, acting both as a sentinel who warns of shifts in disease patterns and as a scout who seizes on such shifts to discover their etiology.

For example, by systematically collecting data on the frequency of disorders in populations or subgroups through surveillance programs, epidemiologists can discern changes in the distribution of diseases in the community. Observations of these distributions, and their variation in subgroups, lead to hypotheses concerning the relationship between the disease and variables that may affect its natural history and clinical course. Using different study designs, epidemiologists attempt to measure, reject, or refine the relative significance of such hypothetical associations. The ultimate objective of these studies is to isolate the causal variables of the disease in question. An intermediate goal is to discover a point in the natural history of the disease where intervention might alter its course, even if its etiology remains unknown.

Epidemiologists tend to believe in multifactorial disease models. They assume, that is, that intervention is possible at several points, even in the absence of a known "first cause." The major premise of the multifactorial model is, as the name implies, that a given disease may have a number of causes or antecedents, a combination of which may be needed to produce the disorder. The "web of causes," therefore, may be interdicted at more than one vulnerable point.[2]

The power of the multifactorial model is that it can incorporate any measurable factor relevant to and statistically associated with the disease or disorder of interest. Unlike the reductionist paradigm of the germ theory, the multicausal model embraces a variety of environmental and social factors. The model's strength, however, is also its weakness. The multifactorial model allows the researcher to cast a very wide net. Scientists may attempt to incorporate many possible explanatory variables whose putative causal connections with the disease in question may be plausible for a number of reasons—scientific, logical, historical, experiential, and so forth. Variables may be drawn in (or left out) as a function of the social values of the scientists, the working group, or the society. When included in the model, embraced by the professionals, and published in the scientific press, such value judgments appear to be objective, well-grounded scientific statements.

Epidemiology is an applied science that responds to two kinds of disorder within the community: one caused by the disease directly, and the other the product of the fears it has aroused. Consequently, epidemiology bore the initial responsibility of outlining the direction of research, generating hypotheses, and synthesizing the results. In the face of a fatal disorder of unknown origin and indefinite proportions, epidemiology offered a set of procedures (for example, case definition, verification, and count) that swiftly generated results and then authenticated them, giving the public a sense of definite progress. The content of this science, by providing and naming concepts (for example, "risk groups"), made the epidemic potentially less frightening by making it appear more likely that the disease would eventually be understood and controlled.

CASE FINDING AND SURVEILLANCE

The initial discoveries heralding a new disorder of unknown origin were made by physicians treating patients in Los Angeles hospitals. Michael Gottlieb and his colleagues alerted the CDC that between October 1980 and May 1981 five young, previously healthy homosexual men had been treated for biopsy-confirmed *Pneumocystis carinii* pneumonia (PCP). PCP is a protozoan-produced condition that occurs almost exclusively in persons with severely suppressed or defective immune systems. On June 5, 1981, a short paper describing the patients was published by the CDC in its *Morbidity and Mortality Weekly Report (MMWR)*.[3]

Gottlieb's communication to the CDC was closely followed by another from New York City and San Francisco, which reported that, in the thirty months prior to July 1981, Kaposi's sarcoma (KS) had been diagnosed in twenty-six male homosexuals between twenty-six and fifty-one years of age.[4] A rare cancer in the United States, KS occurred in this country primarily in elderly males and immunosuppressed transplant recipients. Its manifestation in a relatively large number of young men was considered highly unusual.

An editorial note in the issue of *MMWR* that had published Gottlieb's paper hypothesized that "the fact that these patients were all homosexuals suggests an association between some aspect of a homosexual lifestyle or disease acquired through sexual contact and *Pneumocystis* pneumonia in this population."[5] The conjecture that some aspect of homosexuality predisposed the patients to immune dysfunction and infections was made on the basis of only five cases from a single community, a broad generalization to formulate from so small a sample.

The basis for that sweeping hypothesis lay in a rough mixture of analysis and opinion. The CDC had just completed a cooperative study with a number of gay community health clinics. It was a multiyear, multisite study of risk factors for hepatitis B, a disease which can be sexually transmitted and whose prevalence is very high among homosexual men.[6] In analyzing the interrelation of life-style and hepatitis B, the researchers found that blood markers for the disease were significantly associated with, among other factors, a large number of male sexual partners and with sexual practices that involved anal contact.

The CDC-associated study took place against a background of other investigations that pointed to an increase in the incidence as well as the types of sexually transmitted diseases (STDs) in homosexual men.[7] Analysts linked this epidemic of STDs to gay liberation and the attendant life-style of bars, discos, and bathhouses and of anonymous sexual partners.[8]

The combination of the CDC's recent work on risk factors for hepatitis B transmission, which had increased its awareness of gay life-style and sexuality and its knowledge of the epidemicity of STDs among subgroups within the gay community, probably accounts in part for the hypothesis suggested in the *MMWR*. One might fairly infer that the CDC was prematurely ready to find the etiology of this mysterious disorder in an exotic subculture. This inference is strengthened by the ensuing scientific work of epidemiologists within and outside the CDC, who found in gay culture—particularly in its perceived "extreme" and "nonnormative" aspects (that is, "promiscuity" and recreational drugs)— the crucial clue to the cause of the new syndrome.

Part of the reason for the CDC's speedy adoption of the "life-style" hypothesis was, most likely, that in certain previous outbreaks of diseases of uncertain origin (in particular, legionnaires' disease in 1976), CDC officials had been criticized for committing themselves to a microbial hypothesis without having paid sufficient attention to alternative causative theories.[9] Such criticism probably influenced their desire to throw a causative net widely in the case of HIV infection.[10]

A special task force on KS and opportunistic infections was established at the CDC in mid-1981 and charged with the surveillance of all new cases. As a preliminary step, the CDC had to define what constituted a case. It initially described a case as "a person who 1) has either biopsy-proven KS or biopsy-proven, life-threatening opportunistic infection, 2) is under age 60, and 3) has no history of either immunosuppressive underlying illness or immunosuppressive therapy."[11] By September 1982, when the CDC first used the term *AIDS* in the *MMWR,* it refined this description to define an AIDS case as one with "a disease at least moderately predictive of a defect in cell-mediated immunity, occurring in a person with no known cause for diminished resistance to that disease." Included among the diseases were KS, PCP, and a specific list of "other opportunistic infections," a list which the CDC has amended over the years.[12]

On September 1, 1987, the CDC significantly modified its case definition. It not only included new medical conditions such as HIV-related encephalopathy (dementia) and wasting syndrome but, for the first time, counted as cases those who, along with a positive antibody test, have had only a presumptive (that is, non-laboratory-confirmed) diagnosis for certain diseases, such as PCP and KS. Preliminary evidence indicates that 12 percent of cases diagnosed during the four months after September 1, 1987, met only the new case definition.[13]

What caused this disorder? With limited clinical data at hand, the CDC did a "quick and dirty" survey of 420 males attending venereal disease clinics in San Francisco, New York, and Atlanta, with the intention of finding cases with KS or PCP. The thirty-five cases culled from the sample (biased, since such patients are more active sexually than the general population) were interviewed on many subjects in the hope that a lead might be discovered.

The researchers found two patterns of behavior that "fell out": sex and drugs. The cases, all homosexuals, had had many sexual partners in the past year (the median was eighty-seven) and had frequently used marijuana, cocaine, and amyl or butyl nitrite—inhalant sexual stimulants.[14] Were sex and drugs independent of each other, however? The rate of nitrite use, for example, was closely associated with the number of sexual partners, suggesting that nitrite inhalation might be associated with other hypothetical causal variables, including sexually transmitted diseases, the medications used to treat them, or types of sexual behavior.[15] It was also possible that nitrite use was not an etiological factor, but appeared to be one because it was associated with a casual or "confounding" variable such as sex.

Despite the dearth of evidence (the "quick and dirty" survey had found that 86.4 percent of homosexual or bisexual men, whether cases or not, had used nitrite in the previous five years), amyl nitrite (AN) did become one of the first hypothetical causal variables to be investigated.[16] As a clue, amyl nitrite seemed worth pursuing. It appeared to be compatible with the gay life-style thesis posed by the *MMWR* and attractive to epidemiological researchers. Studies in which nitrite inhalant was a variable will be evaluated below.

Scientific papers published in 1981 consisted mainly of case and surveillance reports, in which attempts were made to define the new syndromes and the patients—that is, to formulate what constituted a "case." By describing the population at risk in terms of person, place, and time, and by learning from physicians the clinical details of the disorder, epidemiologists could grope for etiological clues that they might use to design formal studies.

One of the first clinical clues pursued was the possibility that the new syndrome was caused by the cytomegalovirus (CMV), a microbe suspected of being both sexually transmitted and a cause of KS. In September the British medical journal *The Lancet* published a clinical study of KS in eight homosexual men in New York City; the investigation found that all four patients tested were positive for CMV.[17] Three months later Michael Gottlieb and his colleagues reported that four previously healthy men with PCP were infected with CMV and also were suffering from a marked decrease in white blood cells, particularly of a kind known as T4 helper cells.[18] While acknowledging that CMV infection might result from T4-cell deficiency and the reactivation of a dormant infection, Gottlieb and his colleagues, basing their position on previous studies, preferred to hold CMV highly suspect.

The CDC, in its year-end summary on the epidemic, also cited CMV

as one of three possible etiological agents.[19] Other putative causes, perhaps more closely related to the life-style hypothesis, were amyl nitrite
and opiate addiction. (A recent investigation in New York City of eleven
immunocompromised men with PCP had found that seven of the patients, including five heterosexuals, were drug "abusers."[20]) Did any of
these agents bear a relationship to any other? How did CMV fit into
the life-style hypothesis? An editorial in the *New England Journal of
Medicine* addressed these issues in December 1981.

Ignoring the heterosexual cases of PCP and other opportunistic infections, the editorialist noted that "the question of cause is obviously
central. What clue does the link with homosexuality provide?"[21] The
answer was a high incidence of sexually transmitted diseases, including
viral infections such as CMV and hepatitis B, that might cause immunosuppression and KS. But because neither homosexuality nor CMV is
new, the author suggested that a new factor may have modified the
host-agent relationship: recreational drugs, particularly amyl nitrite. On
the basis of this reasoning, he postulated a possible multifactorial disease model.[22] Specifically, he proposed that the joint effects of persistent, sexually transmitted viral infection (presumably from CMV) and
a recreational drug such as amyl nitrite precipitated immunosuppression in genetically predisposed males. From this followed a clinical course
that included minor illnesses, then KS or other neoplasms, and serious
opportunisitic infections. In essence, the model was an elaboration of
the hypothesis originally proposed in the editorial note appended to the
first *MMWR* on the new disease.

THE LIFE-STYLE HYPOTHESIS: EXPERIMENTAL WORK

To refine hypotheses generated by case reports, "quick and dirty"
surveys, and surveillance, researchers compared patients with the new
syndrome to a group of healthy men possessing comparable sociodemographic characteristics, experiences, or behaviors. Such research designs, which begin with outcome (the disease) and attempt to discover
factors retrospectively that can account for the different health status
of the two groups, are known as case-control studies. The early case-
control studies were meant, in part, to test whether suspected agents
such as CMV or amyl nitrite might be causative factors.

One of the first such studies, by James Goedert and his colleagues at
the National Institutes of Health (NIH) and the Uniformed Services

University of the Health Sciences, explored the relationship between KS and amyl nitrite.[23] Goedert attempted to assess the new disorder (the outcome) by collecting clinical, virological, and immunological information on two male homosexuals with KS and fifteen healthy homosexual volunteers. The researchers hypothesized that CMV hyperinfection and/or the chronic use of amyl nitrite might be causal variables. In presenting their results and assessing the implications, the investigators suggested that amyl nitrite inhalation may predispose homosexual men to immune deficiency.

This investigation had some serious limitations. The small number of subjects in the study, for example, deprived it of the power to find statistical significance if significance existed. Moreover, though amyl nitrite was correlated with immune defects, the researchers did not report controlling for the effects of possible "confounders"—that is, alternative causal variables, such as number of sexual partners or history of infectious diseases. Notwithstanding its defects, this study was cited by others as evidence for the plausibility of amyl nitrite as a causal variable, a tribute, in part, to the power of the life-style hypothesis.[24]

Almost simultaneously with the investigation by Goedert and his colleagues in Bethesda, Michael Marmor and his colleagues in New York City interviewed twenty gay men with biopsy-confirmed KS and forty gay male controls, matched for age and race, eliciting information on sociodemographic characteristics, medical history, sexual practices, and drug consumption. The cases were twenty of the twenty-one males with KS, aged fifty-two or younger, admitted to New York University Medical Center between March 1979 and August 1981. Controls were selected from the private patients of a Manhattan physician. (Since one-third of those asked to be controls refused, it is possible that the control group was skewed in some indeterminate way.) Using multivariate analysis, the investigators found that, of all the study variables, only amyl nitrite and "promiscuity" (as measured by number of different sexual partners per month in the year before onset of disease) appeared to have an independent, statistically significant association with KS.[25]

In October 1981, approximately when the Marmor study began, the CDC undertook a multisite case-control investigation to identify risk factors for KS and PCP in gay men who lacked presdisposing clinical factors for either.[26] The CDC chose as controls male homosexuals without KS or PCP, matched to the cases by age, race, and area of residence. Mindful that private-practice controls might not be drawn from precisely the same population as the cases, the researchers used, where possible, multiple controls—that is, patients from both private practice and STD clinics.

Published in August 1983, the study found that KS and PCP were associated with certain aspects of male homosexuality—in particular, numerous sexual partners per year. Other significant variables were attendance at bathhouses, a history of syphilis, the use of illicit drugs (except nitrites), and exposure to feces during sex. The strong implication was that a subgroup of the male homosexual population, those who were most sexually active, was at greatest risk for KS or PCP. Taking into account the fact that AIDS had by then appeared in other segments of the U.S. population, including hemophiliacs, the authors concluded that an infectious agent might be the necessary cause of the syndrome.

Nonetheless, the CDC was unwilling to dismiss the life-style hypothesis and to commit itself completely to a microbe theory. In the second part of the study report, the authors summarized that position: "Although the cause of the acquired immune deficiency syndrome in homosexual men remains unknown, the study presented here and in the companion paper has identified a distinctive lifestyle as an important risk factor."[27]

The first heterosexual patients, including the first woman, were reported by the CDC in August 1981.[28] The first clinical descriptions of immunosuppression in heterosexual intravenous (IV) drug users appeared in December 1981.[29] By June 1982 the *MMWR* reported that 22 percent of patients with KS and/or PCP were heterosexuals, the majority IV drug users.[30] Almost one-third of the heterosexual patients were women. Despite the early appearance and growing number of heterosexual patients, epidemiological studies of this group were significantly underrepresented in the literature prior to 1984.[31]

Would investigations of heterosexual patients, paralleling those of gays, have offered a different cast to the life-style model? We will never know for certain. Perhaps chemical toxicity or the immunosuppressive power of heroin, nitrites, and other drugs might have had more significance, at least at the start. But inasmuch as women—some of whom were *not* IV drug users—were among the first cases, investigators might have hypothesized much earlier that a microbe was *the* direct cause of the new disorder in all affected groups.

Why, we might ask, were heterosexual intravenous drug users not studied? There is no simple answer. One reason, a structural one, is that at the federal level the National Institute on Drug Abuse (NIDA) had principal responsibility for investigating issues related to intravenous drug use and had a staff of epidemiologists just for that purpose. NIDA's traditional focus, however, was only on drug abuse; it eschewed investigations of diseases such as hepatitis B and endocarditis, which were endemic or epidemic in its target population. The leadership of NIDA decided that AIDS would be treated like any other disease, thereby leaving the research initiative to other centers at NIH or the CDC.[32] Unfortunately, the CDC, lacking previous experience and expertise, shied away from studying the drug-using population, leaving a lacuna.[33]

Another reason drug users were not studied is that only a relatively small number of research subjects were available, particularly outside the New York metropolitan area.[34] That problem was alleviated, however, by the development during the summer of 1984 of a blood test measuring antibodies to the HIV. The test created a much larger pool of potential research subjects by identifying individuals who were infected but who did not have AIDS or serious related illnesses.[35]

A final answer to the question posed is that epidemiologists were unwilling to study this group.[36] Partly justified by the disinclination of addicts to cooperate in interviews and with follow-up, their unwillingness may also, in part, be explained by a feeling among many clinicians and researchers (in this respect reflecting the attitudes of the public at large) that addicts are of less social consequence than other patients.[37] In a striking reflection of that lack of interest, at all levels of government and in the universities few epidemiologists had expertise in drug addiction when the HIV epidemic began.

Despite its appeal, the life-style hypothesis was eventually undercut as a sufficient explanation. During 1982 epidemiological surveillance and case reports clearly indicated that others besides homosexual males were at risk. As an article in the *Journal of the American Medical Association (JAMA)* observed in September of that year, "if lifestyle is the key, the question still remains: Why has AIDS also occurred in heterosexual men (84 cases so far), women (32 cases so far), mostly heterosexual Haitians, and hemophiliacs?"[38] A new model was required.

AN UNKNOWN TRANSMISSIBLE AGENT

On March 4, 1983, after a year of suggestive data, a Public Health Service Inter-Agency Report (published in the *MMWR*) marked a major shift in the conceptualization of the disorder.[39] That shift was caused in part by the kind of evidence cited by *JAMA:* case reports to and surveillance by the CDC made it clear that the disease was more than a syndrome of homosexual men and promiscuous life-style.

On July 9, 1982, the CDC had reported that thirty-two Haitian immigrants to the United States, seven of them women, showed immunological, morbidity, and mortality patterns similar to those in homosexual men and intravenous drug users.[40] Although the *MMWR* had previously published two general updates on the increased incidence of the new disease—updates that had included data on heterosexual patients—the article on Haitians constituted the first complete report focusing directly on persons outside the "homosexual" category.

A week later, and again in December 1982, the *MMWR* alerted its readers that patients with hemophilia but no other underlying disease had contracted PCP.[41] What the hemophilia patients shared was a dependence on Factor VIII, the clotting substance they lacked, usually derived from the pooled blood of two thousand to nearly twenty thousand donors.[42]

The possibility of blood as a vector for AIDS was heightened by a CDC report of unexplained immunodeficiency and opportunistic infection in a twenty-month-old infant who had received multiple transfusions from a donor subsequently diagnosed with AIDS.[43] The sibling of the infant was in good health, and his parents were described as "heterosexual non-Haitians" without a history of intravenous drug use.

Summing up the new cases, the March 4 *MMWR* observed that, according to current epidemiological data, four groups were at increased risk of AIDS: homosexual men with multiple sexual partners, users of intravenous drugs, Haitians who had emigrated to the United States in the previous few years, and hemophiliacs. In addition, unexplained immunodeficiency and life-threatening opportunistic infections had occurred in the female sexual partners of bisexual or intravenous drug-using men and in the children born of their unions.

Instead of life-style, the report suggested that the cases shared exposure to a transmissible agent. Though the agent was unknown, the pattern of cases mimicked that of a known pathogen, one that epidemiology had studied and helped control in the years before AIDS.[44]

> The distribution of AIDS cases parallels that of hepatitis B virus infection, which is transmitted sexually and parenterally. Blood products or blood appear responsible for AIDS among hemophilia patients who require clotting factor replacement. The likelihood of blood transmission is supported by the

occurrence of AIDS among IV drug users. Many drug abusers share contaminated needles, exposing themselves to blood-borne agents, such as hepatitis B virus.[45]

In adopting the hepatitis B analogy, epidemiologists posited an alternative organization of known variables, one that stressed a biological agent whose vector was blood and/or its constituents. Although life-style factors could be incorporated, they had lost some of their cachet. In the CDC national case-control study, for example, Harold W. Jaffe and his colleagues, reporting their results in August 1983, suggested that life-style factors are indirect causes of AIDS, with a microbe, probably a virus, as the direct cause.[46]

Although epidemiologists had not identified an agent, the model of hepatitis B supported the introduction of public health measures. That is, the model offered a putative point of intervention in the multifactorial "web of causes," even in the absence of a known pathogen. Applying recommendations developed for hepatitis B, the Public Health Service suggested that people avoid sexual contact with persons suspected or known to have AIDS. In addition, members of groups at risk were asked not to donate blood or plasma, and doctors were encouraged to recommend autologous transfusions to their patients. Finally, the Public Health Service called for the development of blood-screening procedures.

On March 4, 1983, for the first time in the *MMWR,* the CDC referred to high-risk groups, attesting to the spread of AIDS into multiple segments of the U.S. population and to the relationship between the concept of high-risk group and hepatitis B. High-risk groups were those whose members were at a greater risk of infection *and* of infecting others, carrying a microbe that was capable of spreading through sexual and blood-borne traffic. The *MMWR* underscored that "each group contains many persons who probably have little risk of acquiring AIDS."[47] Nonetheless, no calibration of degree of risk was introduced, so that no distinction could be drawn. Since no microbe had been isolated, risk designation was, in effect, regarded—even among scientists, not to speak of the news media and among the general public—as synonymous with carrier state.

Some months later the CDC justified its use of risk groups, arguing that classification of individuals is intrinsic to any epidemiological investigation.[48] Classification should not be taken to mean, however, that groups at higher risk for AIDS could transmit the disease through nonintimate contact, since casual transmission was a view unsupported by available evidence. To use the likelihood of casual transmission as a basis for social and economic discrimination was unfair.

The apology of the CDC missed the point. Grouping individuals may be traditional in epidemiology, both as a means of intervention and as an analytic prerequisite. The political or social consequences of such grouping are rarely examined. In this instance, even if the fear of casual transmission could be eradicated, the groups identified would still be seen as bearing a strong negative relationship to the life-sustaining blood supply. They were created, qua groups, to signify their potential status as carriers of tainted blood and as contaminators. Moreover, the analogy with highly contagious hepatitis B reinforced the association of casual transmission, particularly for health care providers, because hepatitis B is a disease in which a virus is transmitted through close personal contact, through all secretions, and through wounds and lacerations.[49]

A further consequence of creating high-risk groups was to reinforce the relationship between the disease and "marginal" members of the population. In the case of HIV, although each of the groups ostensibly threatened the remainder of the community through the medium of blood or sex, public health recommendations would inhibit such contamination. Consequently, the disorder could be contained at the boundaries, among people who were "different" from the majority but undifferentiated within each of the high-risk groups.

One of the dangers of a scientific classification of people based on stereotypes was that it defined the questions raised and thus answered. Such categorization created a procrustean mind-set that was evident from the beginning of the epidemic. For example, in early 1982 researchers, in an act of political and scientific oversimplification, designated the new disorder by the acronym GRID (gay-related immunodeficiency), even though the CDC and the *New England Journal of Medicine* had published reports of heterosexual IV drug users with the new syndrome. At a major conference Michael Gottlieb and his colleagues could report, in a paper entitled "Gay-Related Immunodeficiency (GRID) Syndrome: Clinical and Autopsy Observations," that of the ten adult males in the study with the syndrome, two were exclusively heterosexual.[50]

Ultimately, the hepatitis B metaphor assumed the existence of an infectious agent, probably a virus. Though some favored a new variant of the cytomegalovirus, others, including James W. Curran of the CDC Task Force, supported the notion of a new infectious agent.[51] In the long run, either hypothesis rested on the detection of a pathogen that had hitherto proved elusive.

AIDS: "THE STORY OF A VIRUS"

From 1981 until the isolation of a new virus, epidemiology played a central role in the characterization of HIV infection. That discipline, using specific case definitions, surveillance, and case-control studies, identified high-risk groups and offered suggestive models and similes. Although epidemiology formulated the social context and morphology of the new disorder, it could not discover its microbial cause. That function was filled by virologists at the Pasteur Institute in Paris and in laboratories in the United States, at the National Cancer Institute (NCI) in particular.

In May of 1984 the journal *Science* published four reports authored by Robert C. Gallo of the NCI and his colleagues and a fifth by Luc Montagnier of the Pasteur Institute.[52] These reports established a strong case for a causal link between AIDS and a newly discovered retrovirus that the NCI called HTLV-III and the French called LAV. Later an international agreement was made to call the retrovirus human immunodeficiency virus (HIV).

With the isolation of the HIV, the relative importance of epidemiology in the definition of the disease lessened. Epidemiologists continued to play an important, although somewhat more peripheral, role, providing supporting evidence for the viral hypothesis and developing information in areas outside the reach of microbiology and its techniques.

Increasingly, the "bench" scientists—virologists, immunologists, cancer researchers—determined the definition of HIV infection. In effect, they redefined AIDS as a set of biomedical problems open to a chemical resolution in the form of drugs and vaccines. These scientists removed the disorder to a considerable degree from the stigma of its original social matrix, placing it instead in a context resembling that of the supposedly more purely clinical crusades against cancer or polio.

The change in the types of professionals studying HIV infection and in their defined fields of observation and analysis effected a subtle shift in the characterization of the disorder. The disease was increasingly conceptualized in terms of the infectious agent, the virus. Interest in cofactors or a multifactorial model diminished.

One marker of this shift was the title of a book published by the

Institute of Medicine and the National Academy of Sciences in 1986: *Mobilizing against AIDS: The Unfinished Story of a Virus.*[53] Four years earlier, an article in *JAMA* had observed that "it seems unlikely that a virus alone is inducing AIDS."[54] Another marker was the dearth of studies of cofactors, of events or states independent of the virus but necessary to cause HIV infection in general or AIDS in particular. In early 1987 an article evaluating cofactors for HIV could cite only one published report on cofactors after 1984.[55] A few months earlier, another volume by the Institute of Medicine and the National Academy of Sciences, although acknowledging the importance of cofactors, suggested that "there are no data to support the concept [of cofactors], with the possible exception of genital ulcers in Africa."[56]

The increasingly biological definition of the disease was reinforced by the successful development of serological procedures for the detection of antibodies to the virus. These tests—the enzyme-linked immunosorbent assay (ELISA) and the Western blot technique—allowed epidemiologists and other scientists to outline the biological boundaries of the new disorder.

In July 1986 the CDC reported that epidemiologists, using the new blood tests, had confirmed that persons in the previously defined groups at higher risk of AIDS showed a greater prevalence of HTLV-III/LAV viral antibody.[57] Epidemiologists also found that AIDS and a number of less full-blown conditions, including lymphadenopathy and AIDS-related complex (ARC), had the same underlying viral cause. In addition, antibody tests demonstrated the existence of the virus in persons without clinical symptomatology, a not unusual pattern in infectious disease epidemiology. These data suggested to the CDC a wide spectrum of human response to the virus, requiring careful study.[58]

Standardized blood tests thus initially provided a biological justification for the previously defined high-risk groups. At the same time, antibody testing could determine which individuals within the risk groups were seropositive and which were not. As a result, group membership and carrier status could theoretically be separated. Given the logic of the biological model, moreover, the concept of high-risk membership should actually have withered away, replaced by the notion of *high-risk activities* that made infection more likely. Despite logic, a shift in emphasis from "status" to "act" did not occur until "mainstream" heterosexuals were targeted as a population at risk.[59]

Since1984 epidemiologists have also contributed to knowledge of the natural history and transmission of HIV infection. The particular strength of epidemiology in these areas has derived in part from the "bench" scientists' inability to uncover suitable nonhuman animal models and in part from epidemiologists' technical ability to transcend the ethical limitations on human experimentation by studying disease patterns occurring in populations.

Overall, these epidemiological studies are attempting to enlarge our knowledge of the biological and clinical dimensions of HIV infection, but to develop that knowledge, wherever possible, within the social matrix or behavioral history of the populations involved. By so doing, epidemiologists are maintaining the vitality of a multifactorial, social conception of AIDS in the face of a narrower biological definition.

To date, some of the most important epidemiological studies have prospectively followed defined cohorts of individuals—at first cohorts of homosexual men, but more recently cohorts of hemophiliacs, intravenous drug users, women, and children.[60] The purpose of these investigations has been to establish the risk factors for HIV infection; the rate of, and time required for, seroconversion; the progression of pathology in those infected; and the proportion of the infected who eventually develop AIDS. In addition to defining the natural history of the disorder, the researchers aim to find determinative variables that may be open to clinical or social intervention. Finally, epidemiologists continue to develop more extensive and sophisticated means to measure the incidence and prevalence of HIV infection across subgroups in the American population.

For example, a number of studies that followed gay or bisexual men over time in New York City,[61] Holland,[62] and San Francisco[63] isolated several possible risk factors for HIV infection. These included sexual contact with a person known to have AIDS and participation as the receptive partner in anal intercourse,[64] a risk that increased with the number of persons with whom one acted as the anal receptive partner.[65] These behaviors heightened the chance of viral transmission. Implicated as well was a history of anal douche use.[66] In the population studied, therefore, HIV infection is an STD in which anal mucosa appears to be an inefficient barrier to infection, especially when traumatized by frequent contact. These results, consistent over many epidemiological studies, offered the possibility of behavior intervention strategies.

When epidemiologists have researched the natural history of HIV-associated disorders in infected persons, they have provided information on incidence and prevalence rates and, in the main, on biological markers and disease status. Their attempts to isolate cofactors for HIV infection and progression have yielded, at best, some suggestive leads that must be interpreted with great caution. In addition, these investigations, like those discussed above, suffer from design flaws and biases. For example, most studies cannot specify the dates of HIV infection in their subjects. Consequently, endpoints (lymphadenopathy, for example, or AIDS) cannot be linked to and measured from precisely defined initiatory events. This lacuna often inhibits comparisons of findings across studies and prediction of time-measured outcomes. Recently, however, investigators have attempted both, using as their point of departure the few cohorts (primarily patients infected by blood products) with known or well-estimated dates of seroconversion.[67]

One of the first epidemiological studies of the course of HIV infection was that of Harold Jaffe and his colleagues, which followed a cohort of 6,875 male homosexuals and bisexuals recruited originally between 1978 and 1980 from STD patients at San Francisco City Clinic.[68] The researchers found that, by 1984, 87.4 percent of a putative random sample[69] of the cohort were seropositive. More recently investigators have estimated that 54 percent of those seropositive for at least ten years will progress to AIDS.[70] These results suggest that without effective treatment a majority of those infected with HIV will eventually develop the last, usually fatal, stage of the disease.

B. Frank Polk and his colleagues, unlike Jaffe and his colleagues, attempted to define predictors of AIDS in seropositive men by studying a cohort of 1,835 male homosexual volunteers recruited by centers in four cities: Los Angeles, Chicago, Pittsburgh, and Washington/Baltimore.[71] When each of the fifty-nine AIDS cases (developing over a median of fifteen months) was matched to five seropositive controls from the same study center, the researchers found three independent predictors of AIDS: a decreased number of T helper cells, a low level of HIV antibody, and a history of sex with someone who subsequently developed the syndrome. The first two predictors, however, are probably biological markers of disease progression to AIDS rather than determinants or causes of that progression. The last predictor may in fact be a marker of an infection longstanding enough for AIDS to develop in both partners. More recent epidemiological investigations of HIV-infected homosexual men and men with hemophilia have identified additional laboratory markers of progression to AIDS.[72]

Cohort studies have also provided the basis for estimates of the "latency period," the median time between an initial infection and frank AIDS. In seropositive homosexual men, transfusion recipients, and hemophiliacs, the latency period is an estimated seven to eleven years; and half of those infected are free of AIDS for an indefinitely longer term.[73] This highly variable latency period will probably be extended further, moreover, with the prophylactic administration of AZT.[74]

In fact, new evidence appears to show that for some individuals the period between HIV infection and the appearance of persistent antibodies to HIV may be even longer than previously suspected. For some years, the normal period was thought to be three months or less.[75] Investigators in Los Angeles, however, have recently reported multiple instances of delayed seroconversion.[76] Although HIV was isolated from 31 of 133 homosexual men, 27 of the 31 had no antibodies to HIV during the next thirty-six months of follow-up when their sera were tested by the ELISA and Western blot methods. Confirming the results of previous investigations,[77] this study suggests that for an unknown number of individuals a "silent HIV infection," undetectable by conventional blood assays, may be, in fact, part of the latency period.

These recent results carry several further implications. They raise questions about the limitations of current serum antibody tests, particularly worrisome if those with "silent" HIV infection can still transmit the virus. On a more positive note, these results suggest that some infected individuals have immune systems that successfully suppress the replication of HIV indefinitely. This finding has potentially profound implications for future drug research and therapy.

Why does HIV disease have such a variable incubation period? This question intrigues researchers and has renewed their interest in cofactors—exogenous or endogenous exposures that might modulate the rate of HIV-induced immunodeficiency.[78] Investigators have also hypothesized that cofactors may promote initial HIV infection. For example, some have suspected that a history of microbial infections, leading to immunological alterations, may put individuals at greater risk of HIV infection and of disease progression.[79] There is growing evidence that sexually transmissible infections—particularly those that produce genital ulcerations, which, like douching and enemas, facilitate invasion of HIV—may be important cofactors.[80] Evidence is also accumulating that, for reasons not yet understood, lack of circumcision in African men may be a cofactor for HIV infection.[81] According to some researchers, the simultaneous existence of genital ulcers in HIV-infected women and lack of circumcision in their partners may potentiate female to male transmission of the virus.[82] There are also epidemiological indications that age-related variables may be cofactors for disease progression, since infants and older homosexual men have higher rates of disease progression than other groups.[83]

The possible role of cofactors testifies to the terrible complexity of HIV infection and justifies the reluctance of epidemiologists to reduce AIDS and related conditions to an agent-host phenomenon. Epidemiological researchers have consistently held up the possibility of nonviral factors to the "bench" scientists. Since 1981 they have rooted biological or clinical events in the matrices of human behavior and social experience. In one study of the role of cofactors in HIV infection, the authors put the epidemiologists' position quite well.[84] Citing the viral etiology common to all patients with AIDS, they stressed the multiple determinants probably responsible for HIV infection and disease progression, including cultural differences, the presence of other endemic illnesses, and host and viral genetic factors. Their position reaffirms the multifactorial model as central to an understanding of HIV infection and to its control.

FROM AIDS TO HIV INFECTION: TRACKING THE EPIDEMIC

While investigating the natural history of HIV infection, epidemiologists have continued to hold responsibility for an apparently mundane task: systematic surveillance. Since 1981 the CDC has both constructed the surveillance case definitions of AIDS and served as the national registry for all cases reported by the states, the District of Columbia, and the U.S. territories.[85] These data are used to monitor the spread of AIDS, project its future incidence and prevalence,[86] and provide the basis for health service planning and health education.

In recent years, however, the systematic surveillance of cases has grown more problematic. Sources within and outside the CDC have observed that the true number of AIDS cases in the United States has been underreported, thereby weakening the epidemiological and policy functions the data serve. In addition, once the HIV virus was isolated, epidemiologists sought strategies to capture population-based information on HIV seroprevalence in general, not only on AIDS, the last stage of the disease. Methods developed by epidemiologists—the CDC in particular—to survey HIV prevalence put them at odds with other quantitative research workers and, for the first time, threatened the monopoly previously enjoyed by epidemiologists over the population-based definition of the disease.

In an editorial note in the *MMWR* of August 18, 1989, the CDC admitted that its AIDS case count was subject to error: "Because of the combination of underdiagnosis and underreporting of AIDS cases and severe manifestations of HIV infection that do not meet the CDC AIDS surveillance case definition, reported AIDS cases underestimate the number of persons severely affected by HIV since 1981."[87] Since the completeness of the case count varied by geographical region and patient population, the CDC surveillance system had captured only 70 to 90 percent of HIV-related deaths.

In a separate assessment of the CDC's system for reporting AIDS cases, the Committee on AIDS Research and the Behavioral, Social and Statistical Sciences of the National Research Council (NRC) highlighted two problems: only 85 to 90 percent of cases are reported within one year of diagnosis, with a further decline expected; and the reliability and validity with which the mode of transmission of infection is established in each case have not been evaluated.[88] Flaws in the CDC's methodology for establishing mode of transmission could affect the degree to which subpopulations are over- or underrepresented in the national surveillance system; such misreporting might have serious implications for identifying or tracking shifts in the spread of infection.

Indeed, in a recent study the sociologist E. O. Laumann and his colleagues concluded that some segments of the U.S. population are systematically underrepresented. Arguing that the national reporting system is subject to systematic distortions because of "overt manipulations by interested parties" and the stigmatizing nature of HIV infection itself,[89] the investigators used instead the 1988 General Social Survey (GSS), a national household survey in which respondents were asked to identify all those within their network of acquaintances who had either been a victim of homicide or had AIDS. When the GSS results were compared with official national statistics on homicide, the two were congruent. When a similar comparison was made between GSS survey data and those of the CDC, the investigators found that the national surveillance system significantly underestimated the prevalence of AIDS in white middle-class populations and in those living in the Midwest, while overstating the prevalence of that disease in blacks and latinos and in those living in the East. The researchers called for more prevalence studies independent of the CDC's surveillance network, in order to ensure a more accurate assessment of the social epidemiology of AIDS.

The most critical evaluation of the national AIDS surveillance system is that of the U.S. General Accounting Office (GAO).[90] The GAO has found that the system substantially undercounts the number of AIDS cases in the United States. It attributes that problem to essentially four sources, some already identified above. In essence, these sources are (1) the CDC's surveillance definition, which specifies those illnesses that qualify a case as AIDS and thereby excludes a considerable number of fatal HIV-related cases—in particular, young intravenous drug users—who never contract the required diseases;[91] (2) the CDC's test criterion, which excludes from the national surveillance system all cases of AIDS diagnosed without HIV test results—despite the fact that such presumptive diagnoses are not rare and are increasing as physicians become more experienced with AIDS and as patients insist that no test results be attached to their medical charts; (3) physician error, as a consequence of which AIDS cases go undiagnosed or are diagnosed late; and (4) surveillance system breakdown, in which diagnosed cases are never reported or are reported late.

The GAO estimates that, because of these and other sources of error, the national surveillance system may have counted only two-thirds of the cases of AIDS and other HIV-related fatal illnesses in the United States—an estimate that is lower than the CDC's own estimate of 70 to 90 percent. Whatever the precise shortfall, the combined results of the GAO and other studies suggest that the current AIDS case count may be sufficiently flawed to affect health planning or estimates of future cases, particularly for subpopulations or specified regions of the country. Unfortunately, similar, though perhaps more profound, flaws may be vitiating the recent HIV surveillance projects.

The need to monitor HIV infection rather than only AIDS was clearly adumbrated by the Committee on AIDS Research and the Behavioral, Social and Statistical Sciences of the NRC:

> Counts of AIDS cases are out-of-date indicators of the present state of the epidemic. There is a long, asymptomatic latency period between HIV infection and the development of AIDS (in most persons). Consequently, the statistics on *new* AIDS cases reflect *old* cases of HIV infection. . . . [In addition,] persons whose life spans are significantly shortened by HIV infection do not always manifest sufficient symptoms to be captured by the AIDS reporting system. . . . [Finally,] the future magnitude of the AIDS epidemic will be determined primarily by the current extent and future spread of HIV infection in the population.[92]

The CDC recognized the need for HIV seroprevalence data quite early. In the fall of 1985, six months after the ELISA was licensed, the CDC proposed that selected "sentinel" hospitals across the country provide sera for "blinded" seroprevalence surveys—surveys that use anonymous samples of blood and therefore do not require informed consent, so that they are relatively free of self-selection bias.[93]

Once initiated, this plan was followed by another, outlined in September 1987 and implemented thereafter,[94] to develop a "comprehensive family of complementary HIV surveys" that would capture seroprevalence information on pregnant women, those at high risk of HIV infection, and selected subgroups within the general population.[95] Specifically, the CDC agreed to provide technical and financial support to thirty large metropolitan areas across the United States.[96] In each of these urban areas, the federal government, in collaboration with state and local agencies, selected in a nonrandom fashion one or more of six types of health care institutions or groups: sentinel hospitals, newborn infants, tuberculosis clinics, STD clinics, drug treatment centers, and women's health centers. Only "blinded" surveys are conducted in the first three; "blinded" and "unblinded" studies in the last. (Such "unblinded" studies allow investigators to ask in-depth questions, but they require informed consent of the respondents and run the risk, as recent studies have shown, of self-selection bias—the nonrandom refusal of some, perhaps those at greatest risk, to participate.[97]) According to the CDC, the family of surveys is central to defining and managing the problems presented by HIV infection: "Information on current levels and trends of HIV infection is needed to follow the course of the epidemic, to help project future trends in AIDS incidence, and to target and evaluate the impact of AIDS/HIV preventive programs."[98]

The CDC has elected to use health care institutions to capture prevalence information, a traditional epidemiological strategy. The types of facilities selected allow it to obtain seroprevalence data on those at greatest risk of infection: the sexually active (STD clinics), intravenous drug users (drug treatment and tuberculosis clinics), and childbearing or reproductive-age women in lower socioeconomic strata (newborn screening and women's health centers). The CDC admits that the survey design for each of these subpopulations is flawed. It hopes, however, to analyze and evaluate the biases in each design and to compensate for them statistically, so that it can provide accurate prevalence estimates.[99]

The Committee on AIDS Research and the Behavioral, Social and Statistical Sciences of the NRC, advised by a panel of statisticians and demographers, has examined the six surveys in depth. It found that, contrary to the CDC's expectations, the "comprehensive family of surveys" is sufficiently flawed in research design to prevent it from accurately measuring, with knowable margins of error, the incidence or prevalence of HIV infection in the subpopulations of interest. Central to the committee's criticism is that the CDC is using nonrandom samples—samples of convenience—in all surveys except newborn screening.[100] The committee's subsequent conclusions are unequivocally critical of the CDC:

> The committee has listened with interest to arguments that population-based estimates of HIV incidence and prevalence are unnecessary from a public health perspective. Rather, it has been suggested that targeted samples of convenience could suffice to provide "sentinels" that could be used to guide the nation's response to the AIDS epidemic. *The committee concludes that it would be a serious mistake for the Public Health Service to continue to "make do" with estimates derived from convenience samples.* ... Now is the time to prepare for the future, and good data will be indispensable in future efforts to control the epidemic. No postponement should be accepted.[101]

To meet its objections, the committee suggests that the CDC reconstitute each of the seroprevalence surveys as probability samples, despite the administrative, political, and financial difficulties involved. In reformulating the surveys, the committee urges the CDC to draw on the expertise of the National Center for Health Statistics (recently made a part of the CDC), which employs statisticians, demographers, and other social scientists.[102] The committee does not comment, however, on another significant limitation of the "comprehensive family of surveys." These surveys are limited to groups historically at risk of HIV infection and to a special subgroup, the hospitalized sick, which only in part includes those at low risk. The CDC's surveys do not, however, measure seroprevalence in the population at large and therefore cannot estimate, with known margins of error, the prevalence of HIV in the United States. In addition, the surveys cannot monitor the incidence of HIV in new, previously unknown, risk groups.[103]

Responding to the need to measure HIV prevalence in the general population, the National Center for Health Statistics (NCHS) has sponsored a National Household Seroprevalence Survey (NHSS), contracting with a private research organization, the Triangle Research Institute (TRI), to conduct feasibility tests. The ultimate objective of the NHSS will be to survey 50,000 anonymous household respondents concerning factors that might put them at risk for HIV infection and to take a blood sample from each participant. These respondents are to be randomly selected on the basis of probability sampling; the result should be an estimate of HIV prevalence in the total U.S. population. Before the government approves the survey, however, a pilot stage must successfully demonstrate that the study is feasible and can generate new and useful data.[104] Specifically, the pilot involves a careful evaluation of all field procedures and research methodologies, including sampling strategies, protection of the respondents, blood collection methods, survey design, and development of community support.

After an aborted start in Washington, D.C., where local officials and community groups rejected the project, TRI successfully piloted the NHSS in Allegheny County, Pennsylvania, in January 1989; it initiated a second study in Dallas in September of the same year. The results from Pennsylvania show that, of 308 randomly selected households with an eligible respondent (a civilian, permanent resident, eighteen to fifty-four years of age), 85 percent agreed to participate in the study.[105] In Dallas a survey of 1,715 eligible households, completed in December 1989, achieved an overall response rate of 84 percent (90 if one includes those who completed the questionnaire but refused to be bled). Reaching that number proved somewhat more difficult than anticipated, because the leading gay political and service organization in the city, the Dallas Gay Alliance, actively campaigned against the survey.[106]

With the feasibility studies completed, the CDC, along with other federal bodies, must now decide whether a national seroprevalence survey is technically and politically possible. The fierce local controversies in Washington and Dallas make political considerations important; so, too, do actions in Congress, where in July 1989 conservative members of the House Appropriations Committee were able to delete the $11 million required to fund a Public Health Service survey of sexual behavior in the United States.[107] However, the CDC reportedly has an antipathy to the NHSS that predates and is independent of these political considerations.[108] The epidemiologists of the Centers for Disease Control had argued early on that the study, requiring blood samples and a survey of sex- and drug-related behaviors, would be vitiated by nonresponse bias; it would be bad science. They also insisted that the NHSS was politically untenable, in that it needed substantial outreach in the face of community opposition. Finally, the NHSS would consume funds that were better spent on the family of surveys, which, with its use of "blinded" seroprevalence studies, was unbiased (good) science.

The arguments raised by the CDC regarding the scientific and political feasibility of the NHSS are somewhat disingenuous, in that they hide a struggle on the part of the CDC to maintain the hegemony of its own mission and culture over the HIV "territory."[109] The CDC has dominated the population-based study of AIDS since 1981. It has defined the disease for surveillance purposes, directed the national AIDS-reporting system, and designed the "comprehensive family of surveys" to expand that system to the whole spectrum of HIV infection. That design was based on traditional medical epidemiology; to measure rates of disease, the CDC has used patient data captured within health care institutions. After almost a decade of work and achievement, "accomplished in the face of considerable adversity on a number of fronts—physical, diplomatic, political and administrative"[110]—it would be strange if the CDC did not feel that if "owns" to a large degree the population-based study of HIV (as does epidemiology, through it). It would be surprising for the CDC to easily relinquish its funding, political power, and high visibility.

The CDC experiences as an incursion the criticism and critical work of quantitative social scientists, most of whom are relatively new to AIDS research. These social scientists' insistence on population probability sampling—the General Social Survey or the NHSS, for example—as the basis of good science at least temporarily excludes the CDC. The CDC has little experience with the methodologies involved, and the CDC staff in Atlanta includes no sampling statisticians and precious few quantitative social scientists on the Ph.D level.[111] To alter course now requires the CDC to change both corporate strategy and corporate culture and to allow non-epidemiologists, with their own mission and culture, to participate in the population-based definition of HIV. The CDC is loath to share this territory, and a certain degree of inflexibility, even dogmatism, has followed. For example, the leadership of the CDC has made its calculation of 1 to 1.5 million HIV seropositive individuals in the United States an article of faith, despite the fact that the figure is only an estimate, based on much-criticized parameters.[112]

The social scientists who criticize the manner in which the CDC defines cases or collects the data are demanding something more than greater methodological purity—although that is important. They are also frustrated by the dominant role played by the CDC and other epidemiologists in defining and managing the HIV epidemic. Their criticism of the CDC is only the most public expression of anger at the power and apparent insensitivity of epidemiologists, who are seen as excluding, devaluing, or co-opting social science methodologies and objectives. Social scientists argue there are sound reasons for multiple approaches to studying the epidemic. Such approaches would, for example, enable researchers to analyze with greater sophistication the personal (particularly the sexual) behavior of individuals; to measure the unique, local configurations and manifestations of the HIV epidemic; and to develop models of the political economy of that epidemic.[113] In brief, social scientists want badly to broaden the theoretical and empirical basis for the study and management of the epidemic. Such a change, in which they would have a greater voice in defining public policy, would enhance the power and prestige of these professionals and might (although this is not certain) increase the amount of research dollars available to them.

Is the role of epidemiology, of the CDC, in defining HIV infection coming to an end? Most certainly not. That role, however, may be undergoing a subtle shift—not so dramatic as when the HIV was discovered, but still a change of position to make room for the social scientists. The degree of that displacement will depend on a number of issues, not all in the epidemiologists' control. How will the CDC, for example, incorporate the statisticians and social scientists at NCHS into its HIV data collection projects? Will the CDC benefit from the reluctance of political conservatives to survey Americans in their homes about sex- and drug-related activities? Will the growing insistence by clinicians and some public health officials that all pregnant women, surgical patients, and hospital patients undergo "unblinded" serotesting politicize and undercut all seroprevalence studies? Only time, that most confounding of variables, will tell.

CONCLUSION

I have outlined how epidemiologists, drawing on the unique perspectives of their profession, reacted to the outbreak of a new disease of unknown origin. By responding early to the epidemic, epidemiologists defined the syndrome first—an act of scientific acumen and power. Over time, however, investigators using other techniques have challenged the primacy of the epidemiologists' construction of the disorder, both of the disease itself and of the hypothetically infected population. To the extent that these challenges were successful, the definition of the disorder has changed, and with it the relative standing of epidemiologists (the CDC in particular). The history of the epidemic demonstrates that the construction of HIV infection was and is a dynamic process in which different scientific specialties negotiated definitions that, to a degree, reflected their relative power.

In the process, the legacy of epidemiologists remains significant. From the beginning of the epidemic, epidemiologists conceptualized HIV infection as a complex social phenomenon, with dimensions that derived from the social relations, behavioral patterns, and past experiences of the population at risk. On the one hand, the epidemiologists' approach may have skewed the choice of models and the hypotheses pursued and may have offered some justification for homophobia. On the other, by defining HIV infection as a multifactorial phenomenon, with both behavioral and microbial determinants, epidemiologists offered the possibility of primary prevention, a traditional epidemiological response to infectious and chronic diseases. Epidemiologists, in effect, established the basis for an effective public health campaign and—through publications, conferences, and the continuous collection of surveillance data—helped make AIDS a concern of policymakers and the public.

Primary prevention—including blood screening, health education, and behavior modification—is currently the only effective social response to the spread of HIV infection. Evidence from several sites indicates that the rate of HIV infection among some groups of homosexual males and IV drug users has begun to decline, possibly because of a reduction in high-risk activities.[114] These results, hopeful signs, have not yet been linked to a decrease in HIV-associated mortality. They may presage, however, a parallel between HIV and past infectious disease experiences.

Historical epidemiology has shown that medical interventions, both chemotherapeutic and prophylactic, have had little impact on the overall decline in infectious disease mortality in this century. For example, John and Sonja McKinlay found that since 1900 new medical measures have had almost no detectable effect on U.S. disease-specific mortality rates, because such measures usually occurred some decades after significant declines in death rates had already set in.[115] Thomas McKeown and his colleagues obtained similar results in a study of the mortality trends in England and Wales. According to McKeown, the observed secular decline was mainly attributable to community factors, particularly better nutrition and hygiene.[116] It remains to be seen whether HIV-related mortality will also decline as a result of community-directed hygiene (condoms, clean needles, blood screening) before a vaccine or new chemotherapy can be introduced. If it does, the history of HIV infection will offer a powerful vindication of the epidemiologists' multifactorial social definition of disease and of the public health actions that followed from it.

NOTES

This is a substantially revised and updated version of the chapter entitled "In the Eye of the Storm: The Epidemiological Construction of AIDS," in *AIDS: The Burdens of History,* ed. Elizabeth Fee and Daniel M. Fox (Berkeley: University of California Press, 1988), pp. 267–300. This essay has benefited from the generous comments of Ronald Bayer, Ben Brody, Elizabeth Fee, Daniel M. Fox, Robert Padgug, and Anne Stone.

1. Mirko D. Grmek, *Histoire du SIDA* (Paris: Payot, 1989), pp. 58–61. The descriptive term *acquired immunodeficiency syndrome,* or *AIDS,* became synonymous with the new disorder; it has recently been replaced by *human immunodeficiency virus (HIV)* infection. Though, in general, this essay uses the new acronym, in discussing specific studies it will employ whatever term was used by the investigators reporting.

2. Brian MacMahon and Thomas F. Pugh, *Epidemiology* (Boston: Little, Brown, 1970), p. 25. See also John M. Last, ed., *A Dictionary of Epidemiology* (New York: Oxford University Press, 1983), s.v. "multiple causation."

3. U.S. Department of Health and Human Services, Public Health Service, Centers for Disease Control, *Reports on AIDS Published in the Morbidity and Mortality Weekly Report, June 1981 through February 1986* (Springfield, Va.: National Technical Information Service, 1986), pp. 1–2 (hereafter cited as *MMWR*).

4. *MMWR,* pp. 2–4.

5. Ibid., p. 2.

6. David G. Ostrow, "Homosexuality and Sexually Transmitted Diseases," in *Sexually Transmitted Diseases,* ed. Yehudi M. Felman (New York: Churchill Livingston, 1986), p. 210. See also M. T. Schreeder et al., "Hepatitis B in Homosexual Men: Prevalence of Infection and Factors Related to Transmission," *Journal of Infectious Diseases* 146 (1982): 7–15.

7. William W. Darrow, "Sexual Behavior in America," in *Sexually Transmitted Diseases,* ed. Felman, pp. 269–71.

8. Terry Alan Sandholzer, "Factors Affecting the Incidence and Management of Sexually Transmitted Diseases in Homosexual Men, in *Sexually Transmitted Diseases in Homosexual Men,* ed. David G. Ostrow, Terry Alan Sandholzer, and Yehudi M. Felman (New York: Plenum Medical Book Company, 1983), p. 5.

9. See U.S. Congress, House of Representatives, Subcommittee on Consumer Protection and Finance, Committee on Interstate and Foreign Commerce, *Hearings on Legionnaires' Disease,* November 23–24, 1976, 94th Cong. For a defense of the CDC, see Barbara J. Culliton, "Legion Fever: Postmortem on an Investigation That Failed," *Science* 194 (1976): 1025–27.

10. Stephen Schultz, M.D., former deputy commissioner, New York City Department of Health, personal communication, July 22, 1987.

11. *MMWR,* p. 9.

12. Ibid., pp. 18, 95–97.

13. See John M. Karon, Timothy J. Dondero, Jr., and James W. Curran, "The Projected Incidence of AIDS and Estimated Prevalence of HIV Infection in the United States," *Journal of Acquired Immune Deficiency Syndromes* 1 (1988): 542–50.

14. Centers for Disease Control, Task Force on Kaposi's Sarcoma and Opportunistic Infections, "Epidemiologic Aspects of the Current Outbreak of Kaposi's Sarcoma and Opportunistic Infections," *New England Journal of Medicine* 306 (1982): 248 (hereafter cited as Task Force Report); see also Gerald Astor, *The Disease Detectives* (New York: New American Library, 1983), p. 56.

15. Task Force Report, p. 252.

16. *MMWR*, pp. 4–5.

17. Kenneth B. Hymes et al., "Kaposi's Sarcoma in Homosexual Men—A Report on Eight Cases," *Lancet* 2 (1981): 598–600.

18. Michael S. Gottlieb et al., "*Pneumocystis Carinii* Pneumonia and Mucosal Candidiasis in Previously Healthy Homosexual Men," *New England Journal of Medicine* 305 (1981): 1430.

19. Task Force Report, pp. 251–52.

20. Henry Masur et al., "An Outbreak of Community-Acquired *Pneumocystis Carinii* Pneumonia," *New England Journal of Medicine* 305 (1981): 1431–38.

21. David T. Durack, "Opportunistic Infections and Kaposi's Sarcoma in Homosexual Men," *New England Journal of Medicine* 305 (1981): 1466.

22. A model can be defined as "a description, a collection of statistical data, or an analogy used to help visualize often in a simplified way something that cannot be directly observed"; see *Webster's Third New International Dictionary of the English Language Unabridged* (1986), s.v. "model." According to Susser, a model is a system reduced to a set of related variables for the purpose of prediction or representation (Mervyn Susser, *Causal Thinking in the Health Sciences* [New York: Oxford University Press, 1973], p. 32). In the present essay the models discussed perform a representational function in that they "represent existing or postulated relationships in simplified form" (ibid., p. 33).

23. James J. Goedert et al., "Amyl Nitrite May Alter T Lymphocytes in Homosexual Men," *Lancet* 1 (1982): 412–16.

24. As a causal factor, nitrite continues to attract research attention. For a partial list of studies that tested the association of nitrites to AIDS, see Oppenheimer, "In the Eye of the Storm," note 34, p. 295.

25. Michael Marmor et al., "Risk Factors for Kaposi's Sarcoma in Homosexual Men," *Lancet* 1 (1982): 1083–87.

26. Harold W. Jaffe et al., "National Case-Control Study of Kaposi's Sarcoma and *Pneumocystis Carinii* Pneumonia in Homosexual Men: Part I, Epidemiologic Results," *Annals of Internal Medicine* 99 (1983): 145–51.

27. Martha F. Rogers et al., "National Case-Control Study of Kaposi's Sarcoma and *Pneumocystis Carinii* Pneumonia in Homosexual Men: Part 2, Laboratory Results," *Annals of Internal Medicine* 99 (1983): 151.

28. *MMWR*, pp. 4–5.

29. Masur et al., "An Outbreak."

30. *MMWR*, p. 10.

31. For the articles published prior to 1984 on HIV infection in drug users and women, see Oppenheimer, "In the Eye of the Storm," note 51, pp. 296–97.

32. Don C. Des Jarlais, Ph.D., former coordinator for AIDS Research, New York State Division of Substance Abuse Services, personal communication, January 15, 1988. As exceptions to that decision, NIDA funded some internal biomedical work in 1983, the same year it made a single extramural award to New York State to study risk factors for AIDS in drug users. In 1985 NIDA reversed itself and began to fund AIDS research extensively.

33. Stephen Schultz, personal communication, July 27, 1987.

34. Don C. Des Jarlais, personal communication, January 15, 1988.

35. Ibid.

36. Stephen Schultz, personal communication, July 22, 1987.

37. Ibid.

38. Catherine Macek, "Acquired Immunodeficiency Syndrome Cause(s) Still Elusive," *Journal of the American Medical Association* 248 (1982): 1426.

39. *MMWR*, pp. 32–34.

40. Ibid., pp. 12–13.

41. Ibid., pp. 14–15, 24–26.

42. Ibid., p. 47.

43. Ibid., pp. 26–27.

44. W. Thomas London and Baruch S. Blumberg, "Comments on the Role of Epidemiology in the Investigation of Hepatitis B Virus," *Epidemiologic Reviews* 7 (1985): 59–79.

45. *MMWR*, p. 33.

46. Jaffe et al., "National Case-Control Study," p. 149.

47. *MMWR*, p. 32.

48. Ibid., p. 45. Whatever the scientific basis for these high-risk groups, their existence was also open to negotiation. For a short discussion of the successful pressure applied by the Haitian government to have Haitians dropped as a risk group, see Dennis Altman, *AIDS in the Mind of America* (Garden City, N.Y.: Doubleday, 1986), pp. 71–73.

49. Abram S. Benenson, ed., *Control of Communicable Diseases in Man*, 12th ed. (Washington, D.C.: American Public Health Association, 1975).

50. Michael S. Gottlieb et al., "Gay-Related Immunodeficiency (GRID) Syndrome: Clinical and Autopsy Observations," *Clinical Research* 30 (1982): 349A.

51. Jean L. Marx, "A New Disease Baffles Medical Community," *Science* 217 (1982): 619; Robert C. Gallo, "The AIDS Virus," *Scientific American* 256 (1987): 48. James Curran was showing slides demonstrating the plausibility of a viral etiology at scientific meetings as early as February 1982 (Pauline Thomas, M.D., director of AIDS surveillance, New York City Department of Health, personal communication, July 28, 1987).

52. *Science* 224 (1984): 497–508.

53. Eve K. Nichols, *Mobilizing against AIDS: The Unfinished Story of a Virus* (Cambridge, Mass.: Harvard University Press, 1986).

54. Macek, "Acquired Immunodeficiency Syndrome Cause(s) Still Elusive," p. 1425.

55. James J. Goedert et al., "Effect of T4 Count and Cofactors on the Incidence of AIDS in Homosexual Men Infected with Human Immunodeficiency Virus," *Journal of the American Medical Association* 257 (1987): 334.

56. Institute of Medicine and National Academy of Sciences, *Confronting AIDS* (Washington, D.C.: National Academy Press, 1986), p. 45 (hereafter cited as *Confronting AIDS*).

57. *MMWR*, p. 63.

58. Ibid.

59. See, for example, *Confronting AIDS*, pp. viii–ix.

60. For recent results of cohort studies involving one or more of these groups, see papers presented at the Sixth International Conference on AIDS, San Francisco, June 20–24, 1990.

61. Cladd E. Stevens et al., "Human T-Cell Lymphotropic Virus Type III Infection in a Cohort of Homosexual Men in New York City," *Journal of the American Medical Association* 255 (1986): 2167–72.

62. Godfried J. P. van Griensven et al., "Risk Factors and Prevalence of HIV Antibodies in Homosexual Men in the Netherlands," *American Journal of Epidemiology* 125 (1987): 1048–57.

63. Warren Winkelstein, Jr., et al., "Sexual Practices and Risk of Infection by the Human Immunodeficiency Virus," *Journal of the American Medical Association* 257 (1987): 321–25.

64. Stevens et al., "Human T-Cell Lymphotropic Virus," p. 2169; Winkelstein et al., "Sexual Practices," p. 323.

65. Van Griensven et al., "Risk Factors," p. 1055.

66. Winkelstein et al., "Sexual Practices," p. 324. For problems with the early cohort studies, see Oppenheimer, "In the Eye of the Storm," p. 288 and note 95, p. 299.

67. Andrew R. Moss and Peter Bacchetti, "Natural History of HIV Infection," *AIDS* 3 (1989): 56.

68. Harold Jaffe et al., "The Acquired Immunodeficiency Syndrome in a Cohort of Homosexual Men," *Annals of Internal Medicine* 103 (1985): 210–11.

69. About one-third of the sample refused to participate.

70. A. Lifson et al., "The Natural History of HIV Infection in a Cohort of Homosexual and Bisexual Men: Clinical Manifestations, 1978–1989," paper presented at the Fifth International Conference on AIDS, Montreal, June 4–9, 1989.

71. B. Frank Polk et al., "Predictions of the Acquired Immunodeficiency Syndrome Developing in a Cohort of Seropositive Homosexual Men," *New England Journal of Medicine* 316 (1987): 61–66.

72. Andrew R. Moss, "Predicting Who Will Progress to AIDS," *British Medical Journal* 297 (1988): 1067–68; Moss and Bacchetti, "Natural History," pp. 57–58.

73. Andrew R. Moss et al., "Seropositivity for HIV and the Development

of AIDS or AIDS Related Condition: Three Year Follow Up of the San Francisco General Hospital Cohort," *British Medical Journal* 296 (1988): 745–50; Moss and Bacchetti, "Natural History," pp. 56–57; Alvaro Munoz et al., "Acquired Immunodeficiency Syndrome (AIDS)–Free Time after Human Immunodeficiency Virus Type 1 (HIV-1) Seroconversion in Homosexual Men," *American Journal of Epidemiology* 130 (1989): 530–39.

74. Gina Kolata, "Strong Evidence Discovered That AZT Holds Off AIDS," *New York Times,* August 4, 1989, p. A1; Philip J. Hilts, "Drug Said to Help AIDS Cases with Virus but No Symptoms," *New York Times,* August 18, 1989, p. A1.

75. Moss and Bacchetti, "Natural History," p. 55.

76. David T. Imagawa et al., "Human Immunodeficiency Virus Type 1 Infection in Homosexual Men Who Remain Seronegative for Prolonged Periods," *New England Journal of Medicine* 320 (1989): 1458–62.

77. Steve Wolinsky et al., "Polymerase Chain Reaction (PCR) Detection of HIV Provirus before HIV Seroconversion," paper presented at Fourth International Conference on AIDS, Stockholm, June 12–16, 1988; M. Loche and B. Mach, "Identification of HIV-Infected Seronegative Individuals by a Direct Diagnostic Test Based on Hybridisation to Amplified Viral DNA," *Lancet* 2 (1988): 418–21.

78. *Confronting AIDS,* p. 193.

79. Thomas C. Quinn et al., "Serologic and Immunologic Studies in Patients with AIDS in North America and Africa," *Journal of the American Medical Association* 257 (1987): 2617–21.

80. Peter Piot et al., "Serum Antibody to *Haemophilus Ducreyi* as a Risk Factor for HIV Infection in Africa, but Not in Europe"; Edward E. Telzak et al., "A Prospective Cohort Study of HIV-1 Seroconversion in Patients with Genital Ulcer Disease in New York City"; and Robert Cannon et al., "Syphilis Is Strongly Associated with HIV Infection in Baltimore STD Clinic Patients Independent of Risk Group"—all presented at Fifth International Conference on AIDS, Montreal, June 4–9, 1989. See also Jacques Pepin et al., "The Interaction of HIV Infection and Other Sexually Transmitted Diseases: An Opportunity for Intervention," *AIDS* 3 (1989): 3–9.

81. Jean L. Marx, "Circumcision May Protect against the AIDS Virus," *Science* 245 (1989): 470–71; J. Bongaarts et al., "The Relationship between Male Circumcision and HIV Infection in African Populations," paper presented at the Fifth International Conference on AIDS, Montreal, 1989.

82. D. William Cameron et al., "Female to Male Transmission of Human Immunodeficiency Virus Type 1: Risk Factor for Seroconversion in Men," *Lancet* 2 (1989): 403–7.

83. Angelos Hatzakis et al., "Age at Time of HIV Infection as Cofactor of Progression to Advanced Immune Dysfunction and AIDS," paper presented at the Fifth International Conference on AIDS, Montreal, 1989; J. Roy Robertson et al., "Progression to AIDS in Intravenous Drug Users, Cofactors and Survival," paper presented at the Sixth International Conference on AIDS, San Francisco, 1990.

84. Quinn et al., "Serologic and Immunologic Studies," pp. 2617, 2620.

85. AIDS has been a reportable condition since 1983, when the Council of State and Territorial Epidemiologists passed a resolution to that effect.
86. James W. Curran et al., "Epidemiology of HIV Infection and AIDS in the United States," *Science* 239 (1988): 610–16; Karon, Dondero, and Curran, "Projected Incidence of AIDS."
87. *MMWR* 38 (1989): 562.
88. Charles F. Turner, Heather G. Miller, and Lincoln E. Moses, *AIDS, Sexual Behavior and Intravenous Drug Use* (Washington, D.C.: National Academy Press, 1989), pp. 32–33.
89. E. O. Laumann et al., "Monitoring the AIDS Epidemic in the United States: A Network Approach," *Science* 244 (1988): 1186. By "overt manipulations" the authors mean that the highly decentralized CDC reporting system allows individual physicians and hospitals considerable opportunities to hide cases of AIDS if they have an interest in doing so (John H. Gagnon, personal communication, August 31, 1990).
90. U.S. General Accounting Office, *AIDS Forecasting: Undercount of Cases and Lack of Key Data Weaken Existing Estimates* (Washington, D.C.: General Accounting Office, June 1989). A study published some months later, albeit based on the experience of only one state, found that only an estimated 60 percent of AIDS cases in South Carolina were reported to the state's registry in 1986 and 1987. See George A. Conway et al., "Underreporting of AIDS Cases in South Carolina, 1986 and 1987," *Journal of the American Medical Association* 262 (1989): 2859–63.
91. Rand L. Stoneburner et al., "A Larger Spectrum of Severe HIV-1 Related Disease in Intravenous Drug Users in New York City," *Science* 242 (1988): 916–19.
92. Turner, Miller, and Moses, *AIDS,* pp. 31–32.
93. Ronald Bayer, L. H. Lumey, and Lourdes Wan, "The American, British and Dutch Responses to Unlimited Anonymous HIV Seroprevalence Studies: An International Comparison," *AIDS* 4 (1990): 283–90.
94. U.S. Department of Health and Human Services, Public Health Service, Centers for Disease Control, *Human Immunodeficiency Virus Infections in the United States: A Review of Current Knowledge and Plans for Expansion of the HIV Surveillance Activities,* a Report to the Domestic Policy Council (Washington, D.C.: DHHS, November 30, 1987).
95. Timothy J. Dondero, Jr., Marguerite Pappaioanou, and James W. Curran, "Monitoring the Levels and Trends of HIV Infection: The Public Health Service's HIV Surveillance Program," *Public Health Reports* 103 (1988): 213–20.
96. Of the thirty large metropolitan areas, twenty are cities that report 75 percent of the current cases of AIDS; the remaining ten were selected from cities with moderate to low prevalence of AIDS.
97. Harry F. Hull et al., "Comparisons of HIV-Antibody Prevalence in Patients Consenting to and Declining HIV-Antibody Testing in an STD Clinic," *Journal of the American Medical Association* 260 (1988): 935–38.
98. U.S. Centers for Disease Control and National Institute on Drug Abuse, "Proposal for Monitoring HIV Seroprevalence in Intravenous Drug Users in

Treatment, National HIV Seroprevalence Surveys," CDC Protocol No. 840, 1988.

99. Karon, Dondero, and Curran, "Projected Incidence of AIDS," p. 547.

100. Turner, Miller, and Moses, *AIDS*, pp. 52–62.

101. Ibid., pp. 68–70.

102. Ibid., p. 7.

103. Other federal agencies measure seroprevalence in segments of the general population—for example, civilian applicants for military service, active-duty military personnel, and Job Corps entrants; but the results obtained are flawed by self-selection bias.

104. Research Triangle Institute, "National Household Seroprevalence Survey, Pilot Study Summary Report," Contract No. 200-88-0605, Research Triangle Park, N.C., April 1989, p. 1.

105. Ibid., p. 7.

106. On the Dallas survey, see National Center for Health Statistics, "Report on the Dallas County Household HIV Survey," Hyattsville, Md., May 1990; and Bruce Lambert, "Dallas AIDS Survey Is Begun amid a Furor over Its Worth," *New York Times,* September 27, 1989, p. A1.

107. Michael Specter, "Funds for Sex Survey Blocked by House Panel," *Washington Post,* July 26, 1989, p. A3.

108. Privileged communication.

109. Privileged communication.

110. Turner, Miller, and Moses, *AIDS,* p. 70.

111. Ibid., p . 24.

112. Privileged communication. In 1986 the CDC estimated that 1 to 1.5 million people in the United States were infected with the HIV, a range that it modified the next year to between 945,000 and 1.4 million; see Institute of Medicine and National Academy of Sciences, *Confronting AIDS: Update 1988* (Washington, D.C.: National Academy Press, 1988), p. 51. Early in 1990 the CDC changed the estimate slightly to between 800,000 and 1.3 million.

113. John H. Gagnon, personal communication, August 31, 1990.

114. Marshall A. Becker and Jill G. Joseph, "AIDS and Behavioral Change to Reduce Risk: A Review," *American Journal of Public Health* 78 (1988): 394–410; Andrew Moss et al., "Seroconversion for HIV in Intravenous Drug Users in Treatment in San Francisco, 1985–1990," paper presented at the Sixth International Conference on AIDS, San Francisco, 1990.

115. John B. McKinlay and Sonja M. McKinlay, "The Questionable Contribution of Medical Measures to the Decline of Mortality in the United States in the Twentieth Century," *Milbank Memorial Fund Quarterly* 55 (1977): 425.

116. Thomas McKeown et al., "An Interpretation of the Decline of Mortality in England and Wales during the Twentieth Century," *Population Studies* 29 (1975): 391–422.

The Mass-Mediated Epidemic: The Politics of AIDS on the Nightly Network News

Timothy E. Cook and
David C. Colby

In June 1981 a rare assortment of opportunistic diseases was first noticed among otherwise healthy gay men. Now, ten years later, the epidemic known as acquired immune deficiency syndrome is one of the
leading political and social dilemmas facing the United States and the
world. Privately experienced illness became not only a public phenomenon but also, as political actors slowly agreed that it demanded public
response, a public problem.[1] How did this happen? We nominate one
key actor: the news media. If Vietnam was the first "living-room war,"
with images broadcast directly into American homes, then AIDS may
well be the first "living-room epidemic." As early as June 1983, when
the first public opinion polls on AIDS were taken, virtually all of those
surveyed were aware of it, even though scarcely 3 percent of them actually reported knowing a person with AIDS.[2] After all, the media help
to determine which private matters, such as disease, become defined as
public events, such as epidemics. Since the reach, scope, and gravity of
problems cannot be fully judged in one's immediate environment, the
media construct the public reality, a reality distinct from the private
world that we inhabit, and provide "resources for discourse in public
matters."[3]

But the process by which AIDS became an epidemic of public proportions is far from value free. Though journalists may claim to reflect
outside reality, news cannot report everything that has occurred in a
given day. News is invariably selective. Not all issues and individuals
seeking to make news are equally favored in the process of determining

newsworthiness.[4] Nobody really knows what news is, but journalists still have to produce a certain amount of this highly perishable commodity every day. They must develop ways to "routinize the unexpected," which push them toward recurring news sources, stories, and concerns. But, unlike most news, AIDS was unforeseen and unintentional. It thus provides unusual insight into the processes of negotiation by which events become structured as news.[5]

The media's identification and definition of public problems work not only on mass audiences but also on policymakers, who are highly attentive to news coverage. They are most likely to respond to highly salient issues, even those that provoke considerable conflict, but largely in the context of the initial frame that the media have provided.[6] The construction of AIDS as a social and political problem thus has influenced not merely our reaction as individuals but also our response as a society and a polity.

Finally, though most attention has separated the scientific study of AIDS from "its metaphors,"[7] the very process of science is affected by the media. Because publicity can influence the allocation of the grants, profits, and prizes that enhance physicians' and scientists' careers, they have incentives to present findings that the media will cover, a situation leading to what has been called "science by press conference."[8] Moreover, since scientific results are fundamentally products of the questions asked, the media's priorities can push medical inquiries in certain directions. Even the answers may be affected by patients' quickness to report those symptoms and behaviors that have been the subject of media coverage.

In short, the media may have played (and may continue to play) a critical role in the public perception of the epidemic and the range of possible social and political responses to it. By their ability to transform occurences into news, the media exert power. After all, "one dimension of power can be construed as the ability to have one's account become the perceived reality of others. Put slightly differently, a crucial dimension of power is the ability to create public events."[9]

We suggest that the addition of AIDS to the political agenda was slow because of the way the problem was defined and the epidemic framed. Many observers have suggested that because the group initially most affected included gay men, the media delayed reporting AIDS, consequently postponing and distorting the governmental response.[10]

Although AIDS had entered public awareness by mid-1983, public opinion polls at that time showed relatively little concern that AIDS would reach epidemic proportions. The issue had been seemingly contained, defined as a distant, not an immediate, threat. Only after the summer of 1985 did a large percentage of the public begin to conceive of the disease as likely to affect their world—and only then was there much pressure on the government to do something about the epidemic.[11] Even then, political response was muted and often confused. AIDS did not become an agreed-upon issue until President Reagan and Vice-President Bush gave their first speeches on the epidemic in 1987, six years after the initial reports.

Systematic studies of media coverage of AIDS have been largely limited to print media, such as newspapers and newsmagazines.[12] Most imply that AIDS was initially ignored because it was regarded as a "gay disease"; but once the possibility of a large-scale epidemic became clear, AIDS evolved into a subject inviting metaphorical and sensationalized treatment. Dennis Altman has conjectured that "from mid-1983 on, AIDS had entered the popular consciousness and was widely discussed. Nor did press attention go away. . . . Medical stories are particularly attractive to the media, and where they can be linked to both high fatalities and stigmatized sexuality, we have all the ingredients for banner headlines."[13] But print coverage was far from consistent. The volatility of the AIDS story is curious, give Edward Albert's claim that "acquired immune deficiency syndrome seemed tailor-made to the who, what, where and when ideology that often accounts for the content of stories which appear as the 'news.' "[14]

The opportunities for sensation, drama, and moralizing notwithstanding, AIDS presented numerous dilemmas for journalism as an institution.[15] First, the earliest identified group at highest risk comprised gay men. The media would have to deal with individuals who had not attained journalistic standards for newsworthiness prior to 1981. Particularly in television, reporters emphasize issues that are thought to affect the majority of their audiences. With the exception of a few event-driven stories—such as the 1975 discharge of Leonard Matlovich from the Air Force for homosexuality, the 1977 referendum organized by Anita Bryant to repeal the Dade County (Florida) gay rights ordinance, and the 1978 assassination of gay San Francisco County supervisor Harvey Milk—homosexuality and homosexuals had not become a news topic of continuing concern.[16] Reporters on the AIDS newsbeat, whether gay or straight, dealt with a group that mainstream news had neglected.

Second, the subject matter of AIDs, mixing as it does references to blood, semen, sexuality, and death, defied traditional notions of "taste."

As Herbert Gans has noted, journalists take the audience into account by considering norms of taste, especially during the dinner hour of the nightly network news.[17] This audience is viewed as a collection of middle-class families. Av Westin, who has been an executive news producer at ABC and CBS, revealed the networks' logic: "I developed a series of questions to determine what should go into a broadcast and what should be left out. Is my world safe? Are my city and home safe? If my wife, children and loved ones are safe, then what has happened in the past twenty-four hours to shock them, amuse them or make them better off than they were? The audience wants these questions answered quickly and with just enough detail to satisfy an attention span that is being interrupted by clattering dishes, dinner conversation or the fatigue of the end of the working day."[18] By making such choices, newspersons may inadvertently censor themselves; issues are thereby avoided or euphemized.

Finally, and perhaps most important, the media were in the unenviable position of seeking to raise public awareness without creating public panic. While the media take seriously their perceived role of educating and alerting, reporters sense that they must also avoid being inflammatory.[19] The reason is simple. Because they believe that they should reflect politics rather than shape it, they are reluctant to appear to be interfering with the natural unfolding of the political process. Reporters attempt to ignore the consequences of their work lest they be in the paralyzing role of having constantly to predict the future impact of their reporting. They prefer either to avoid topics that could touch off panic or to report such topics in a reassuring way. Indeed, the media periodically examine their coverage of AIDS; and, as we shall see, the network news reports often disclose considerable discomfort as they perform the balancing act between education and instilling "AIDS hysteria."[20]

We focus here on television news. Television is perhaps, in Tom Brokaw's curious but pungent phrase, "the most mass of the mass media." Although it is commonly reported that citizens receive the bulk of their information from television news, most Americans do not attend systematically to any single medium but, instead, assemble information in haphazard and casual ways. Television news is only one part of the news environment to which individuals react.[21] Nonetheless, it is a central part of that environment and has become important in its own right as an agenda setter. Daily newspapers have become more analytic as television takes over the role of headline services for breaking news.

And public officials, although they may not often watch the network news for new information, attend to television "to find out what the rest of the nation is finding out."[22]

Studying television as well as print is also crucial because the two versions often diverge and because audiences learn differently from television accounts than from newspaper stories, as recent studies of information about AIDS have confirmed.[23] In each medium the process of newsmaking is essentially the same: go where news is expected to happen, consult individuals who are agreed-upon authoritative sources, and rework these recorded observations into a coherent account that takes advantage of widely shared cultural scripts and storylines. But the product differs. Television presents different kinds of information. Visual images provide more personalized, vivid, and memorable messages, which may differ from those set forth in print.

All newsmaking assembles stories around a particular angle, but newspapers typically conceal this process by the inverted pyramid form, where each succeeding paragraph becomes progressively less essential, so that editors can cut at will. In television, the imperative is to keep the audience tuned in, or at least to ensure that they don't switch channels. Consequently, television news programs are thematic, attempting to flow both between and within stories. Similar subject matters are clustered together, and the half-hour moves gradually from important and serious "hard news" to more contemplative or upbeat feature stories. The reports themselves are miniature narratives, with the anchor's introduction, the correspondent's lead, and a closer that functions as the moral of the story. These stories introduce conflict that is either resolved or left hanging to bring viewers back for more the next day.

As Daniel Hallin has insightfully noted, "Because of their different audiences, then, and because of television's special need for drama, TV and the prestige press perform very different political functions. The prestige press provides information to a politically interested audience; it therefore deals with *issues*. Television provides not just 'headlines' . . . nor just entertainment, but ideological guidance and reassurance for the mass public. It therefore deals not so much with issues as with symbols that represent the basic values of the established political culture."[24] Of course, the symbolic presentation favored by television news may serve either to reassure or to mobilize.[25] Which symbols and which visuals are chosen can have a considerable influence on the public construction of the epidemic.

We begin our investigation of AIDS coverage with the nightly news broadcasts by the three major commercial networks. Despite the proliferation of news into the morning and nighttime hours, the nightly news remains the flagships of the three major networks, ABC, CBS, and NBC. Moreover, since 1968 these broadcasts have been videotaped, archived, and indexed by Vanderbilt University's Television News Archive. For our analysis we made a search of all AIDS news stories listed in the archive's abstracts and indexes through December 1989. We then viewed and analyzed all stories from January 1981 through April 1, 1987, when President Reagan made his first major speech about the epidemic.

THE AIDS "ATTENTION CYCLE"

First of all, we should establish a benchmark against which to measure television coverage. In this case there is an easy comparison with empirical measures of the increasing severity of the epidemic. The medical community recognized the first cases in 1981. The number of new cases of AIDS per year, as estimated by the Centers for Disease Control (CDC), rose—at first exponentially and then more gradually (see fig.1). As for medical attention, a count of articles on AIDS and related subjects in *Index Medicus* shows similar growth, with a slight drop in 1986, from twenty articles on AIDS in 1981; the medical community sustained regularly increasing interest in the problem (see fig. 2). If the media were merely reflecting either a growing problem or a professional concern, the trajectory of television coverage would follow similar lines as the exponential increase in morbidity rates.

Such was not the case (see fig. 3). There were few stories on AIDS as long as it was identified as a disease that affected only gay men. The CDC had first reported evidence of the disease in June 1981, and the *New England Journal of Medicine* carried three original articles and an editorial on AIDS in its December 10, 1981, issue. Although major newspapers did report this news,[26] there was no nightly news coverage in 1981 and only six stories in 1982. With the exception of the three initial stories about the disease that attacked gay men, the nightly news did not cover AIDS until it spread beyond groups that could be held complicitous in their own illness—gay men and intravenous drug users.[27]

As the risk groups proliferated, the amount of news time devoted to AIDS rose in 1983 but *declined* in 1984 and early 1985, even as the morbidity rate dramatically rose, until Rock Hudson's trip to Paris to receive an experimental treatment against AIDS. Hudson's illness revi-

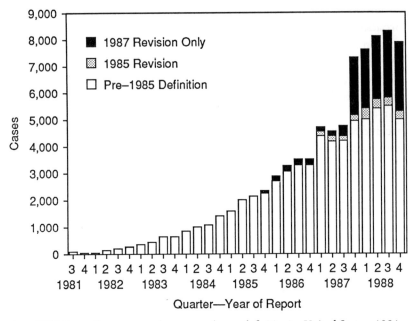

1. AIDS Cases (by quarter of report and case definition)—United States, 1981–1988

SOURCE: *Morbidity and Mortality Weekly Report* 38, no. 14 (April 14, 1989): 230.

talized and legitimized the media's interest in ways we shall shortly describe, but again the attention slackened off after Hudson's death in October, only to rise to a new height in 1987 with increasing attention to the possible heterosexual transmission of the human immunodeficiency virus (HIV) [28] and with Reagan's and Bush's first pronouncements on AIDS. Since that peak AIDS has become routinely reported news, with especially heavy concentration on the International AIDS Conferences that have been held generally in June.

What accounts for this remarkably variable interest of network news programs in AIDS? In particular, how can we understand that their coverage actually declined at the same time that the severity of the epidemic continued to rise and as medical interest increased? One possibility is provided by Anthony Downs's famous "issue-attention cycle." [29] In the first stage of the cycle, the condition exists but is not constructed as a social problem; in the second stage an event triggers awareness of the problem and the public's demand that it be solved; in the third stage the public discovers the political and/or economic costs of solving the problem; and, finally, the revelation of these costs forces

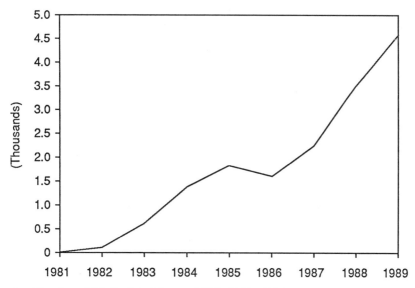

2. Number of Medical Articles on AIDS, 1981–1989

a decline in public interest. But Downs recognized that not all problems are likely to go through a cycle, and there is no evidence that the public beginning in late 1983 saw any costs to doing something about AIDS.

Another possible explanation has to do less with the public than with institutional dynamics of journalism. In particular, while some argue that AIDS was a perfect subject for newspersons, we contend that the epidemic caused newspersons less to sensationalize than to reassure, particularly following their apparent realization that their initial reporting had touched off "an epidemic of fear." News organizations therefore decreased their attention to the disease, which was, in any event, rapidly becoming so familiar that it was "old news." Thus, beginning in late 1983, coverage was sporadic, dictated more by events than by topics. Yet the cycle could begin again if it were refreshed by dramatic new developments that synopsized the reach and extent of the epidemic—and such were the effects of the disclosure of Rock Hudson's illness in July of 1985 and later of the evidence from abroad, particularly Africa, of a heterosexual epidemic.

PHASES OF THE CYCLE

The dynamics of the media's attention to AIDS are further revealed in the themes that characterized the coverage. From 1981 to 1985 the

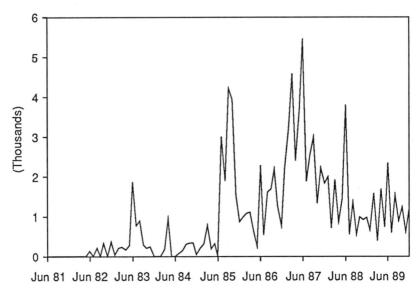

3. Seconds of Nightly News Time on AIDS, June 1981–December 1989

nightly news developed, in sequence, five major clusters of themes on AIDS. The first saw AIDS as largely a gay disease, implicitly blaming gay men and their "life-styles" for the disease. This "mysterious" disease became "deadly" only when it went beyond the initial risk populations, but the media then bypassed openly gay persons with AIDS while pursuing other angles and only eventually legitimized gay spokespersons as accepted authorities. The spread of AIDS beyond the originally demarcated risk groups was the second theme. The "epidemic of fear" about AIDS provided a third theme. The fourth sought scientific breakthroughs and potential cures that provided hope along with hype— reassurance to calm the fears resulting from the reports of the spread of the disease. The fifth theme, news about the most famous AIDS patient, Rock Hudson, provided a new legitimacy for the issue.

Although these themes do not fall into distinctly separable phases, there is a recognizable time sequence to their initial development. The gay stories appeared at the outset in 1982. They were quickly followed by the stories emphasizing the spread beyond gay men, focusing in particular on hemophiliacs, children, and recipients of blood transfusion.[30] In May 1983, following Dr. Anthony Fauci's speculation that HIV might be transmitted by recurring personal contact, the news began to battle the "epidemic of fear," a phase that overlapped with the search on the part of the media to locate scientific breakthroughs. At this point attention was paid to the isolation of HIV and the development of blood-screening tests, and only occasionally to angles that diverged from the media's stereotype of an illness affecting gay men in New York and San Francisco. Interest declined until the illness of Rock Hudson, which, in effect, certified the newsworthiness of the disease and provided an opportunity for the networks to investigate other aspects of AIDS. And the cycle began anew.

THE MYSTERIOUS DISEASE

Scientists at the National Center for Disease Control in
Atlanta today released the results of a study that shows
that the life-style of some male homosexuals has trig-
gered an epidemic of a rare form of cancer.
NBC, June 17, 1982

Anchor Tom Brokaw's lead-in to Robert Bazell's report in June 1982 introduced a new topic to nightly network news audiences. Both stressed the possibility that gay men's behaviors were directly responsible for the disease. Bazell noted, "Investigators have examined the habits of homosexuals, looking for clues," and then switched to a clip of a gay man, Bobbi Campbell, saying, "I was in the fast lane at one time in terms of the way that I lived my life. And now I'm not." After soliciting a comment from another gay man, Billy Wilder, that the disease itself was worse than dying, Bazell ended on a pessimistic note: "Researchers are now studying blood and other samples from the victims, trying to learn what causes the disease. So far they have had no luck."

A similar angle characterized ABC's first report, on October 18, 1982. George Strait began with a profile of a gay man, Phil Lanzaratta, who had been hospitalized several times in the previous months and who said, "I was walking around like a time bomb." In introducing the report, anchor Max Robinson had referred simply to "a mysterious disease," and the signals that Strait gave on the gravity of the disease were also mixed. After showing graphic photographs of lesions from Kaposi's sarcoma (KS) and emphasizing that it was spreading at "an alarming rate," the worst epidemic since polio in the 1950s, he also noted that Lanzaratta's doctors thought he would likely survive. Most prominent was the link of the epidemic to gay men and then to their sexual practices. Indeed, Lanzaratta's body became a signifier for the disease; a shot on the left half of the screen of him walking down the street—with close-cropped hair, mustache, tight-fitting jeans, and cowboy boots—was juxtaposed with the words "acquired immune deficiency syndrome" on the right. And after listing the established high-risk groups, Strait returned to the connection between sexuality and disease: "Hotlines in New York and other cities are handling up to fifty calls a day from homosexuals who fear their sexual intimacy may make them especially vulnerable to immune deficiency syndrome." Yet, although his report was more vivid than Bazell's initial report, complete with graphics of the states affected and lists of the diseases that affected individuals contracted, Strait ended with a reassuring touch, noting that medicine and government were both hard at work trying to figure out the syndrome.

The first AIDS story on CBS, by Barry Petersen on August 2, 1982, diverged in many ways from Bazell's and Strait's reports. Unlike its counterparts, CBS did not initially entrust AIDS coverage to its medical or science correspondents and consequently presented a more overtly political report. Petersen paid less attention to the life-style hypotheses circulated by epidemiologists; instead, he was the most critical of the government's slow response and treated the men who had been diagnosed with the disease as tragic figures, fighting nobly against the odds, rather than as pathetic, helpless victims. Starting with a filmed quote from, again, Bobbi Campbell about his "devastation," the report featured gay activist Larry Kramer complaining that Kaposi's sarcoma was unknown because it was a "gay cancer"; it also included sound bites from physicians such as James Curran and Marcus Conant, who noted that spending on KS could also lead to an increased understanding of cancer. The report closed, "For Bobbi Campbell, it is a race against time. How long before he and others who have this disease finally have answers, finally have the hope for a cure?" But even here, Petersen seemed to be less concerned about its initial outbreak than about its spread: "It appeared a year ago in New York's gay community, then in the gay communities of San Francisco and Los Angeles. Now it's been detected in Haitian refugees. No one knows why." He continued to list its presence among hemophiliacs and intravenous drug users, again asking why; but, tellingly, he never asked why KS appeared among gay men. Even the angriest and least judgmental of these three reports did not find the first identification of the epidemic among gay men to be a puzzle.

All three reports—by starting with the experiences of Campbell, Wilder, and Lanzaratta and then broadening out—followed the networks' tradition of placing disaster in its human-interest context,[31] but they referred to the outbreak simply as "mysterious" and "fascinating." Only later would it turn "deadly." Implicitly, these reports characterized gay men—because of their "habits" or their "sexual intimacy"—as responsible for their illness.

These themes were not surprising. Much of the early speculation by scientists came from epidemiology, which studied stereotyped social behaviors thought prevalent among the initially affected group—behaviors such as the use of poppers (the drug amyl nitrite), multiple sexual partners, and the like.[32] Defined primarily as a venereal disease, AIDS drew on an old and familiar stigma in American culture.[33] Even when a gay man with AIDS was interviewed in respectful terms, shot in the close-up "touching distance" favored by human-interest stories that personalize and individualize the subjects, some images stressed the "otherness" of the group. Strait's report showed two men walking to the camera's right shot from above, so that the viewer can see only their legs. As the men pass the camera, it pans up when their faces cannot be seen, while the voiceover tells us, "The only clue to this disease are the types of people caught in this epidemic." The New York location, the shots from above and the back, and the shoulder bag of one man provide a visual shorthand that would be repeated in later reports as a symbol of the anonymous, potentially dangerous urban gay man.

But the most striking aspect of this first phase is how short-lived it was. In contrast to the thorough popular-magazine coverage at this time, the initial network reports on AIDS were the only stories to emphasize the "gay plague." In their next stories all three networks concentrated on the spread beyond gay men, "needle-using drug addicts," and Haitians to hemophiliacs, children, and recipients of blood transfusions. Yet the early framing did not disappear. Instead, by stating in each story that the syndrome was first seen among homosexuals—and by often accompanying such a statement with stock footage of gay-pride marches shot from above[34] or a gay couple from the back[35]—the media reinforced the portrayal of AIDS as something emanating from the anonymous gay "other" and striking "innocent victims." And no other persons with AIDS were depicted in such an advanced state of the disease as were gay men. In its grisliest version, an NBC report on April 29, 1983, showed a skeletal man in a hospital bed lamely saying, "Dying at thirty-five isn't so bad. Maybe I'm being given a break," with the voiceover informing us that shortly after this was filmed, the man did indeed die.

Many stories blamed the sick in subtle ways. The first story on the
AIDS "Haitian connection" (shown on NBC, June 21, 1983) concluded
that AIDS cannot be blamed on Haitians but "is transmitted among
Haitians just as it is in the United States." The narration tells us that
poverty, poor health practices, and prostitution are related to the transmission. But then the reporter takes the viewer via a hidden camera into
a Haitian bar that caters to foreign gay men—with the implication that
AIDS came to the United States from Haiti via an infected gay man who
had sex with a Haitian "boy prostitute." The Haitian connection thus
became subsumed under the already existing storyline of gay responsibility for the disease. The tendency to blame gay men was apparent even
years later. On May 6, 1985, for example, when NBC reported on a
hemophiliac who gave AIDS to his wife and child, the anchor referred
to this family's plight as a "tragedy that goes beyond numbers," and
noted that these people "live in a mobile home in central Pennsylvania,
far from the gay bars in New York and San Francisco." The tragedy of
those who live near the gay bars in those cities—for, as this report also
noted, three-quarters of all persons diagnosed with AIDS were gay men—
was ignored, since their disease was no longer news.

In short, gay men were shown more often as carriers than as victims.
Yet at the same time, gay spokespersons were occasionally identified as
authoritative sources, if only where they reacted to events initiated by
others.[36] Thus, a March 2, 1983, ABC report on proposals to exclude
all gay men from giving blood quoted Virginia Apuzzo of the National
Gay Task Force protesting such a move and urging that more attention
be paid to research. Gay spokespersons could also be included if they
participated in an official event that intersected with already established
newsbeats and legitimated the networks' use of their comments. Thus,
on August 1, 1983, two networks, ABC and CBS, reported on congressional hearings with numerous gay witnesses; both included Roger Lyon's
quote, "I came here today to hope that my epitaph would not read that
I died of red tape." In the first several years of coverage, gay men were
asked to talk about discrimination; gay health issues; and, to a lesser
extent, other gay problems, such as being closeted. By 1985 gay spokespersons were quoted on screen fifteen times in the network news—far
less frequently than the ninety-five times that non-gay authoritative
sources, such as politicians and doctors, were quoted but more often
than the initially negative portrayal would have predicted.[37]

How do we explain this turning to gay sources for comments in the
midst of often negative reporting? One clue is provided by earlier television news coverage of homosexuality, which tended to be respectful

as long as the subject matter concerned individual gay men or (much more rarely) individual lesbians. But in the initial stages of the epidemic, when gay men were categorized as a high-risk *group,* the ambivalence of the media toward homosexuality as a social phenomenon became clear.[38] Only when the individualistic emphasis could return would the media's assessment be less condemning. Second, because the gay movement was well organized and, once AIDS first hit, its members became convinced that the news media had to be pursued, reporters were provided with willing and easily accessible sources.[39] These sources, of course, may have unwittingly enabled the media to frame AIDS as a largely gay disease.[40] But at a later point, once the threat to the innocent was downplayed, gay men moved from being persons responsible for the spread of the illness to "owners" of the problem, legitimate authorities to be interviewed. As Altman has noted, the gay movement may have thereby attained legitimacy, but at a terrible price.[41]

THE THREAT TO THE INNOCENT

An unknown and mysterious disease is spreading. It
has killed more people than toxic shock syndrome and
legionnaires' disease combined. It first struck homosexual men; but, as Robert Bazell reports, others are getting it.

                                        NBC, October 6, 1982

After the intermittent coverage when gay men and other minorities were deemed the sole persons with AIDS, the media dramatically reported the spread to the "general public."[42] In July 1982 the CDC had noted thirty-four Haitians with opportunistic infections similar to those discovered in gay men, but the networks did not emphasize the spread until the CDC reported AIDS in hemophiliacs and infants. The December 10, 1982, reports of all three networks emphasized the spread of AIDS by blood transfusions, with two noting the CDC's recommendations that those in the high-risk groups not give blood. Two reports fed the fears about the spread. ABC ominously concluded, in an invasion-of-the-body-snatchers tone, that "blood banks cannot know who to look out for if they cannot know what to look out for." CBS suggested that the virus also might be transmitted by saliva, sperm, and mucus in addition to blood. Stories about transmission by blood continued throughout the period under study and were pushed farther forward in the broadcast, even well after the development of the blood test. Other potential transmission modes—such as saliva, tears, mucus, urine, dirty needles, and even close contact—were alluded to, though with lesser frequency than blood. These stories, unlike their predecessors, could have proved alarming to viewers. For one, they could easily slip from the conditional "could" to the more inevitable "would." And, among those infected, gays were shown in ways that emphasized their roles as patients or as others, whereas hemophiliacs and children were portrayed as ordinary individuals who happened to be in the wrong place at the wrong time. The gay men interviewed in the first three reports, for instance, were shown alone, either in public places such as parks and cafes or in doctors' offices. In contrast, the hemophiliacs appeared at home surrounded by family members. The reports stressed the fact that hemophiliacs could not adjust their behavior to avoid exposure to AIDS—thereby implying that gay men *could* adjust their behavior.

Typical in this regard was a CBS story from February 26, 1983. Anchor Bob Schieffer began by noting, "Some doctors suspect that blood banks and plasma centers may be spreading a new and mysterious disease called AIDS." The report dealt with hemophiliacs, which the correspondent, David Dow, labeled a "small but vulnerable part of the population." The networks never reported on gay men in similar terms, though those terms would have been accurate. In the CBS report Dow interviewed one hemophiliac:

DOW: The unaffected are beginning to worry. . . . For college professor
            Charles Bell and many other hemophilia patients, the plasma con-
            centrate they can store at home and inject themselves is not just a
            lifeline; it is their key to an active, somewhat normal life.

BELL: I really don't have an option. I really have to continue using the
            plasma, or the concentrate as it's called. The thought of abandon-
            ing the kind of life I have as a result of the concentrate is almost
            unthinkable. . . .

DOW: For now, no one is flatly declaring that the nation's blood supply
            is in danger. Too little is known about AIDS itself—what it is and
            how it spreads. But until those questions are answered, other
            questions will persist among those Americans who depend on the
            blood of others for their own life and health.

The demarcation between "innocent victims" on one hand and the gay men and IV drug users on the other, which implicitly characterized early AIDS reporting on television, became explicit later on, when virology took over from epidemiology and the stress on behaviors became downplayed. On September 18, 1985, in a revealing passage during the Rock Hudson saga, CBS anchor Dan Rather introduced one sequence:

"It's not at all what people first thought—a mysterious killer that seemed to strike beyond the bounds of respectable society. People thought AIDS was something you caught in alleyways from a dirty needle or picked up in gay haunts doing things most people don't do. But now science knows it is a deadly virus that makes no moral or sexual distinctions. And it's making its way very slowly toward Main Street."

The networks could find little assurance in the statistics about the spread, with the exception of the decreases in syphilis infection rates among gay men.[43] At the outset all that reporters could do was to draw some reassurance from their setting—usually a hospital laboratory or, as in George Strait's first report, the Capitol building. Posing in front of the Capitol, Strait closed his report with these words: "In Phoenix and in labs around the country, researchers are trying to solve the mystery around AIDS and the disease it causes. To help, Congress has just appropriated a half a million dollars for more research, reflecting the growing national concern about the spread of this immune deficiency syndrome" (ABC, October 18, 1982). In contrast to Bazell's downbeat presentation in the first report on NBC, later reports sought to depict people hard at work unraveling the mysteries of the mysterious and now "deadly" disease.

THE "EPIDEMIC OF FEAR"

Fighting the fear of AIDS, it seems, is as important as
fighting the disease itself. . . . As researchers attempt to
conquer this disease called AIDS, public officials attempt to conquer the epidemic of fear. . . . It is a deli-
cate balancing act, raising the level of concern for the
disease on the one hand, while reducing the level of
panic on the other.

                                              ABC, June 20, 1983

Anchor Max Robinson's lead-in and Ken Kashiwahara's voiceover adroitly captured the dilemma for journalists covering AIDS. Already, in noting the spread beyond gay men, they had fallen into a typical approach to a potential disaster, best indicated by a study of how newspapers covered (and how the population responded to) predictions of earthquakes after the discovery of the Palmdale bulge north of Los Angeles. News fell into "an alarm-and-reassurance pattern. . . . [S]tories began with dramaticized accounts of worst-possible scenarios, as though to shake readers out of their lethargy, and concluded with reassurances about the seismic resistivity of most local construction . . . as though to quiet the alarm so deliberately generated."[44] As these authors note, such a pattern, derived from journalists' attempts to show two sides to an issue, could easily leave audiences confused or able to read in their own (possibly incorrect) conclusion. In television, alarm could easily dominate, even when the final tagline attempted to reassure.

For newspapers AIDS became front-page news in May 1983, after Dr. Anthony Fauci's editorial in the *Journal of the American Medical Association* noting cases of children with AIDS and raising the hypothesis that recurring household contact could be a mode of transmission. The networks did not initially rush to cover this new story. Indeed, only ABC, in a twenty-second throwaway, made any mention of it at all. However, the potential of contamination by casual contact provoked fearful responses, which, in turn, were ambiguously covered by reporters, who partially condemned the "hysteria" but also instilled fears about the potential for a pandemic.[45]

CBS reported the first epidemic-of-fear story on May 18, 1983. Dan Rather introduced the segment, which was placed early in the broadcast to signal its importance,[46] with an overview of the exponential climb in AIDS cases. He continued: "Those of course are frightening figures, and Barry Petersen tonight reports that in some places fear of the disease is itself becoming epidemic." In the report San Francisco police officers were shown demanding special masks and gloves; health care and sanitation workers were shown, concerned about contamination; and blood banks were shown turning away donors whose "life-style fits that of AIDS victims." Yet, in his closing words, Petersen left open the possibility that such fear was warranted: "Doctors say they do not yet know how far and how fast the disease could spread."

Petersen's report on fear of AIDS was perhaps the most alarming. Later reports, starting with NBC's May 24 story, explicitly attempted to calm these fears. In mid-June all three networks aired lengthy stories about "AIDS hysteria" within a day of each other. The news had piqued interest in the spread of the disease, which had gone from being "mysterious" to being "deadly." Now the attention shifted from the threat to would-be innocent bystanders caught by circumstance to social institutions. Most prominent among these institutions were, of course, blood banks and hospitals; but prisons, the military, and schools were all shown as undergoing considerable anxiety, with the possibility of infected or exposed inmates, soldiers, or schoolchildren. Such locales often provided, whether advertently or not, an opportunity to spread misinformation as frightened individuals made emotional statements.

Take CBS's prison story from June 19, 1983. Anchor Morton Dean introduced the lengthy story by quoting Edward Brandt, assistant secretary of the Department of Health and Human Services, to calm concerns with factual information about the only known modes of transmission. But the report had other effects. Reporter Joan Snyder said that AIDS was probably not spreading rapidly in prison: "But what has spread rapidly is fear." She illustrated this statement by showing an emotional correctional officer shot in dramatic close range and yelling, "Get these people out of the jails! It's gonna cost people's lives one way or another. Either we're going to die of AIDS or these people are going to kill us or something. Get 'em out of the jails! That's the answer." Snyder could not counteract this vivid quote with a bland statement from what she termed "a correctional officer at a meeting called by state prison officials to try to relieve anxiety among prison workers with medical information." Her indication of no evidence for transmission by casual contact was again counterbalanced by inmate liaison Pedro Soto arguing, "Once you have AIDS, you're gonna die. . . . There is no way that they can tell you how to catch AIDS. They have ideas. They're checking 'em out. But they cannot say," followed by an inmate endorsing the idea of quarantine.

These stories often showed persons-in-the-street commenting in ways that defied scientific understanding, even at that time, of how the disease would spread, or expressing doubts that one could be absolutely sure. Reporters, hewing to the strategic ritual of objectivity, never specifically rebutted these misleading statements, apparently considering it sufficient to mix alarm with reassurance from public officials.[47] The report could then inadvertently reinforce and authenticate the viewers' doubts.

Ironically, although journalists sided with those who were trying to calm the fear, their reports about it may have served not to exorcise but to heighten it. The emotionally charged quotes from upset individuals would in all likelihood have overridden the cool statistics proffered by the authorities. Other vivid film excerpts portrayed reactions that may have (incorrectly) seemed legitimate: police officers donning surgical gloves and masks, prison guards putting on futuristic "special protective outfits should they have to subdue a prisoner with AIDS," and television technicians refusing to fit a microphone on a person with AIDS.[48]

In later stories the news would recount the various impacts of fear:

discrimination against AIDS patients; discrimination and violence against gay men; shortage of blood supplies after incorrect rumors that people could contract AIDS by donating blood; anxiety among health care workers, police, and prison guards; refusals to adopt AIDS children; and, most frequently of all, the attempts to keep children with AIDS out of public schools. Only a few stories presented segments showing cool, deliberate reactions from the public: the townspeople who allowed a child with AIDS to attend school without protests; the young playmates of an HIV-positive child.[49] Vividness alone does not explain this preference. Witness a moving NBC story of a teacher with AIDS who had been transferred out of his classroom for the hearing-impaired and who won a suit that returned him there; his press conference in the school library was interrupted by several beaming students who embraced him (November 23, 1987). But such a story evaded the usual priority of television media for setting forth an easily reported either-or conflict, preferably in continuing sagas, such as those of schoolchildren struggling to stay in school: Ryan White in Kokomo, Indiana, in 1985; or the Ray brothers in Arcadia, Florida, in 1987. In search of the balance between being informative and being interesting, network news tended to offset the bland reassurances of government health officials with the dramatic emotions of those who feared the worst. The epidemic of fear was far from stemmed.

Faced with an impossible balancing act, the news media seem to have decided to turn their attention elsewhere. As long as a story had to involve two distinct sides that often talked past each other and were rarely directly rebutted by reporters, calling attention to the potential gravity of AIDS provoked fearful responses, whose coverage simply made matters worse. The epidemic had not played itself out, but the topic as a news story had, and journalists would now await authoritive scientific and political sources to let them know when news on AIDS would happen.

THE SEARCH FOR THE BREAKTHROUGH

There may be a dramatic breakthrough in the treatment of AIDS tonight. Maybe. Everybody is anxious for some encouraging news.

NBC, October 29, 1985

Tom Brokaw, in his lead to a story about the promising effects of Cyclosporin A, typifies reports on scientific research and treatments for

AIDS. After emphasizing the spread of this disease to "innocent" victims and the consequent fearful reaction, the networks proceeded, beginning in 1983, to express cautious hope, reassuring the audience that scientists were inexorably progressing toward a treatment, cure, or vaccine.[50] As with newsmagazines, the focus of coverage shifted from a preoccupation with life-style and contagion to reports on science and medicine.[51] Such attempts to reassure had been evident in news reporting since Strait's October 1982 ABC story, but the search for a breakthrough began in earnest in mid-1983. For example, on April 29, 1983, NBC reported that the isolation of a virus was the "best lead yet" and, three months later (on July 12, 1983), that research on Interleukin-2 provided "encouraging news tonight—not enough to call it a breakthrough, but encouraging news nonetheless."

This phase differed from the preceding ones. Coverage was no longer topic-driven, whereby enterprising reporters dug up new aspects of a continuing story. Instead, it was event-driven; that is, reporters routinely awaited event summaries or pseudo-events, such as news conferences or demonstrations, to discuss the otherwise less than newsworthy subject.[52] Reporters consequently became even more dependent on authoritative sources, such as political officials, prestigious doctors, or drug companies' spokespersons, to create such events and allow an opportunity to cover the issue. In the absence of new developments announced by these sources, the only news about AIDS that would develop were occasional odd angles, such as the death of a great-grandmother from AIDS (NBC, February 27, 1985).

Such authoritative sources also had reason to look for a breakthrough and to provide reassurance. At the very least, governmental officials and scientists were more likely to call a press conference when progress and promising news would occur.[53] Moreover, the Reagan administration was eager to limit the damage near an election year. Thus, in a July 12, 1983, story on Interleukin-2, NBC quoted Health and Human Services secretary Margaret Heckler: "It's the first glimmer of light. It's not the whole answer, but it is promising." The most notable example of the media's being misled was Heckler's prediction that, with the isolation of the virus, a vaccine was only a few years away. The reporters added some caution, but the optimism of the authoritative source dominated the reports. Meanwhile, scientists downplayed dead ends and stressed advances—findings that the news media would cover and that would boost the scientists' credibility and their careers. Given the interest on the part of both political officials and scientists to call attention only to progress, if not breakthroughs, much reporting on AIDS went from alarming to soothing.

To be sure, many reports on cures were often interwoven with stark data on the spread of the disease. In an August 17, 1984, report on the isolation of the virus by San Francisco scientists, NBC introduced the story with the following statement: "No one knows for sure what causes AIDS. But what both scientists and researchers know is that it attacks homosexuals mostly and that invariably it kills. Tonight Robert Bazell tells of one more step in the search for clues to the disease and a new and sinister element in the AIDS equation." As with many of the stories, NBC first alarmed and then assured the audience—by raising anxieties that can be resolved. Thus, the media created a "strong" science story that reaches the "boundaries of truth." [54]

Sometimes they offered only faint hope, but virtually no reports were as downbeat as Bazell's original story in 1982. On March 1, 1984, in one of its several reports on simian AIDS, CBS interviewed a researcher who described his findings as follows: "There is no immediate signifi-cance, in terms of therapy. However, there is great significance in terms of hope." Most stories carried caveats, such as "Officials warn against premature expectations of a quick cure"; "Scientists caution that even when they are certain of the cause of AIDS, it will probably take years of more research before they develop a vaccine"; and "The next step: a vaccine. But that's a big step, and researchers say that it could take years." [55]

This tendency from mid-1983 until mid-1985 is important because dead ends in research were not considered newsworthy by any of the actors involved in making news—neither the sources (whether politi-cians or physicians) nor the journalists—even though gay spokesper-sons were then vocal in their denunciation of government inaction. And even more than most sources, the networks stretched to the boundary of truth, looking for a breakthrough that would reassure. Reports on tongue sores, a plant fungus, feline AIDS, and experimental drug treat-ments provide examples.

This attempt to be the first to report a breakthrough is, of course, common to many science stories, as the flap over "cold fusion" in 1989 clearly illustrates. But not only does this penchant exaggerate prelimi-nary or mixed results; it also leads to omissions, so that certain stories (or parts of stories) are not covered. [56] Breakthroughs are key, because if events are not perceived to move the process along, then by definition news did not occur. [57] We have already noted that television failed to report the AIDS story until more than a year after the disease was first noted. And when it did cover the AIDS story, it overlooked a number of significant events: the development of a clinical case definition of AIDS in September 1982; the voluntary guidelines developed by the American Red Cross and others advising against accepting blood from high-risk groups in January 1983;[58] the discovery in May 1983 by scientists from Harvard, the Pasteur Institute, and NIH that HIV infected at least some AIDS patients; Interleukin-2 clinical testing that began in March 1984; the First International Conference on AIDS in Atlanta in April 1985; and the May 1985 NIH study showing that health care workers have a low risk of contracting HIV.

The event-driven storyline not only tended to discourage access of gay spokespersons to the media, who could not point out the lack of progress that they perceived; it also meant that the story of how the gay community was responding to the crisis went almost unreported. From mid-1983 to mid-1985, most events concerning AIDS were not included in the news, and larger assessments of the epidemic and the responses to it were all but nonexistent. In this event-driven phase of routine journalism, the news media may have continued intermittently to sound the alarm, but the alarm was now at least equally balanced by reassurance. Consequently, AIDS stories not only declined in number but also became less urgent and tended to imply that the situation, however grave, was largely under control.

ROCK HUDSON AND THE LEGITIMATION OF AIDS

Hudson's condition has brought AIDS back into the
headlines, but after all it is an ongoing emergency.
NBC, July 24, 1985

The illness and death of a famous actor with a masculine image, "the most well-known victim yet" (CBS, July 25, 1985), legitimized the media's attention to this disease as a continuing story instead of sporadic breaking news. Indeed, it would not be too far-fetched to describe AIDS coverage in television as falling into two phases: before and after Rock Hudson. Some of this new attention can be attributed to Rock Hudson's status as a celebrity. But the replayed visuals of his scenes with Doris Day, Elizabeth Taylor, or Linda Evans tended to reinforce Hudson's powerful image as the epitome of heterosexuality—an image that the networks, presumably concerned about privacy, did not contest, since they kept largely silent about Hudson's sexual preferences in real life. Little wonder that the new image of AIDS was that it was at last hitting home.

Yet what is most striking about this phase of reporting is the new legitimacy accorded to topic-driven stories about AIDS and to sources, notably in the gay movement, that had been absent in the preceding several months. This new concentration also provoked agencies, such as the National Institutes of Health, to be more proactive than reactive.[59] Not only did the new legitimacy allow the networks to develop longer stories and special segments on AIDS; it also pushed AIDS stories earlier in the broadcast, thus according them more importance, and allowed the "old news" story of gay men with the disease to reappear.

The initial reports, on July 23, 1985, described Hudson's hospitalization in Paris and reported speculation of his having AIDS. On the second day of this story, two networks, in rare lead stories, not only confirmed reports that he had AIDS but also used the opportunity to report broader aspects of the AIDS story.[60] CBS developed the story of experimental drugs, using, as the rationale, Hudson's attempt to be treated in Paris with HPA-23. NBC further broadened the story by presenting an extensive report on the stress experienced by health care workers and AIDS patients in the clinic at San Francisco General Hospital. For the first time in months, instead of reporting primarily on hemophiliacs or other people with AIDS from atypical locales or groups, the networks showed gay people with AIDS—and treated them with respect. On July 25 all three networks led with the news confirming Hudson's diagnosis of AIDS and also examined other aspects of the AIDS story: ABC reported on the development of experimental treatments; this report was followed by a lengthy question-and-answer session between anchor Peter Jennings and medical editor Timothy Johnson on the transmission of AIDS. CBS reported on the development of experimental treatments. NBC reported on fund-raising efforts in Hollywood, and Tom Brokaw interviewed Dr. Paul Volberding, the AIDS clinic director at San Francisco General Hospital, on AIDS transmission. On July 26, after perfunctory reports on Hudson's condition, ABC described the AIDS clinic at San Francisco General Hospital, and NBC recounted the development of experimental drugs. Then, on July 28, ABC described fund-raising efforts such as a ten-kilometer walkathon in Hollywood. In late September ABC presented a week-long series of reports on the origins, extent, transmission, cures, and treatments of AIDS and, even more unexpectedly, on AIDS-related complex (ARC), which had been previously unmentioned by the networks.[61] Even on the day of Rock Hudson's death, October 2, NBC recapitulated general information about AIDS.

To be sure, in many ways coverage merely revived a wealth of familiar storylines. CBS's Dan Rather resuscitated "an epidemic of fear that seems to be spreading faster than the disease."[62] The principal stories were related to schoolchildren with AIDS: an unidentified second-grader in Queens and, what was better for the news, the ongoing saga of Ryan White.[63] But coverage of fear also included people with AIDS who were barred from nursing homes; unwanted and thus unadoptable foster children of AIDS-afflicted mothers; and even extraordinary precautions at the Rajneeshpuram community in Oregon.[64]

But the epidemic-of-fear story now concentrated less on frightened heterosexuals, particularly parents pulling their children out of school, than on gay men who were subjected to discrimination and violence. Thus, in one report CBS not only showed conventional incidents of fear—Houston police wearing rubber gloves when frisking gay suspects, a school board meeting in New Jersey—but also interviewed a man with AIDS who was suing to regain his job as a budget analyst in Florida.[65] In an NBC story gay men in Colorado expressed their concern about losing insurance coverage after a law was passed requiring blood banks and doctors to report HIV-positive individuals by name; and a CBS story reported discrimination against gay actors in Hollywood in the wake of Hudson's illness.[66] ABC broadcast a "special segment" on violence against gay men and lesbians, with Jennings noting, "There's always been prejudice and violence against homosexuals and lesbians [sic]. But the public concern about AIDS and its connection to homosexuals has made it a more serious problem."[67]

The illness of Rock Hudson recertified AIDS as a newsworthy topic suitable for stories beyond breaking news. The authoritative sources that had dominated the coverage of AIDS prior to the revelation of Hudson's illness no longer held the upper hand, and the reappearance of AIDS as a newsworthy issue allowed gay spokespersons to add their perspective. But instead of maintaining a continuing high attention, the networks' interest again would decline in late 1985 and early 1986. In effect, the cycle may have begun again. After Hudson's death AIDS became old news, and reporters relapsed to an event-driven mode. Although Hudson's illness ushered in a new phase of AIDS reporting, notable for its thoroughness and for its new sympathy to both gay persons with AIDS and gay-movement spokespersons, it did not last.

THE CYCLE AGAIN, BUT WITH A DIFFERENCE

Hope and despair. Those are the conflicting emotions
evoked by two stories tonight.
                                        CBS, September 18, 1986

Anchor Dan Rather's lead-in to two stories, one about the drug AZT and the other about the epidemic in Africa, shows how the AIDS attention cycle replayed itself with a difference. Already, in the fall of 1985, there had been a spate of epidemic-of-fear stories, but by the beginning of 1986, the topic-driven coverage provoked by Rock Hudson's illness had once again been replaced by a largely event-driven routine approach. And once again, news organizations relied on political officials and authoritative medical and scientific sources to indicate when an AIDS story was newsworthy.

But five linked characteristics distinguished the post-Hudson coverage. First, although the number of stories declined from the 1985 level, they were presented earlier in the news flow, and items were placed among the top stories—a status that had rarely occurred prior to the revelations about Rock Hudson.[68] More telling, the networks' complete neglect of AIDS as recently as the month before Hudson flew to Paris would never be repeated. Second, as AIDS became more generally recognized as newsworthy, more approaches were brought to bear; thus, stories in 1986 were covered not only by medical and science correspondents but increasingly by law reporters, political reporters (both foreign and domestic), and regional stringers who sought new angles and spoke to new sources. Third, there was thus less consensus about how best to cover the epidemic. The medicalization of the epidemic was no longer complete. The networks' confusion is best revealed by the contrasting logos placed behind the anchor announcing the story—ABC using two overlapping faces of uncertain gender in 1986 and, beginning in March 1987, the word *AIDS* against two crumbling male and female symbols; CBS using the medical symbol to replace the "I" in AIDS; and NBC varying the graphic for medical stories (e.g., a hand holding a test tube of blood) or for items emphasizing social ramifications (e.g., a man and a woman silhouetted against the letters AIDS). Fourth, this lack of consensus meant that a variety of storylines would be revived—the continuing preoccupation with the safety of the blood supply, or the Rock Hudson angle applied to other famous people with AIDS, such as pro football star Jerry Smith—and would continue to reinvigorate the media's attention to the epidemic on a variety of dimensions.[69] Fifth and most important, the increased prominence of AIDS and the new variety of approaches allowed more authoritative sources to be heard. And now these sources were in disagreement, whereas from late 1983 to mid-1985 they had converged on a storyline that reassuringly noted science doggedly at work to master the epidemic. Although the First International AIDS Conference in Atlanta in 1985 went unnoticed by the networks, its 1986 counterpart in Paris became the first of periodically recurring events that attracted enormous coverage.

As the number of cases in Europe and Africa grew, sources outside the United States—at an international conference on AIDS in Africa held in Brussels in November 1985, at the Paris conference in June 1986, and later at the World Health Organization—began providing information. Significantly, these sources, drawing from African data, were more likely than their American counterparts to raise the possibility of an epidemic among heterosexuals. As AIDS gained attention, scientists and physicians who were not directly involved in research or treatment spoke out. These sources, instead of talking primarily about progress and breakthroughs, pointed to the rising number of cases and to what became a lead story on both ABC and NBC—the National Academy of Sciences report of a "woefully inadequate" response. Within the Reagan administration, too, there was disagreement; in addition to confusion in the Justice Department over the reach of antidiscrimination laws to people with AIDS and HIV-positive individuals, the outwardly united front was publicly broken by Surgeon General C. Everett Koop, who tersely called for massive education of adults and children with the words "We're talking about death because of our reticence. . . . This silence must end" (ABC, October 22, 1986).

Early in 1986 the networks were still trying to maintain a balance between alarm and reassurance. In February, for example, Dan Rather announced new evidence about "how the AIDS virus works with terrifying speed," and science reporter Susan Spencer used this evidence to add a more upbeat closer: "A major development in basic science does not mean that a cure for AIDS is around the corner. But the virus has given up another secret and scientists have a new weapon in the fight against it" (CBS, February 12, 1986).

But as the sources expanded, even the most reassuring of journalists, such as ABC's George Strait, changed tone. Strait was the first to report about the potential for the drug AZT as an area where "great progress is being made," with footage of AIDS patient John Solomon in what Strait termed "the midst of a remarkable recovery."[70] But, along with his colleagues, he too would note "the latest disturbing news about the spread of the disease" from the Paris conference in June.[71] By the spring of 1987, when governmental sources began suggesting testing for those in high-risk categories (including recipients of blood transfusions), Strait showed clinics with heterosexuals seeking to be tested. Then, segueing from a shot of a New York street scene to one of a man and a woman in a rural field, walking and nuzzling, he added, "For most people, the likelihood *is* low, *but* even small-town America is not completely safe." The woman in this story had AIDS. After running a quote from her, in which she wondered how many people might be infected without being aware of it, the report froze the frame, and Strait noted, "Last January, two years after these pictures were taken, Amy Sloan died" (ABC, March 19, 1987).

Even with the September 1986 announcement of the dramatic results of AZT, the first effective treatment against AIDS, and with the lead stories allocated to the Food and Drug Administration's approval of AZT in March 1987, the networks balanced only muted reassurance with alarm, either noting the toxicity and uncertain duration of AZT's effect or pointing to areas where AIDS was seemingly out of control. Similar storylines emerged once more. Blaming the victims occurred in curious ways. An otherwise bland ABC report on anonymous tests by the CDC to gauge the spread of HIV shifted its visuals from CDC headquarters to a back shot of two jeans-clad men holding hands when Mike von Fremd intoned his close: "Those testing positive cannot and will not be told" (January 10,1987).

But the stories now used less file footage of the Castro district and more of New York telephoto street scenes or of heterosexual couples shot from behind as they walked down the streets. Some of the reports emanated from bars frequented by single heterosexuals, who now responded with the same caution about multiple partners that the networks had elicited from gay men in 1983.[72] The epidemic-of-fear stories—noting again that "the AIDS virus is spreading rapidly, but even more contagious are the fears of the worried well" (NBC, March 17, 1987)—began to fuel not just reaction against high-risk groups and people with AIDS but also a seemingly growing concern from that general population itself that it, too, might be infected. The epidemic, as far as the nightly news was concerned, had been heterosexualized.

The increased diversity of newsbeats, journalists, and sources brought to bear on the AIDS epidemic after Rock Hudson's death was responsible for the upward spiral of stories that peaked in the spring of 1987. When President Reagan finally delivered a major address on AIDS on April 1, 1987, before the College of Physicians in Philadelphia, he briefly halted this climb, since there was a hiatus of several days on each network before they reported another AIDS story. But in the process the president also guaranteed that all authoritative sources now agreed about the place of the epidemic on the political agenda.

CONCLUSION

We cannot agree that "media response to AIDS has generally been irrational."[73] The ebb and flow of AIDS reporting reflects considerable rationality, *but by the standards of "media logic."* After all, journalists used authoritative sources, presented ostensibly balanced reports (which, as we have seen, may not have been so evenly balanced as the reporters thought), moved away from stories seen as repetitive "old news," and sought to avoid subjects that present too many complexities for the audience. Each of these strategies represents a journalist's rational adaptation to the uncertainty and vulnerability of trying to figure out what's news. Merely arguing that the media should be more objective or more rational overlooks the possibility that objectivity and rationality led us to the inadequate picture of AIDS that television presented.

Our evidence supports the conclusion that the media did not merely reflect outside events but, instead, profoundly recast the epidemic for both public and governmental audiences. The media played a crucial role in agenda setting on AIDS, particularly at the time of problem definition. First, the lag time between the first identification of the syndrome and the earliest television reports may have caused or allowed delay on the part of government officials, who could overlook the gravity of the epidemic. More important, the evidence from television network news suggests that—in contrast to the expectation that coverage of AIDS would tend to be sensational—the networks attempted to reassure at least as much as they played up the story. After they discovered the "epidemic of fear" set off by reports of AIDS in mid-1983, the networks quickly searched for a breakthrough, particularly in progress toward the development of a vaccine, and turned away from AIDS stories unless government officials and high-ranking doctors presented them with breaking news, which itself was likely to be taken as an indication of progress against the disease. In short, the media did not maintain consistent pressure after AIDS was brought to public attention in the summer of 1983. The access of the gay movement was highly conditional and was low during the period before Rock Hudson's illness became known. When the media did cover the issue, they defined the problem not as the lack of a cure for those already afflicted but as the lack of a vaccine that would control the spread to the "general population." Overall, media coverage was more inclined to reassure than to criticize.

The initial coverage, with its emphasis on gay life-styles and "innocent victims," made AIDS a much more controversial matter than it would have been if the initial coverage had addressed purely medical problems. As Barbara Nelson has noted, only when child abuse was packaged as a medical question rather than a moral question did government action proceed.[74] A similar conclusion could emerge from the evidence on AIDS.

Even here, television did not do a stellar job, partially because of its squeamishness not only about disease but about sexuality in general and homosexuality in particular.

But AIDS reporting was primarily shaped by a routine that was, on its face, neutral. The epidemic hit first and hardest a stigmatized group that the media considered to be distinct from their audience at large. As long as AIDS was defined as a disease that largely affected gay men— who were depicted as anonymous, often foreboding, carriers of the illness—media attention was marginal. As NBC's Robert Bazell admitted in February 1983, "It would be dishonest not to say we couldn't sell the AIDS story early on because it was about gays."[75] Moreover, the access of gay-movement spokespersons to television news was lower than that of scientific or political authorities, whose "event needs" favored reassurance about the progress to a breakthrough. Television news, if it were to find a way to cover AIDS, had to sell the story to the general public—hence the early focus on hemophiliacs and children—in ways that enlightened without panicking and that violated none of the taste taboos prominent in television. This was, as it turns out, an almost impossible task; little wonder that after each of the upswings in 1983, 1985, and 1987, the networks receded from covering it.

In 1985 television would eventually accord AIDS the ultimate status of a social problem—a made-for-TV movie, NBC's acclaimed *An Early*

Frost. As with network news, the producers faced considerable difficulty in selling the story to the network's broadcast standards department. One source pointed out, "The NBC censor said to the producer,
'I thought we were doing a film about AIDS, not about homosexuality.'
And the producer said to him, 'What planet have you been living on?'
If this were a heterosexual AIDS movie, there would have been no problems at all."[76] This temptation to make a movie about AIDS without
making a movie about homosexuality is much the same as the temptation to ignore AIDS as legitimate news when it appeared to affect only
homosexuals. The consequences to us seem far-reaching indeed.

POSTSCRIPT: THE HIV EPIDEMIC AND
THE NETWORKS IN THE 1990s

By mid-1987 President Reagan and Vice-President Bush broke their
silence on the epidemic, and AIDS entered the political agenda not as a
sporadically recurring problem but as a permanent matter, to which
politicians would be expected to respond. Indeed, the cycles of television coverage that followed after the three peaks—in June 1983, with
the first concentration on the epidemic reaching beyond the four risk
groups then classified; in September 1985, with a gay actor's illness
symbolizing, paradoxically, the long reach of AIDS; and in the spring
of 1987, with the warnings about a heterosexually transmitted epidemic—may well have played themselves out in the absence of new
evidence of a more rapid or widespread expansion of the epidemic that
challenges the current understanding. AIDS has become a routinely reported matter, no longer subject to fluctuations inherent in crisis reporting.

As with prior periods following the peaks, reporting since mid-1987
has slackened off.[77] Once again, it has become event-driven, focusing
above all on occasions that can be planned for well in advance, especially the annual international AIDS conferences. But in contrast to the
earlier phases, in which spokespersons for the gay movement or for
people with AIDS were consulted only when stories were cued by scientists or by politicians, the post-1987 coverage has been shaped by the
routine ability of these sources to make news on their own, particularly
as they anticipate and plan for just such long-scheduled events. These
sources have hailed not only from more mainstreamed groups such as
the National Lesbian and Gay Task Force or the Names Project but
also from confrontational organizations such as the AIDS Coalition to

Unleash Power (ACT UP). ACT UP, particularly in its earliest stages, often received respectful coverage, which is striking given its members' penchant for disrupting speeches, conducting sit-ins (or "die-ins"), and getting arrested. But ACT UP's more radical and far-reaching critique that science and medicine were inherently political may have been blunted. Though ACT UP received air time, journalists either framed its agenda as reformism favoring anti-bureaucratic, clear-cut good-government solutions or reported the demonstrations as political theater in, of, and for itself.[78]

In the 1990s, then, the coverage of the HIV epidemic, though avoiding the extraordinary focuses of its peaks in 1983, 1985, and 1987, should continue to be a routine and relatively constant news item. There are, to be sure, some drawbacks to routine coverage, insofar as saturation of the airwaves may be necessary to keep individuals vigilant about proper prevention, such as safer sex. But it avoids the on-again, off-again cycle of alarm and reassurance that proved debilitating in the first years of the epidemic.

Yet the future coverage of the epidemic will be far from problem free. The network news lagged in realizing that the epidemic has slowed among the initial high-risk group of gay men but continues to rage within the population of intravenous drug users, and primarily through them into urban minority communities and to women. Such sectors are even less organized and less legitimated to speak for themselves than were gay men in the early 1980s, and their ability to influence the future progress of the epidemic may be seriously harmed. If journalists are to play a virtuous part in stemming the HIV epidemic, they must take care to reflect a democratic variety of voices, whether or not these voices are connected to the usual authoritative sources and whether or not their concerns can be linked to the supposed "general population." But given the constraints on journalism that push it toward elite sources and away from democratized news, we cannot be optimistic that such reporting will indeed occur.

NOTES

Earlier versions of this essay were presented at the annual meetings of the American Political Science Association, Chicago, September 1987, and the International Communication Association, San Francisco, May 1989. Portions of this essay appeared in the *Journal of Health Policy, Politics and Law* (16 [1991]) and are reprinted with permission of Duke University. We are indebted to many individuals, whom we will thank personally for advice and suggestions; but particular thanks go to Timothy Murray for his exemplary research assistance and coauthorship of the earliest version; Martha Roark for additional research assistance; Michael Kolakowski for advice and suggestions on poll data; Brenda Laribee for helping to process the charts; Williams College for several Division II grants and the University of Maryland Baltimore County for financial support; the Vanderbilt University Television News Archives for its excellent services; and Edward Brandt, Ellen Hume, Jim Lederman, and Keith Mueller for detailed critiques of earlier drafts.

1. On public problems see Joseph R. Gusfield, *The Culture of Public Problems: Drinking-Driving and the Symbolic Order* (Chicago: University of Chicago Press, 1981), and John W. Kingdon, *Agendas, Alternatives and Public Policies* (Boston: Little, Brown, 1985). Our perspective has been heavily influenced by the literature on construction of social problems; for an overview see Joseph W. Schneider, "Social Problems Theory: The Constructionist View," *Annual Review of Sociology* 11 (1985): 209–29.

2. These and other data through 1986 are reported in Eleanor Singer, Theresa F. Rogers, and Mary Corcoran, "The Polls—A Report: AIDS," *Public Opinion Quarterly* 51 (1987): 580–95. See also James W. Dearing, "Setting the Polling Agenda for the Issue of AIDS," *Public Opinion Quarterly* 53 (1989): 309–29.

3. Harvey Molotch and Marilyn Lester, "News on Purposive Behavior: On the Strategic Use of Routine Events, Accidents and Scandals," *American Sociological Review* 39 (1974): 101–12, at p. 103.

4. The most important studies of the processes of newsmaking in national media include Edward J. Epstein, *News from Nowhere: Television and the News* (New York: Random House, 1973); Leon V. Sigal, *Reporters and Officials* (Lexington, Mass.: Heath, 1973); Gaye Tuchman, *Making News* (New York: Free Press, 1978); and Herbert J. Gans, *Deciding What's News* (New York: Vintage, 1979).

5. "We take accidents to constitute a crucial resource for the empirical study of event-structuring processes" (Molotch and Lester, "News as Purposive Behavior," p. 103).

6. For a fuller discussion of the media's role in elite agenda setting, see Timothy E. Cook, *Making Laws and Making News: Media Strategies in the U.S. House of Representatives* (Washington, D.C.: Brookings Institution, 1989), chap. 6.

7. For example, Susan Sontag's influential and thought-provoking books *Illness as Metaphor* (New York: Farrar, Straus and Giroux, 1978) and *AIDS and Its Metaphors* (New York: Farrar, Straus and Giroux, 1989) tend to adopt a positivist approach that separates scientific discourse from its literary versions.

8. Jay A. Winsten, "Science and the Media: The Boundaries of Truth," *Health Affairs* 4 (1985): 15. For a fuller account see Sharon M. Friedman, Sharon Dunwoody, and Carol L. Rogers, eds., *Scientists and Journalists: Reporting*

Science as News (New York: Free Press, 1986), and Dorothy Nelkin, *Selling Science: How the Press Covers Science and Technology* (New York: W. H. Freeman, 1986).

9. Harvey Molotch and Marilyn Lester, "Accidental News: The Great Oil Spill as Local Occurrence and National Event," *American Journal of Sociology* 81 (1975): 235–60 (quoted passage, p. 237).

10. See for example, Dennis Altman, *AIDS in the Mind of America* (Garden City, N.Y.: Doubleday, 1986), pp. 16–21.

11. In addition to the results presented by Singer et al., "The Polls—A Report: AIDS," this conclusion is based on Gallup poll data from the releases of July 7, 1983, and August 18, 1985; *Newsweek,* August 8, 1983, p. 33; *Newsweek,* August 12, 1985, p. 23; *New York Times,* September 12, 1985, p. B11; and the Harris poll released September 19, 1985.

12. The central systematic studies of news content in print media published thus far include Edward Albert, "Illness and Deviance: The Response of the Press to AIDS," and Andrea Baker, "The Portrayal of AIDS in the Media: An Analysis of Articles in the *New York Times*," both in *The Social Dimension of AIDS: Method and Theory,* ed. Douglas A. Feldman and Thomas M. Johnson (New York: Praeger, 1986), pp. 163–94; Edward Albert, "Acquired Immune Deficiency Syndrome: The Victim and the Press," *Studies in Communications* 3 (1986): 135–58; William A. Check, "Beyond the Political Model of Reporting: Nonspecific Symptoms in Media Communication about AIDS," *Reviews of Infectious Diseases* 9 (1987): 987–1000; and Sandra Panem, *The AIDS Bureaucracy* (Cambridge, Mass.: Harvard University Press, 1988), chap. 8. On journalists covering the AIDS beat, see James Kinsella, *Covering the Plague: AIDS and the American Media* (New Brunswick, N.J.: Rutgers University Press, 1989). The only examination to our knowledge of television news coverage of AIDS is Everett M. Rogers, James W. Dearing, and Soonbum Chang, "Media Coverage of the Issue of AIDS," a paper submitted to the Media Studies Project of the Wilson Center, Washington, D.C., 1989, but its primary concern is with the timing of stories rather than the interpretive frameworks provided therein.

13. Altman, *AIDS in the Mind of America,* p. 19. See also Warren Burkett, *News Reporting: Science, Medicine, and High Technology* (Ames: Iowa State University Press, 1986), p. 145: "The story of AIDS contained all elements necessary for sensational reporting: sex, threat to health, mystery, and high probability of death."

14. Albert, "Acquired Immune Deficiency Syndrome," p. 136.

15. Kinsella, in *Covering the Plague,* presents numerous portraits of individual journalists and shows how their individual perspectives and experiences shaped their approach to the epidemic, but he neglects the impact of standard practices of journalism as a whole. As we shall argue here, the high points and valleys of AIDS coverage was due to more than individual journalists' attributes or failings.

16. Ransdall Pierson, "Uptight about Gay News," *Columbia Journalism Review,* March–April 1982, pp. 25–33; Timothy E. Cook, "Setting the Record Straight: The Construction of Homosexuality on Television News," paper pre-

sented to the Inside/Outside conference of the Lesbian and Gay Studies Center at Yale University, New Haven, October 1989.

17. Gans, *Deciding What's News*, pp. 242–46. He notes three other considerations for journalists seeking to protect their audience: shock, panic, and copycat behavior.

18. Av Westin, *Newswatch: How TV Decides the News* (New York: Simon and Schuster, 1982), p. 62.

19. See, for example, David Paletz and Robert Dunn, "Press Coverage of Civil Disorders: A Case Study of Winston-Salem, 1967," *Public Opinion Quarterly* 33 (1969): 328–45.

20. For example, Don Colburn, "Pursuing the Disease of the Moment," *Washington Post,* February 10, 1987, Health Section, p. 7; Eleanor Randolph, "AIDS Reporters' Challenge: To Educate, Not Panic, the Public," *Washington Post,* June 5, 1987, p. D1.

21. Doris A. Graber, *Processing the News* (New York: Longmans, 1984); John Robinson and Mark Levy, *The Main Source: Learning from Television News* (Beverly Hills, Calif.: Sage, 1986).

22. Michael J. Robinson and Maura Clancey, "King of the Hill," *Washington Journalism Review* 5, no. 6 (July–August 1983): 49.

23. A survey in Washington, D.C., comparing television-reliant and newspaper-reliant citizens, and an experimental study in New England, estimating learning from television, magazine, and newspaper accounts, both point to significantly lower amounts of information about AIDS among television viewers. See Carolyn A. Stroman and Richard Seltzer, "Mass Media Use and Knowledge of AIDS," *Journalism Quarterly* 66 (1989): 881–87; and W. Russell Neuman, Marion Just, and Ann Crigler, "Knowledge, Opinion, and the News: The Calculus of Political Learning," paper prepared for delivery at the annual meeting of the American Political Science Association, Washington, D.C., September 1988.

24. Daniel C. Hallin, *The "Uncensored War": The Media and Vietnam* (New York: Oxford University Press, 1986), p. 125. Emphasis in original.

25. The best statement on symbolic presentations continues to be Murray Edelman, *Politics as Symbolic Action: Mass Arousal and Quiescence* (New York: Academic Press, 1971).

26. For example, the *New York Times* carried stories on July 3, July 5, and August 29; the *Chicago Tribune,* on July 4; the *Washington Post,* on August 30 and December 11; the *Los Angeles Times,* on June 5, July 3, and December 10; and the *San Francisco Chronicle,* on June 6 and August 29.

27. The initial indications of AIDS among heterosexual intravenous drug users appeared in early 1982; the CDC first reported AIDS infections among Haitians in July 1982.

28. Although the virus was named differently at different times, we choose to call it by the terminology agreed upon in 1987.

29. Anthony Downs, "Up and Down with Ecology: The Issue-Attention Cycle," *Public Interest* 28 (1972): 38–50.

30. It is worth noting that until very recently intravenous drug users have been mentioned only in passing as a high-risk group.

31. Av Westin, in a memo to ABC News correspondents, suggested, "If we are covering a hurricane, begin by concentrating on some wind-swept birds ('the gulls knew Clara was due. They felt the wind early. . . .'), then move on to the general panorama of impending disaster." Westin explained his logic as follows: "[A] viewer has to grasp the main points of a story quickly before they are embellished with supporting elements. Starting 'small' and then broadening out helps maintain clarity in the short time usually available" (*Newswatch*, p. 44).

32. Gerald M. Oppenheimer, "In the Eye of the Storm: The Epidemiological Construction of AIDS," in *AIDS: The Burdens of History*, ed. Elizabeth Fee and Daniel Fox (Berkeley: University of California Press, 1988), pp. 267–300; Meyrick Horton and Peter Aggleton, "Perverts, Inverts and Experts: The Cultural Production of an AIDS Research Paradigm," in *AIDS: Social Representations, Social Practices*, ed. Peter Aggleton, Graham Hart, and Peter Davies (New York: Falmer Press, 1989), pp. 74–100.

33. Allan Brandt, *No Magic Bullet: A Social History of Venereal Disease in the United States since 1880* (New York: Oxford University Press, 1987). Horton and Aggleton, in "Perverts, Inverts and Experts," note that a blood-borne disease, such as hepatitis B, is actually a more accurate comparison for AIDS than venereal diseases such as syphilis, let alone leprosy and plague.

34. For example, ABC, December 10, 1982.

35. For example, ABC, March 3, 1983.

36. The analysis in this section is based on the following broadcasts: (1) ABC: October 18, 1982; March 2 and June 26, 1983; October 23 and November 23, 1984; March 2, July 28, September 16, October 2, and October 21, 1985. (2) CBS: August 2, 1982; March 23, June 26, and August 6, 1983; April 23 and October 9, 1984; March 2, August 27, September 18, September 19, September 24, October 2, October 15, November 7, and December 12, 1985. (3) NBC: June 17, 1982; June 21, June 26, and October 13, 1983; March 15, August 17, and October 9, 1984; March 2, May 6, July 25, September 18, and October 2, 1985. The first network story that was clearly pegged to a media event by a gay group was CBS's coverage of an ACT UP demonstration on Wall Street on March 24, 1987.

37. Baker, "Portrayal of AIDS in the Media," finds a similar pattern in 1983 in the *New York Times*. We should be cautious about interpreting these figures too literally, however, since the gay movement may have sought out non-gay individuals (such as Mathilde Krim, researcher from Sloan Kettering Cancer Center) to serve as authoritative sources. The most important conclusion we can derive is that until mid-1985 the gay movement was not a salient aspect of television coverage.

38. See Cook, "Setting the Record Straight," for a further discussion.

39. Altman, in *AIDS in the Mind of America*, points out that the governmental response to AIDS probably would have been even slower if AIDS had been first identified in less organized groups, such as Haitians or intravenous drug users. Social movements face difficulty in making news, not only because of reporters' doubts about their authority (and hence their newsworthiness) but also because they are often either insufficiently organized to constitute a news-

beat or are ambivalent about the priority of making news. See especially Edie N. Goldenberg, *Making the Papers: The Access of Resource-Poor Groups to the Metropolitan Press* (Lexington, Mass.: Heath, 1975). Presumably, the professionalization within AIDS activism—what Cindy Patton has termed the move from grass roots to business suits—has contributed to a greater willingness on the media's part to rely on sources within the gay movement. For a good study of this shift, see Donald B. Rosenthal, "Dilemmas in the Institutionalization of AIDS Service Organizations in Upstate New York," paper presented at the annual meeting of the American Political Science Association, San Francisco, August 1990.

40. The media attention may have been a double-edged sword for the gay movement in the early stages; even if negative, it alerted audiences both to the importance of the disease and to the presence of gay organizations. John D'Emilio, in *Sexual Politics, Sexual Communities: The Making of a Homosexual Minority in the United States* (Chicago: University of Chicago Press, 1983), notes that, paradoxically, even negative reporting in the 1950s and 1960s spurred the development of a gay minority by alerting audiences to the presence of a community they had not known existed before.

41. Dennis Altman, "Legitimation through Disaster: AIDS and the Gay Movement," in *AIDS: The Burdens of History,* ed. Fee and Fox, pp. 301–15. On owning a problem, see Gusfield, *Culture of Public Problems.*

42. The analysis in this section is based on the following reports: (1) ABC: December 10, 1982; March 2, July 14, and September 7, 1983; August 16, August 29, September 5, September 11, September 19, October 21, November 13, and November 14, 1985. (2) CBS: December 10, 1982; February 26, March 23, July 26, August 30, and November 9, 1983; April 26, August 2, September 1, November 23, and November 29, 1984; July 29, July 30, July 31, August 27, September 5, September 11, September 18, November 14, December 12, and December 13, 1985. (3) NBC: October 6 and December 10, 1982; March 1, July 14, August 22, August 30, and November 2, 1983; October 9, October 10, November 9, and November 29, 1984; February 27, March 15, April 26, May 6, May 7, July 30, August 15, August 16, August 29, August 30, September 5, September 11, September 19, October 17, November 7, November 8, November 13, November 14, November 21, December 5, and December 8, 1985.

43. For example, NBC, June 13, 1983.

44. Ralph H. Turner, Joanne M. Nigg, and Denise Heller Paz, *Waiting for Disaster: Earthquake Watch in California* (Berkeley: University of California Press, 1986), pp. 58–59.

45. The analysis in this section is based on the following reports: (1) ABC: June 20, 1983; August 2, August 26, September 9, September 13, and September 25, 1985. (2) CBS: May 18, June 19, August 6, and August 11, 1983; March 2, August 9, August 25, August 30, September 9, September 10, September 11, September 12, September 18, September 19, October 3, and November 7, 1985. (3) NBC: May 24, June 20, July 14, September 4, and October 13, 1983; August 26, September 9, and September 12, 1985.

46. This story appeared six minutes after the broadcast began; it was the

first story after the first commercial break. By contrast, the three original stories appeared after twenty-two (NBC), fifteen (CBS), and fourteen (ABC) minutes.

47. Kashiwahara's June 20, 1983, story on ABC, for example, followed images of discrimination with the statement "Politicians and health officials have declared war on AIDS hysteria," with sound bites by New York mayor Edward Koch, CDC scientist James Curran, and Health and Human Services secretary Margaret Heckler.

48. See ABC, June 20, 1983; CBS, June 19, 1983; NBC, June 20, 1983.

49. ABC, September 13, 1985; CBS, January 22, 1986.

50. The following broadcasts are examined in this section: (1) ABC: July 12, August 1, and October 26, 1983; April 4 and April 23, 1984; January 10, January 11, March 2, and July 26, 1985. (2) NBC: January 14, April 29, July 8, and July 12, 1983; March 15, August 17, and December 14, 1984; January 17, February 8, March 2, July 24, July 26, October 29, and November 11, 1985. (3) CBS: July 12, 1983; March 1, April 4, April 19, April 20, and April 23, 1984; January 5, January 10, February 20, March 1, March 2, May 5, May 6, May 10, July 25, September 4, September 12, September 18, November 14, and December 13, 1985.

51. Albert, in "Acquired Immune Deficiency Syndrome: The Victim and the Press," notes that life-style/contagion stories in newsmagazines peaked in May–July 1983 and fell behind science/medicine stories in May–July 1984.

52. For discussion of these issues, see G. Ray Funkhouser, "The Issues of the Sixties: An Exploratory Study of the Dynamics of Public Opinion," *Public Opinion Quarterly* 37 (1973): 62–75. This split is similar to the contrast between enterprise and routine journalism provided by Sigal, in *Reporters and Officials*.

53. A recent example occurred in 1989, when HHS secretary Louis Sullivan appeared before the news media to announce the government's finding that the drug AZT worked to slow the reproduction of HIV among infected asymptomatic individuals. According to Sullivan's spokesman, had the news not been so upbeat, his boss would likely not have appeared (Robert Schmermund, comments in panel "NIH Announces AZT," at the Harvard School of Public Health, April 1990).

54. Winsten, "Science and the Media", pp. 11, 9.

55. Respectively, NBC, July 12, 1983; NBC, March 15, 1984; CBS, April 20, 1984.

56. In the story of Baby Jane Doe, an infant with multiple birth defects, the major distortion, according to Klaidman and Beauchamp, was not inaccuracies but incomplete reporting. See Stephen Klaidman and Tom L. Beauchamp, "Baby Jane Doe in the Media," *Journal of Health Politics, Policy and Law* 11 (1986): 271–84.

57. Mark Fishman, in *Manufacturing the News* (Austin: University of Texas Press, 1980), has suggested that reporters at a governmental newsbeat decide what to cover by referring to a "phase structure," or an idealized version of how that institution's process unfolds; newsworthy points occur when the process moves from one phase to the next. The same may be true of science

correspondents, but here the idealized process may well be science marching on.

58. NBC briefly mentioned this, but ABC and CBS did not.

59. According to Ann Thomas, director of public information at NIH, "After Rock Hudson, instead of responding to reporters, we were so nicked by the criticism why weren't we doing more that we decided to give more backgrounders and send out more press releases." At this point Fauci was designated as the principal source for reporters (Thomas, comments on panel "NIH Announces AZT," Harvard School of Public Health, April 1990).

60. CBS, July 24, 1985; NBC, July 24, 1985.

61. September 23, 24, 25, 26, and 27, 1985.

62. September 9, 1985.

63. The first Ryan White story appeared on CBS on July 31, followed by ABC on August 2 and NBC on August 16. All three covered the first day of school in Kokomo on August 26.

64. Respectively, ABC, August 2, 1985; CBS, August 2, 1985; ABC, September 5, 1985.

65. October 7, 1985.

66. NBC, September 18, 1985; CBS, September 19, 1985.

67. October 21, 1985.

68. Indeed, during 1986, when the number of stories dipped, AIDS was the top story on NBC on June 12 (announcing federal forecasts of 170,000 cases). It was also the top story on ABC on June 23 (reporting the Justice Department's announcement that laws barring discrimination against the handicapped did not extend to HIV-positive individuals—this announcement occurring on the same day that the international AIDS conference was held in Paris). Finally, AIDS was the top story on ABC and NBC on October 29 (quoting a National Academy of Sciences report, which charged that the response to AIDS was "woefully inadequate").

69. Rogers, Dearing, and Chang, in "Media Coverage of the Issue of AIDS," identify thirteen "sub-issues" of AIDS, whose individual ebb and flow actually allowed the epidemic to continue to be in the news on a regular basis.

70. ABC, March 13, 1986. Strait was then still searching for the breakthrough, as an interview with Samuel Broder revealed. Strait, with urgency in his voice, asked Dr. Broder, "Is this a breakthrough?" and Broder cautiously responded, "It's not a breakthrough, but it's a dent."

71. ABC, June 23, 1986. On CBS Dan Rather noted, "Just how shocking and widespread is the disease is the subject of Susan Spencer's report" (June 25, 1986); on NBC anchor Chris Wallace pointed to "the alarming spread announced in Paris" (June 22, 1986).

72. For example, ABC, March 11, 1987.

73. Albert, "Acquired Immune Deficiency Syndrome: The Victim and the Press," p. 155.

74. Barbara J. Nelson, *Making an Issue of Child Abuse: Political Agenda Setting for Social Problems* (Chicago: University of Chicago Press, 1984).

75. Quoted in Altman, *AIDS in the Mind of America*, p. 16.

76. Stephen Farber, "A Drama of Family Loyalty, Acceptance and AIDS," *New York Times*, August 19, 1985, p. 23.

77. A search of the Nexis data base showed that the number of stories was halved between 1987 and 1989. See Larry Thompson, "Commentary: With No Magic Cure in Sight, Dramatic Epidemic Loses Luster as News Story," *Washington Post Health*, June 13, 1989, p. 7.

78. Future scholars will want to study the development of ACT UP as it interacted with the news media, since those interactions seem to be subject to the same dynamics that Todd Gitlin identified for the New Left in *The Whole World Is Watching: The Mass Media in the Making and Unmaking of the New Left* (Berkeley: University of California Press, 1980).

PART II

Law, Ethics, and Public Policy

The Politics of HIV Infection: 1989-1990 as Years of Change

Daniel M. Fox

A decade after AIDS emerged in the United States, most of the people who made health policy perceived it as a stage, at present the end stage, of a chronic disease that was spreading most rapidly among the disadvantaged, especially among blacks and Hispanics. This perception was the latest, and certainly not the last, chapter in a story that has changed repeatedly since 1981. As the story has changed, so has the debate about proper policy. This essay is a history of the politics of making policy for preventing the disease and caring for the majority of those who acquire it.

THE POLITICS OF AIDS TO 1989

The brief history of the epidemic has been dominated by four interacting factors: fear and fascination; the identity of those who have the disease and those to whom it seems to be spreading; the endemic problems of our social policy; and the impact on policy of advances in scientific knowledge. These factors created the political context for the perception of AIDS as a chronic disease that is increasingly a burden for the disadvantaged and, therefore, for all of us.

AIDS, more accurately if ponderously called HIV infection and related diseases, has been a public issue out of proportion to its cost or mortality relative to such other contemporary afflictions as cancer, alcoholism, and automobile injuries. The standard, and probably accurate, explanation for the high public salience of the epidemic, especially as revealed in coverage by the media, is that it evokes fascination and fear—fascination with a disease that kills celebrities and those with homosexual life-styles; fear of transmission through blood transfusion or sexual intercourse.[1] Moreover, as the incidence of the infection spread among urban blacks and Hispanics, fear of HIV intensified white people's dread of random aggression by darker-skinned males.

The public salience of the epidemic was also a result of longstanding problems of social policy in the United States. Nationally and in most of the states, there is no consensus on how to educate the public about sexual behavior and what (and how much) to do about drug addiction. Our employment-based private health insurance is least comprehensive in providing outpatient and long-term care and prescription drugs, which are growing costs of treating HIV infection. Medicaid eligibility and coverage vary widely among the states; as a result, many persons who have HIV infection are left without effective entitlement to care. Moreover, states and local governments have enormous financial and political problems in serving as the health care payers of last resort.

These problems of social policy were exacerbated by both the politics of the 1980s and the epidemic of HIV infection. When the first cases of the syndrome to be called AIDS were reported in 1981, cost containment had become the priority of public policy for health financing, both for employers and for the insurance industry. A new national administration was determined to reduce federal domestic spending, including funds to assist the states in providing health care and social services to the poor. By the mid-1980s, when the Congress and many of the states took new initiatives in health policy, AIDS was already a financial burden for several states, especially New York, New Jersey, California, and Florida, and was an emerging problem in most others.[2] Each new case represented a burden of about $100,000 in direct costs.[3] As the number of cases increased among blacks and Hispanics, and as the number grew among women and children, these costs became a heavier burden on state and local government. By 1989 perhaps half the costs of caring for persons with HIV infection had been paid by state and local government, through their share of Medicaid; by insurance pools and indigent care programs; and by operating subsidies to public hospitals and clinics.[4]

The politics of HIV infection changed in 1989 for two reasons. The first reason was that infection and disease had spread rapidly among members of disadvantaged minorities. Moreover, the incidence of infection with the virus among blacks and Hispanics was growing faster as a result of a newly observed causal relationship that linked AIDS to crack, sex, and venereal disease. This new source of infection augmented to an ominous but unmeasurable extent its diffusion by needle sharing, by intravenous drug addicts having unprotected sex, and by women with the virus having children.

The second reason for this change in the politics of HIV infection was that many health professionals and people who made policy now agreed that HIV infection must be considered a chronic disease. From 1981 to the summer of 1989, the consensual view of the epidemic employed the historical model of plagues that Elizabeth Fee and I describe in the introductory essay in this volume. Many experts argued, using the plague analogy, that AIDS required an emergency policy response because it was both an unusual and an unusually severe infliction.

The first challenge to the plague model of policy for the HIV epidemic derived from politics and policy analysis rather than from medical science and its applications. The challenge came from people who were absorbed with the problems of financing the epidemic. From the point of view of insurance executives, state Medicaid officials, and legislators addressing problems of the uninsured and hospital deficits, AIDS was similar to a chronic disease that was compressed into a period of less than two years. Like other chronic diseases, AIDS was characterized by relatively brief acute episodes, requiring hospitalization, and longer periods when patients could be cared for in nursing facilities or at home. Like persons with other chronic diseases, persons with AIDS needed considerable social support, either from friends and families or from public agencies.[5] Unlike most people with expensive chronic diseases, however, most people with AIDS were not eligible for Medicare, either because they were under sixty-five or because they did not live long enough to become eligible for Social Security Disability Insurance.[6]

This financially driven analogy to chronic disease was unpopular until the summer of 1989. Many advocates for persons with AIDS, especially gays, feared that defining the syndrome as a chronic infectious disease would lead to its "normalization." If AIDS became just another of the long list of killer diseases, it would cease to evoke fear and fascination and, therefore, cease to have as large a claim on public attention and funds. Some scientists attacked the chronic disease model as defeatist. A few others, notably William Haseltine of Harvard, endorsed it.[7] Critics insisted that a disease that was spread by sex and drugs could not be considered another chronic disease.[8]

The chronic disease model became central to policy as a result of two clinical trials sponsored by the National Institutes of Health, one terminated in the spring and the other in the summer of 1989. The first trial justified the use of aerosolized pentamidine for persons who had an episode of the most common complication of HIV infection, *Pneumocystis carinii* pneumonia. The other validated the use of AZT to postpone the onset of symptoms of disease secondary to HIV in certain patients. Both drugs resembled cancer chemotherapy more than the romantically misnamed "magic bullets" that cured many infectious diseases of bacterial origin, or the vaccines against major infections. Like cancer chemotherapy, the anti-HIV drugs inhibited the progress of disease but did not prevent or cure it.

The new drug treatments created a new imperative and a new burden for policy. The imperative was that, for the first time since the beginning of the epidemic, persons who had engaged in risky behavior had a powerful incentive to be tested and, if infected, to receive prophylactic treatment. The burden was that treatment would be more expensive, but nobody could predict precisely how much more expensive, because it was based on new drugs. Moreover, the new drugs made the duration and course of the disease considerably more uncertain than before.

By the late summer of 1989, physicians and an increasing number of people who made health policy were describing HIV as the cause of a chronic illness with a long and lengthening course between infection and death. New diagrams that experts used to describe the disease to audiences of health and policy professionals exemplified the new perception of HIV infection. Throughout the 1980s medical scientists had drawn an iceberg, with only the tip susceptible to treatment, to depict the disease. They now offered a time-line intersected by numerous and increasing opportunities for intervention.[9]

While this shift of perception was occurring, the incidence and prevalence of HIV infection were increasing disproportionately among the disadvantaged. HIV infection and its consequences were therefore becoming a problem of American policy and politics as they affect minorities and the poor. AIDS had been normalized, but in a somewhat different way than advocates for according it higher priority had expected. The response to the disease was now part of the normal fragmentation and frustration created by our health policy and disproportionately shared by the forty to fifty million Americans who lacked minimal health insurance coverage and by the health and policy professionals who addressed their needs.

PERCEIVING HIV INFECTION AS A PROBLEM OF THE DISADVANTAGED

The HIV epidemic offers elegant proof of the proposition that scientific evidence, especially statistics, contributes to but does not drive public policy. In the early 1980s, when most media attention and most advocacy for policy focused on AIDS as a disease of homosexuals, hemophiliacs, and recipients of transfused blood, overwhelming statistical evidence revealed that the epidemic was a serious problem for blacks and Hispanics and that most of the people at risk of infection in these groups were of relatively low socioeconomic status. In 1982, the second year in which the federal Centers for Disease Control counted cases of AIDS, blacks and Hispanics comprised just under half of the males, almost 80 percent of the females, and almost two-thirds of the children diagnosed with the disease in the United States. In subsequent years the percentage of black and Hispanic men with AIDS ranged between 30 and 40 percent; the percentage of black and Hispanic women and children was always considerably more than half.[10]

More important for gauging the impact of the disease on populations, and therefore on politics and policy, the number of cases per 100,000 population was always higher among blacks and Hispanics than among whites. By 1988 the cumulative total of cases per 100,000 was almost three and a half times higher among black men and two and a half times higher among Hispanic men than among whites. The rate among females was fourteen times higher among blacks and seven times higher among Hispanics. For children the cumulative rates were four times as high among blacks and twice as high among Hispanics.[11]

There was, moreover, considerable evidence of undercounting of cases among blacks and Hispanics. In particular, intravenous drug users were reported as dying at higher rates in these years from tuberculosis and other diseases that were, most likely, secondary to HIV infection, for which they had not been tested.[12]

By 1988 the rate of increase in reported cases was highest in cities with large black and Hispanic populations. This increase followed the pattern that had been observed earlier in the gay communities of San Francisco and New York and in other countries. As epidemiologists writing about Latin America described this pattern, once the virus was "introduced into a population, indigenous transmission soon became established and propelled the epidemic at an alarming rate."[13] For example, in Newark, New Jersey, a predominantly black city, the rate of

cases increased from 39 per 100,000 in the twelve months ending February 1988 to 56.5 a year later, a growth of 31 percent. In San Juan,
Puerto Rico, the rate of reported new cases increased by 78 percent to
66.5 per 100,000 in the same period. But in San Francisco, which has a
predominantly white population, new cases increased by only 12.7 percent in the same year. Published data reveal similar, though less dramatic, contrasts across the country.[14]

It is easier to describe than to account for the gradualness of the
realization of the political and policy problems that result from the disproportionate impact of HIV infection on the disadvantaged. Several
factors seem important in explaining what happened. One factor involves the politics of epidemiological evidence; the others involve the
intersection of special-interest politics with larger issues of social policy
during the Reagan years.

The most important data about any epidemic, indeed about any
problem, for most public officials and health professionals are the number of people clamoring for scarce resources in a particular fiscal year.
For the first eight years in which cases of AIDS were counted, the largest
number of cases occurred among white males. The numbers of women
and children, among whom the disadvantaged were an overwhelming
majority, remained relatively low for most of the 1980s; the cumulative
number of cases reached only 1,000 among women in 1986, and 500
among children in 1989. Prudent political professionals logically accorded priority to financing care for white males.

The second most important data about any problem for health professionals and public officials are those that project its consequences
into the practical future. The practical future for most elected officials
is the year before and, sometimes, the year after the next election. For
officials in the executive branch of state or local government, the practical future is the fiscal year after the one for which agencies prepared
their most recent budget request. Most health professionals, especially
those who treat patients or manage hospitals, have even shorter practical futures. They are trying to get through a day, a week, a few months,
or a fiscal year. For both public officials and health professionals, projections of the incidence and demography of HIV infection three to five
years into the future were ominous but not a problem for the practical
future.

Official projections of the future number and demography of cases
of AIDS had three characteristics that reduced their political salience:
they were controversial; they were based on statistical reasoning rather

than on field research; and most projections were not targeted to particular jurisdictions.

Much of the controversy has been unavoidable. It is a result of ignorance about people's sexual behavior and drug habits, of congressional and White House opposition to or reluctance about asking people to describe these activities to interviewers paid with government funds, and of disputes among social scientists and biostatisticians about the accuracy of survey questions on matters about which many people are inclined to be evasive or dishonest. Moreover, strong opposition to mandatory testing for HIV or reporting the names of people who test positive has come from civil libertarians, ethicists, gay advocates, and health professionals. These people have feared that mandates would, contrary to intent, persuade many people at high risk to avoid testing from fear of punishment or discrimination.[15]

As a result of this controversy, projections of future cases of HIV-related disease have been based on statistical reasoning according to competing methods. When experts disagree about the future, even when, as in projections of the number of people with HIV infection, the range of their disagreement is narrower than their area of agreement, prudent public officials are highly motivated to temporize.

An even better excuse for officials to temporize has been the lack of credible projections for specific political jurisdictions. By 1989, only the cities and states with the highest number of cases had adopted any of the competing methods of projection for local use. Moreover, both AIDS activists and their adversaries frequently challenged the accuracy of these numbers. Credible and frightening data about the impact of HIV in minority communities came mainly from New York and New Jersey, states that are not normally regarded by people in other jurisdictions as harbingers of their social problems. Most states had relatively few cases of diagnosed AIDS (half had counted 200 or fewer through the first six months of 1989) and hence no political incentive to sponsor local projections of controversial data.

The general condition of social policy and special-interest politics reinforced the willingness of public officials to interpret data in ways that made it possible for them to avoid stark confrontation with the steady increase in AIDS cases among the disadvantaged throughout the country. There was little sympathy for expanding social programs in Washington or the states during the first Reagan administration. What sympathy existed was directed mainly at poor children, at working-age adults whose health insurance lapsed when they lost their jobs or whose employers were too marginal to purchase insurance, at people with disabilities who became ineligible for Social Security Disability Insurance as a result of new administrative procedures, and at the elderly who could not pay the catastrophic costs of illness or of long-term care. State officials were preoccupied in these years with policies to reduce the rate of increase in hospital costs in order to address competing pressures for new programs in health care, environmental regulation, welfare, and housing.

This picture of social policy is deliberately overdrawn. There were still many advocates for more health care for the disadvantaged. The people who managed health services that were traditionally aimed at black and Hispanic populations—clinics, health centers, hospitals, drug treatment programs—continued to lobby vigorously and effectively. Hospital leaders, alarmed by the growing cost of care for the poor and by the unwillingness of private insurance executives (themselves pressed by employers to reduce costs) to maintain traditional cross-subsidies, clamored for public funds to relieve their deficits. State government proposals to curtail Medicaid benefits or eligibility for coverage were strongly opposed by associations of health professionals concerned about their earnings.

Nevertheless, for the first few years of the HIV epidemic, the states with the highest number of cases, especially New York and California, assumed that they would receive little additional assistance from the federal government and that most expenditures for AIDS—especially for testing, treatment, and support services—would be made as the result of state budgetary politics. In the politics of AIDS in New York State and California in the early and middle 1980s, "doing it yourself" meant taking action mainly in response to pressures from the white gay population and the health professionals who treated them. Special-interest politics reinforced the way public officials had chosen to interpret the epidemiological data.

Two special interests were involved: gays and blacks. Gay leaders in New York City and San Francisco built effective coalitions that leveraged funds for programs to prevent HIV infection, offer anonymous testing, and provide services for people with symptoms of disease. The coalitions led by gays were not opposed to helping poor blacks and Hispanics. Many of the service programs they established (notably the Gay Men's Health Crisis in New York City) provided considerable assistance to the disadvantaged. But they had other priorities: to promote safe sex among gays and, as both a goal and a shrewd political tactic,

among white heterosexuals; and to provide better health and social services to people with the disease, the majority of whom were still white
and gay. Understandably, too, they wanted to help gays who were also
black and Hispanic; many of these people were not economically poor,
but most of them were discriminated against by other blacks and Hispanics.

At the same time, many black leaders were unwilling to advocate
that special attention or funds be given to the problem of HIV infection
in their communities. Their refusal to become advocates for particular
interventions to prevent the spread of infection, especially for the interventions urged by most white public health leaders, reinforced the disproportionate attention to HIV among white gays.

The reluctance of many black leaders to become special-interest lob-
byists on behalf of HIV infection had complicated, overlapping causes.
In a recent essay Harlan Dalton explains the political and cultural logic
of reticence about AIDS among African Americans. He isolates five
"overlapping factors": wariness about acknowledging "our association
with AIDS so long as the larger society seems bent on blaming us as a
race for its origin and initial spread"; the "suspicion and distrust many
of us feel whenever whites express a sudden interest in our well-being";
the "pathology of our own homophobia"; the "uniquely problematic
relationship we as a community have to the phenomenon of drug abuse";
and "difficulty transcending the deep resentment we feel at being dictated to once again." [16]

Some of these factors also influenced the behavior of Hispanic leaders in the early years of the epidemic. Most accounts (in the press and
by other politicians) stress homophobia as the most important reason
for the unwillingness of these leaders to be perceived as special-interest
advocates on behalf of AIDS.

The politics of the epidemic changed quickly late in 1989, especially
in the cites and states with the highest incidence of cases. The priorities
in fighting a plague are learning where it came from, taking emergency
action to protect endangered communities, and creating crash programs
to experiment with vaccines and potential cures. The priorities in managing a chronic disease are different. These priorities are familiar to
everyone who has followed the recent history of lung cancer, heart disease, stroke, or renal disease. Preventing new cases of chronic disease is
a difficult and expensive process. Fear and education are effective; but
there is no consensus about how much of each to use and what techniques have which effects on particular people. Treatment is expensive

and arduous. Moreover, effective treatment means incremental improvement, not cure.[17] Plagues are fought; chronic diseases are managed.

By the end of 1989, the coalition demanding more resources for HIV infection had changed, and its membership remained in flux. Prominent blacks were becoming part of the HIV lobby, joining leadership coalitions in several cities and nationally. Dalton, for example, was appointed by Congress to the new National AIDS Commission. Advocates for spending more to prevent and treat HIV were included in the constituency for President Bush's drug abuse initiative. Black and Hispanic advocates for persons with HIV infection (and for minority physicians) were demanding new roles in the politics of research as NIH prepared to award the first contracts for community-based clinical trials. The organizers of these trials made special efforts to increase the enrollment of disadvantaged people. The increasing cost of care for people who were chronically ill with HIV infection was bringing new pressures on federal and state officials to pay for prescription drugs and increase access to outpatient and long-term-care services for members of minority communities. In addition, these new political alignments were occurring when, for the first time in almost two decades, many leaders of state government, industry, and labor were beginning to talk about rethinking our customary arrangements for financing health care, including the care of the poor.

POLICIES FOR HIV INFECTION AMONG THE DISADVANTAGED

The coalition on behalf of people with the chronic disease of HIV infection will probably be most effective in obtaining incremental changes in existing policies. More fanciful scenarios will be proposed, but there is little reason to expect that fundamental changes in our national health policies, or in those of the states, will be more than talk for the next several years. It is therefore useful to describe what the dominant policies are, how they affect the increasing proportion of people with HIV infection who are disadvantaged, and what incremental changes seem feasible. Four areas of policy are important: surveillance, prevention, research, and financing.

Surveillance is becoming more aggressive and less responsive to the concerns of civil libertarians and advocates for minority groups. Surveillance means both counting the number of people with infection and

among people without private health insurance. In the summer of 1990 Congress authorized the expenditure of $2.9 billion over five years for planning and services in the cities and states with the highest incidence of HIV infection. The act was named for Ryan White, the Indiana teenager whose exclusion from school had attracted national media attention in 1985, and who had died in the spring of 1990. But naming the act for White did not disguise the fact that it provided services mainly for the disadvantaged in a tough budget year that was also an election year for the Congress. In the budget compromise of 1990, the Ryan White Act received only a token appropriation.

The most important impediment to successful political advocacy for additional federal financing of treatment for HIV disease may be that it is one among many areas of inadequacy in health care financing and organization. Only a few political leaders, even in the states with the most cases of AIDS, are willing to risk being accused of trying to solve the AIDS problem while they neglect others. Many state political leaders and representatives of health care interest groups who say that they would join a coalition to promote federal legislation to address access to care for the uninsured, the underinsured, and the poor are refusing to support legislation that is limited to HIV.[19]

Moreover, few states are likely to legislate comprehensive solutions to the problems of financing treatment for HIV infection. Not surprisingly, in the epidemic to date, state financing policies have been a result of past and present health politics, particularly the politics of Medicaid, rather than of the number of cases of disease. In the HIV epidemic, as for most other illnesses, equality of access to health care is not yet an attainable entitlement. For Americans of working age and their children, where they live and for whom they work continue to be the major determinants of what care they can have and how it will be financed.

There have been three stages in state responses to the epidemic, each stage a result of the interaction of politics and the incidence of disease. In the first stage, a state relied on its existing policies for financing health care and regulating the institutions that provide it. Toward the end of the first stage, states earmarked appropriations to pay for care of persons with AIDS. New York was the first to earmark funds. By 1986 states that earmarked funds included, among others, California, New Jersey, New Mexico, and Ohio.

In the second stage, states made deliberate decisions about how to adapt their Medicaid policies and regulations and often initiated state-only programs to address some of the problems of financing and organizing care for persons with HIV-related diseases. The most frequently implemented policies concerned "waivers," a ruling by the Health Care Financing Administration (HCFA) that a state may make a particular mix of Medicaid services available to some but not all beneficiaries on the condition that the proposed services will not add to federal costs. By the end of 1988, HCFA had granted waivers to six states to reimburse care for persons with AIDS in homes or community facilities as a substitute for acute hospital care. Other states obtained waivers in 1989 and 1990. Several states—Illinois and North Carolina, for example— financed treatment for persons with AIDS as part of a broader grant of waiver authority (for the aged and disabled) from HCFA.

Other states decided not to seek a waiver. Several did not apply, either because they wanted to avoid potential costs or because officials believed that the problem of financing care for HIV-related disease was not yet pressing. In other states—New York and Michigan, for example—the decision not to seek a waiver had other sources. In New York officials decided that Medicaid was already covering "almost everything that was waiverable." In Michigan officials also believed that they were already providing a "rich service package," and, in any case, they regarded waivers as difficult to administer.[20]

By 1989 twenty-seven states routinely appropriated funds for patient care for persons with HIV-related diseases in addition to their Medicaid programs. Eighteen of these states also made appropriations for support services. Most of these funds subsidized inpatient care for people with low incomes, but they were also used for hospices, outpatient clinics, and case management services, and, in ten states, to purchase and administer AZT.

In the third stage—reached by 1990 in California, New York, and to a lesser extent Michigan and New Jersey—states, in collaboration with other payers and institutions, adopted policies for organizing and financing care so that populations other than those eligible for Medicaid services could be helped. In New York, for example, the AIDS Treatment Center program, begun in 1986, mandated enhanced reimbursement to hospitals from all payers for inpatient care and for case management of ambulatory and long-term care. New York also provided enhanced reimbursement rates in long-term-care facilities. In California the Department of Health Services funded twenty-six pilot projects to provide home health and attendant care; subsidized hospice services; and established a new institutional category, a "licensed health care facility for persons with AIDS." Late in 1989 New Jersey established a new program, apparently the first in the country, of "assessment centers," to encourage early detection of infection, regular testing for the level of T4 cells, and the use of AZT to retard the onset of symptoms. The state provided the start-up costs for this program; Medicaid and private insurers covered most of the ongoing costs.[21]

By 1990 three states had addressed the problem of financing care for persons with HIV infection as part of the larger problem of access for the uninsured and the underinsured. A 1989 Michigan law required the Department of Social Services to "identify potential Medicaid recipients who test HIV positive and pay their insurance premiums so that they can maintain their health insurance policies." The state of Washington implemented a similar HIV/AIDS insurance continuation program. California had a continuation program, but only for persons who were already eligible for Medicaid. Officials in all three states acknowledge that these programs are pilots for addressing other chronic diseases that lead to financial impoverishment and have high public costs.[22] Efforts to legislate a similar program in New York failed in 1990, mainly as a result of opposition from an aroused insurance industry that was eager to avoid what would be certain losses.

Because it is new, spreads so rapidly, and is expensive to treat, HIV infection reveals—more clearly than most diseases do—the flaws in the collection of laws and customs we call health policy. But recognizing flaws creates both problems and opportunities. There is no lack of clever solutions to the problems of health policy in the United States. There is, however, no politically effective coalition at the present time, either nationally or in any of the states, that is willing to pay the price of legislating any of the more fundamental solutions.

THE FUTURE OF POLICY FOR HIV

Four uncertainties will have a profound influence on the politics of the HIV epidemic. One, discussed above, is how the states and the federal government will address the general problems of paying for the care of people with chronic diseases and of providing access to care for the uninsured and the underinsured. The price of the epidemic of HIV infection will surely increase, whether new strategies to finance treatment are specific to this epidemic or address the fundamental problems of health policy in the United States. What is uncertain, however, is the total price and the politics of paying it.

The other three uncertainties arise at the intersection of politics and policy with biology and human behavior. The first is uncertainty about the natural history of the virus—whether it will mutate and, if so, how it will mutate, and how it will respond to efforts by scientists to produce vaccines to inhibit its infectivity and drugs to reduce or prevent its effects.

The second is uncertainty about the number and distribution of the sexual behaviors that transmit infection with HIV and about the effectiveness of various policies to persuade people to modify these behaviors. There is little evidence about the number, distribution, race, ethnicity, and socioeconomic class of homosexuals, of bisexuals, and of heterosexual people who practice unprotected anal intercourse. Moreover, there is little research-based knowledge about the relative effectiveness of various methods of inducing fear and prudence and thereby changing people's sexual behaviors.

The third area of uncertainty concerns the number of people who use addictive drugs and the effectiveness of measures to change their behavior. Estimates of the number of people who use intravenous drugs are mainly conjectures based on extrapolation from the number of people who seek treatment. Moreover, little is known about the linkage of crack, heightened sexual activity, venereal disease, and HIV infection. There is impressionistic evidence that drug-using behavior among more affluent people is linked to HIV infection in areas as diverse as the suburbs of New York and rural Georgia.[23] Evidence about the effectiveness of programs to persuade drug users to change their needle-using and sexual practices has, to date, been more persuasive to advocates than to political leaders.

These uncertainties, taken together, make impossible any predictions, or even very many recommendations, about future policies. Numerous alternative scenarios were being debated in late 1990, when this essay was revised for publication in this book. The authors of most of these scenarios assumed that the epidemic would become increasingly expensive to treat, as a result of advances in therapeutics, and that it would continue to have a disproportionate impact on blacks and Hispanics. Thus, most scenarios assumed that the epidemic would make increasing claims on scarce public funds but that it was unlikely that a powerful coalition of political leaders who have white, relatively affluent constituencies would be eager to grant these claims. At the end of 1990, most political leaders seemed to agree that the public attitude (and that of most of their colleagues) toward HIV infection had become "massive apathy," as one powerful state legislator said.[24]

Scenarios are inevitably extrapolated from current events. As recently as 1987, for example, a few serious scenarists were conjecturing a rapid spread of HIV infection among affluent white heterosexuals. By 1989 such a scenario was regarded as alarmist. In 1986 and 1987 most scenarios assumed that AIDS was a disease with a relatively swift and terrible course that would, for the near future, not be treatable. By 1989 most health professionals talked about AIDS as the end stage of a chronic disease of uncertain course that could be modified by chemical therapies. Any scenario is likely to be wrong.

For almost a decade, however, HIV infection has dramatized the dilemmas of health policy in the United States. HIV disease is an expensive disease to manage, but our policies distribute most of the resources for managing expensive diseases through Medicare and Medicaid payments for long-term care for the elderly. Prevention is the most cost-effective intervention, but we know very little about the effectiveness of different strategies and have no routine way to pay for implementing them. We spend an unusually large proportion of our national income on health care, but increasing numbers of people are dependent on the inadequate care that is provided by state and local government as payers of last resort. We generously finance biomedical science, but the results of that effort do not translate quickly into measures that reduce the incidence and pain of disease.

In sum, the epidemic of HIV infection continues to reveal what many people already know about health policy in the United States. By doing so, the epidemic clarifies the difference between knowledge and power, and between concern, even compassion, and effective political will.

NOTES

An earlier version of this essay, with the title "Chronic Disease and Disadvantage: The New Politics of HIV Infection," is reprinted with permission from *Journal of Health Politics, Policy and Law* 15 [Summer 1990]:341–56.

1. See the essay by Timothy E. Cook and David C. Colby in this volume.
2. Daniel M. Fox, "AIDS and the American Health Polity: The History and Prospects of a Crisis of Authority," in *AIDS: The Burdens of History,* ed. Daniel M. Fox and Elizabeth Fee (Berkeley: University of California Press, 1988), pp. 316–43.

3. Daniel M. Fox and Emily H. Thomas, "The Cost of AIDS: Exaggeration, Entitlement and Economics," in *AIDS and the American Health Care System,* ed. Lawrence D. Gostin (New Haven, Conn.: Yale University Press, 1989), pp. 192–94.

4. Dennis P. Andrulis, U. B. Weslowski, and Lawrence S. Gage, "The U.S. Hospital AIDS Survey," *Journal of the American Medical Association* 262 (August 11, 1989): 784–94.

5. Daniel M. Fox, Patricia Day, and Rudolf Klein, "The Power of Professionalism: Policies for AIDS in Britain, Sweden and the United States," *Daedalus* 118 (Spring 1989): 93–112.

6. Fox and Thomas, "Cost of AIDS."

7. William Haseltine, "Prospects for the Medical Control of the AIDS Epidemic," *Daedalus* 118 (Summer 1990): 23–46.

8. Personal communications with Allan M. Brandt and David Rothman, May 1989.

9. The first time-line that I saw was on a slide presented by Deborah Cotton at a workshop sponsored by the United States Public Health Service for state legislative leaders late in August of 1989, the week following the announcement that AZT had prophylactic effects. Dr. Cotton's slide was arresting and seemed to the audience to describe a new perception of the disease. Since then I have seen similar diagrams at national and international meetings. By the spring of 1990, newspapers routinely used time-lines to update the public about HIV infection.

10. "AIDS Cases in the United States, 1982–88," *The Blue Sheet,* March 22, 1989, p. 8.

11. "CDC AIDS Surveillance Data Omits One-Third of Current Cases," *The Blue Sheet,* June 22, 1989, p. 3.

12. Ibid.

13. T. C. Quinn, F. R. K. Zacarias, and R. K. St. John, "AIDS in the Americas: An Emerging Health Crisis," *New England Journal of Medicine* 320 (April 13, 1989): 1005–1007.

14. Centers for Disease Control, United States Public Health Service, *HIV-AIDS Surveillance* (Atlanta: Centers for Disease Control, July 1989).

15. Ronald Bayer, *Private Acts, Social Consequences* (New York: Free Press, 1989).

16. Harlan Dalton, "AIDS in Blackface," *Daedalus* 118 (Summer 1989): 205–28.

17. Daniel M. Fox, "Policy and Epidemiology: Financing Health Services for the Chronically Ill and Disabled, 1930–1990," *Milbank Quarterly* 67, Suppl. 2, part 2 (1989): 257–87.

18. Daniel M. Fox, "Financing Health Care for Persons with HIV Infection: Guidelines for State Action," *American Journal of Law and Medicine* 16 (Spring 1990): 223–47.

19. Ibid.

20. Ibid.

21. Ibid.

22. Ibid.

23. Emily H. Thomas and Daniel M. Fox, "AIDS on Long Island: The Regional History of an Epidemic," *Long Island Historical Journal* 1 (Fall 1989): 92–112. For rural Georgia, personal communication from Charles Konigsberg, Jr., member, National Commission on AIDS.

24. The legislator was David C. Hollister, who chairs the health appropriations subcommittee in the Michigan House of Representatives. Lest anyone mistake his position, I must emphasize that Hollister made this comment in order to emphasize the importance of overcoming this apathy and to underline the difficulty of doing so in difficult economic times. The comment was made at a planning meeting for a USPHS workshop on AIDS.

The AIDS Litigation Project: A National Review of Court and Human Rights Commission Decisions on Discrimination

Larry Gostin

Every major government, medical, public health, and legal organization to issue a report on the HIV epidemic has condemned discrimination because it violates basic tenets of individual justice and is detrimental to the public health.[1] Discrimination based on an infectious condition is just as inequitable as discrimination based on race, gender, or disability. In each case people are treated inequitably, not because they lack inherent ability but solely because of a status over which they have no control. Complex and often pernicious mythologies develop about the nature, cause, and transmission of disease. As the Supreme Court has recognized: "Society's accumulated myths and fears about disability and disease are just as handicapping as are the physical limitations that flow from actual impairment. Few aspects of handicap give rise to the same level of public fear and misapprehension as contagiousness."[2]

Persons infected with HIV must endure not only the archaic assumption that they present a health menace but also moral disapproval of their behavior. The public association of the disease with traditionally disfavored groups—gays, intravenous drug users, and prostitutes—only compounds the bigotry.

The Presidential Commission on the HIV epidemic concluded that "discrimination is impairing this nation's ability to limit the spread of the epidemic." The absence of adequate safeguards against discrimination undercuts the Public Health Service's strategy of early identification of persons infected with HIV.[3] Case identification (testing, reporting, and partner notification) is of growing importance as the benefits of early intervention become clearer. Fears that there will be a breach of confidentiality and subsequent discrimination may discourage individuals from cooperating with vital public health programs.

No studies have yet revealed the scope and kinds of discrimination that have occurred since the beginning of the HIV epidemic. In this essay I review 149 cases of discrimination described in complaints, legal briefs, settlements, and decisions by courts and human rights commissions. (The cases cited are listed at the end of this essay; numbers in brackets in the text refer to these cases.) I also review major reports from federal[4] and municipal[5] antidiscrimination agencies, as well as independent policy analysts.[6] Together these data provide a comprehensive picture of past, current, and potential future patterns of discrimination.

AMERICANS WITH DISABILITIES ACT

In 1990 the U.S. Congress enacted the Americans with Disabilities Act (ADA), the most sweeping civil rights measure since the Civil Rights Act of 1964 with respect to people with disabilities. For the first time, federal legislation will comprehensively extend antidiscrimination protection for people with disabilities, including HIV infection, to the private as well as the public sector, in employment, public services, public transportation, public accommodations, and telecommunications.

The ADA proscribes discrimination against a qualified individual because of his or her disability. "Disability" is construed very widely to include a broad range of physical and mental disabilities "which substantially limit one or more of the major life activities of that individual; a record of such impairment; or being regarded as having such an impairment." The courts have consistently found that all stages of HIV disease—including AIDS, AIDS-related complex (ARC), and asymptomatic infection—are handicaps under the federal Rehabilitation Act of 1973 [15, 84]. That act continues in force and includes an almost identical definition of "handicap" as in the ADA.

Congressional debates demonstrate conclusively that HIV/AIDS comes within the purview of the ADA. The act would make AIDS discrimination unlawful unless the person poses a "direct threat" to fellow workers. "Direct threat" means a "significant risk to the health or safety of others that cannot be eliminated by reasonable accommodation." Particularly controversial was the applicability of the act to food handlers infected with HIV. The ADA instructs the secretary of health to publish a list of infectious or communicable diseases that are transmitted through handling of the food supply. Even though the risk of HIV transmission gave impetus to this amendment, it is unlikely—given the extant epidemiological data—that HIV will appear on the secretary's list.

A disabled person must be "qualified," which means that he or she is capable of meeting all performance criteria of the particular position, service, or benefit. There is, moreover, an affirmative obligation to provide reasonable accommodation if it would enable the person to meet the performance criteria. Accommodation is not reasonable if it involves "undue hardship," which is an action requiring significant difficulty or expense.

The ADA does not cover federal employees, who continue to be protected by the Rehabilitation Act of 1973. Nor does the ADA cover housing. The Federal Fair Housing Amendment of 1989 prohibits private and public discrimination in the sale or rental of accommodation.

All states also have handicap statutes, all but four of which prohibit discrimination in the private as well as the public sector. In more than half the states, courts, human rights commissions, or attorneys general have formally or informally declared that handicap laws apply to AIDS or HIV infection.[7] Courts have reasoned that state handicap statutes closely follow the federal civil rights approach, and should cover HIV as a protected disability [16, 18]. To reinforce the importance of safeguarding persons infected with HIV from discrimination, many states and municipalities have enacted AIDS-specific antidiscrimination statutes.[8]

Discrimination based on an immutable condition such as infection should be so repugnant in our society that it should not be left to the inconsistencies and vagaries of the current legal system; states where people infected with HIV need greatest protection may afford the least.

This essay will review the major areas of discrimination currently being litigated: education, employment, housing, insurance, and health care.

EDUCATION

From the earliest times of the HIV epidemic, exclusion of schoolchildren infected with HIV was an issue debated with great emotion. Parents of children infected with HIV sued school boards for denying children state education [13], giving homebound instruction [3, 12], or making the child wait for inordinate periods while the board developed a policy [9]. In other cases HIV-infected children were permitted to attend school, but they were clearly singled out as different: placed alone in a separate "modular" classroom [4]; required to use a separate bathroom and to be accompanied by an adult on all field trips [14]; or even isolated inside a glass booth [1].

Some school board policies, perhaps reasonably, required disclosure of the child's identity to the school district, faculty, and staff [3]. Others revealed the child's identity throughout the school or even publicly announced to the entire community that the infected child had been admitted to the school [2].

Parents challenging decisions to exclude their children from education at school relied on the Rehabilitation Act, which applies to most schools because of their receipt of federal funding [3], and on the federal Education for All Handicapped Children Act,[9] which gives all school-age handicapped children the right to a free public education in the least restrictive environment appropriate to the case [1, 6].

The courts have not tolerated decisions to exclude HIV-infected children from ordinary schools [3–5, 7, 9]. The courts even found it unlawful to exclude a kindergartner who bit another child and was labeled "aggressive" by the school psychologist [8].

Courts that have safeguarded the right of HIV-infected children not to be discriminated against in their school placement have, nonetheless, required the school, parents, and child to comply with specified safeguards [3, 7, 8], including stringent compliance with CDC guidelines;[10] covering of all sores and lesions; maintenance of elevated standards of personal hygiene; denial of participation in curricular or extracurricular contact sports; and frequent medical examinations by both a private and a school physician. Some courts have gone further and required sexual and drug education for students, parents, and even the entire school system [7, 13].

In cases where the school board believed there was some behavioral or medical reason not to integrate the child fully, some courts have delineated a fair procedure for deciding the case, including parental and medical participation [13].

Most courts have required full integration without any visible barrier between the child and his or her classmates. To do otherwise, the courts reasoned, would cause irreparable emotional and psychological harm to the child [3, 4, 7]. However, a federal district court mandated a "safeguard" that stigmatized the child perhaps more than exclusion from school [1]. The court ordered the school board to construct a cubicle in the classroom with a large picture window to allow sound from the outer area to be heard. The cubicle, to be sure, allowed the child to be in the classroom and avoided the already remote risk of transmission. However, it provided a visible symbol of separation of the child from the rest of her class. The Eleventh Circuit Court of Appeals subsequently vacated the district court's decision, holding that the child must be placed in the least restrictive environment that would allow her to attend school.

The most difficult cases involve decisions to exclude students from educational settings where they may be inherently more likely to cut themselves and expose others to their blood.[11] Illustrative cases involve a dental student excluded because the course of study required performing invasive procedures, such as tooth extractions [122], and a student excluded from a medical assistant program [116].

EMPLOYMENT

The complaints reviewed by courts and human rights commissions provide insight into the kinds of employment disputes that have occurred since the start of the epidemic: dismissal without medical evidence [51, 55], notice [28], or a hearing [16, 18]; demotion to positions of lower experience and skill—for instance, an experienced teacher to an administrator [15], a fire fighter to a janitor [32], and a finance manager to a car salesman [49]; denial of insurance benefits to pay for AIDS-related expenses [36, 49]; reduction in salary [31]; harassment [39]; and a dishonorable discharge from the National Guard after the serviceman refused a reduction in rank solely because he was infected with HIV [52].

Cases were clustered in three areas, which account for the majority of employment disputes: health care workers [47, 48, 117, 118]; workers who provide human services for children—for example, teachers [15, 35, 58, 59], foster parents, and day care workers [34, 50]; and food handlers [21, 27, 37, 41].

Adverse employment decisions did not appear to be based on an assessment of the person's ability to do the job. Subtle abilities to do complicated or safety-oriented tasks were rarely an issue. Indeed, some adverse employment decisions were based merely on rumor [27, 54] or innuendo [37] that the person was infected with HIV; other such decisions were made because the employee appeared to have lost weight or was absent from work for short intervals as a result of pneumonia [44], or refused to be tested for HIV [53], or refused to disclose the results of a test taken at an anonymous site [34]. Employees were dismissed despite the fact that they had received regular salary increases based on merit [30], had been honored for "outstanding" work [56], or had "exemplary" work records [52].

Employers have given many reasons for their decisions. They have contended, for instance, that their establishment was being picketed [45]; that there was a threat of violence to the infected worker [22]; that they received adverse publicity when an employee appeared on television as an AIDS advocate [48]; or that they had to protect their business interests [43] and were facing a significant increase in insurance premiums because an employee was known to have AIDS [29].

Virtually all courts have held that a positive HIV test result or a diagnosis of an HIV-related disease does not provide a sufficient basis for unfair treatment by employers [15, 16, 18] or their agents [21]. If a person infected with HIV is capable of doing the job with reasonable accommodations, then discrimination is prohibited. The employers' decisions, moreover, must be based on reasonable medical judgments [18].

HOUSING AND PROPERTY

People infected with HIV have been denied equal opportunity in the purchase or lease of housing because of an erroneous belief that they pose a health risk, and because they make nondisabled people uncomfortable [63]. The factual pattern of complaints brought under this legislation by persons infected with HIV are varied: evictions from housing [68]; rescission of a contract to buy because the previous owner had AIDS [65]; locking out an infected tenant; and harassment or assault [73].

Numerous cases before human rights commissions involved evictions from premises because a person with AIDS missed monthly rent payments. One court refused to "add to the tenant's misery and suffering" by allowing the eviction [68]. Other cases involved tenants with HIV disease whose health was being affected by landlords' refusal to repair broken plumbing, heating, or other basic services in the building [72, 74].

Where courts or human rights commissions have applied handicap law to housing discrimination, they usually afford relief [65, 68, 73]. Courts have extended this protection to those who were evicted because they were perceived to be infected with HIV, although they actually were not—for instance, a mother and sister of a person with AIDS [71] and a healthy homosexual man [72]. It is reasoned that to discriminate against persons on the basis of a fear that they are infected is contrary to the purpose of civil rights law [64].

Still, serious questions remain about the adequacy of existing law to protect HIV-infected persons from housing discrimination. A particularly important consideration is whether a "life partner" can be protected against discrimination [66, 67]. Where a person with AIDS has in every manner possible made his life partner a member of his immediate family, that partner should be afforded the same rights in law as a spouse [67].

More troubling is the tendency of some courts to rely on contract rather than handicap law. Where contract law is used, courts focus on the failure to disclose a person's serological status, thus voiding the housing contract [109]. Other courts have suggested that if housing contracts were clearer in requiring disclosure of a person's medical condition, the property might not have to be sold to a person with AIDS [65]. The Federal Fair Housing Act may provide a solution by proscribing contract provisions that require disclosure of a person's HIV status.[12]

NURSING HOMES

The federal Office of Civil Rights, in the Department of Health and Human Services, investigating admissions to residential health care facilities, found a general reluctance to provide services for persons infected with HIV. Hospital discharge planners experienced so many admission denials of AIDS patients that many stopped their attempts to place them in skilled nursing facilities.

State human rights commissions have reported the same difficulty in obtaining admissions to skilled nursing facilities. Illustrative cases included a city's refusal to issue a zoning permit for a hospice for terminally ill AIDS patients [63] and a refusal to rent premises for a group home for people with AIDS [69]. Some nursing homes have a fixed policy not to take patients with AIDS, and patients have died before hearings to challenge these rules could be held [100].

PREMISES FOR HEALTH CARE PROFESSIONALS

Professionals who provide health care or social services for persons with HIV disease sometimes have found themselves the objects of housing discrimination. Examples include the eviction of a dentist who listed his name with the Gay Men's Health Crisis to provide services for AIDS patients [101]; refusal to sell property to a social service group that would be serving clients with AIDS [112]; or refusal to allow physicians to move into an apartment because they would be treating persons with AIDS [110].

The courts have protected health care professionals who are not themselves handicapped but are trying to provide vital services for those who are [70, 111]. When the courts balance the equities of such cases, they consider the "enormous public interests involved," because discriminatory practices "injure society as a whole." If professionals were prevented from serving persons with AIDS, "arguably the group most in need of medical treatment would suffer" [110]. Health care professionals who sought to make their services available to "a needy and discriminated against class and who are thwarted in their efforts" would be protected [111].

PUBLIC ACCOMMODATIONS

The right of persons infected with HIV to receive equal treatment in public accommodations has been an ongoing concern of human rights commissions. Complaints of discrimination in physicians' private offices have predominated and are discussed below, in the section on "Health Care Providers' Duty to Treat." Other discrimination complaints in this area concern refusals to provide personal services at a nail salon [75, 77, 82, 83], an airline [81], a television studio [79], and a spiritual retreat [78]. Funeral home owners have refused to embalm the body or to allow an open-casket service [80], or they have charged inflated fees [76]. Courts and human rights commissions have ruled that the protection afforded by handicap legislation persists after death [76].

INSURANCE

There is an irresolvable conflict between standard insurance underwriting and nondiscrimination principles. Health and life insurance policies are written after an assessment of the applicant's risk. The industry's objective is to discriminate against those with higher risk by charging higher premiums, placing a cap on expenses covered [147], or refusing to write the policy [137]. If the actuarial principles of the insurance industry are fully accepted, it follows that persons infected with HIV will be treated differently because of the undoubtedly higher risk they incur. The increased risk of HIV infection is greater than the risk associated with smoking, high blood pressure, or other conditions that are taken into account by insurers. The industry therefore regards persons infected with HIV as uninsurable,[13] and it does not believe that such a position reflects unlawful discrimination [131].

Insurance underwriting, however, is not merely a business, particularly when it provides health coverage. Public policy favors the provision of decent health care for all persons suffering from serious illness. The consequence of systematic refusal to insure persons infected with HIV is that the financial burden shifts to public hospitals that must care for patients without compensation. Many hospitals that serve large numbers of low-income persons with AIDS have encountered moderate to severe financial shortfalls because of their patients' lack of private health insurance coverage.[14] The most advantageous policy would share the health costs equitably among the government, private insurers, and employers.

Several states have sought to regulate the insurance industry by limiting the use of HIV testing in making decisions about insurability. The intention is to ensure that the industry assumes its fair share of the burden of health care costs. The courts, however, have been highly suspicious of such regulation. The Massachusetts Supreme Judicial Court held that the insurance commissioner had no statutory authority to prohibit insurers from using HIV tests in making underwriting decisions regarding health insurance. The court reasoned that the commissioner cannot interfere with an insurer's ability to assess risk [135]. A New York court also limited the regulatory power to require insurers to offer insurance without regard to proven actuarial factors [136].

A federal district court did uphold a District of Columbia statute that proscribed the use of any HIV test for the purposes of issuing insurance or adjusting rates or premiums [131]. The court, however, suggested that the law may well be "inequitable" or "unwise." It also based its decision largely on the unreliability of HIV antibody tests, an argument that may not be valid today.

HEALTH CARE

The HIV epidemic has transformed perceptions about the hazards involved in the practice of medicine, nursing, and associated fields.[15] Documented cases of occupational transmission of HIV have demonstrated that health care professionals can contract their patients' lethal infections.[16] AIDS, therefore, is increasingly being viewed as an occupational disease for health care professionals, despite the evidence that HIV is exceedingly hard to transmit in health care settings. The litigation reviewed in this section examines the duty to treat patients with HIV disease, access to experimental treatments, and the rights and responsibilities of HIV-infected health care professionals.

HEALTH CARE PROVIDERS' DUTY TO TREAT

Health care professionals have an ethical duty to provide treatment for persons infected with HIV.[17] The training, licensure, and professional purpose of health care professionals require that decisions be based on a good-faith clinical assessment of benefit and harm to the patient, and not on the patient's handicap. The risks to health care professionals who take rigorous precautions against contracting infection, moreover, are remote and do not justify deviation from this professional obligation not to discriminate. Certainly, the vast majority of health care professionals provide dedicated and equal treatment for all their patients.[18] In the instances where treatment has been withheld from patients infected with HIV, the courts have enforced the professional obligation to treat HIV-infected patients [84, 88, 89].

The litigation illustrates the harm that can result from treatment refusals. In one case a clinically depressed woman was left unattended in a room where she could lock the door and take an overdose of pills [94]. In other cases medical personnel refused to perform a routine hernia operation;[19] intentionally dropped a gurney after hearing that the person was infected with HIV [97]; or were so late in responding to an emergency call that the patient suffered an aggravated brain injury [100]. In some cases patients allege that excessive force was used [94].

Discriminatory practices may not always cause physical harm but show a lack of respect, empathy, and care that is inexcusable. Patients should not be placed in isolation except in rare circumstances when their medical condition requires it [94, 103, 104]. There is no adequate public health justification for refusing to administer medicine or alter a chest drain [104]; for leaving food trays outside the door [104]; or for excluding the patient from patient activities, including use of the telephone or other hospital amenities [103].

While few health care professionals would condone blatant treatment refusals that cause harm or result in insensitive treatment of patients, some practices are far more subtle; so it is often difficult to distinguish between the valid exercise of clinical judgment and a disguised form of prejudice. Physicians are defending their decisions not to treat, or to refer, HIV-infected patients by arguing that they are exercising clinical judgment and are not practicing discrimination, and that to restrict the physician's right to decide whom to treat or when to refer is to dictate the practice of medicine [102].

It is true that the physician-patient relationship is not easy to regulate by law, and that courts must grant due deference to the good-faith judgments of responsible health professionals [87]. Still, the physician's exercise of clinical judgment cannot render all treatment refusals or referrals immune from review if there is evidence to show they were motivated by prejudice [88]. Consider, for example, physicians' claims in court that they have insufficient expertise to treat any person with AIDS [87, 127]. Certainly, there are some manifestations of HIV disease that require specialized knowledge. However, all physicians are held by law to have a level of expertise commensurate with the standard prevailing in their specialty. As HIV disease becomes more prevalent, primary practitioners such as internists [87] or dentists [88] must be trained in the diagnosis and treatment of HIV disease, with referral where indicated. Specialists such as surgeons, nephrologists [93], and allergists [92] also need to be able to provide services for persons infected with HIV. Failure to maintain basic skills in relation to one disease may be grounds for revocation of a physician's license. A decision not to treat any patient infected with HIV [96, 98] or a refusal even to make a referral is likely to be viewed by the courts as medically unjustified and based on irrational fear or prejudice [102].

Another reason given for refusing to treat patients infected with HIV is a concern about occupational hazards. Legal and ethical obligations of health care professionals require them to endure reasonable risks, for example, where treatment is necessary to save or prolong life [93]. But some health care professionals take a different view when the treatment is elective [92, 98] or cosmetic [107]. The question then becomes whether patient X should receive different treatment from patient Y, not because of clinical differences but because of a perceived occupational risk to the physician. Professionals sometimes refuse to provide treatment because of inadequate equipment, education, or training for infection control [101, 107]. In particular, they claim that the federal Occupational Safety and Health Rules permit employees to refuse to perform assigned tasks because of a reasonable apprehension of serious injury [89].

All patients have a right to expect appropriate treatment. They also have a right to expect that professionals will have available, and will utilize, adequate infection control. Where the necessary equipment or training is not available, the proper response is to seek redress from the health care facility and not to turn the patient away [89].

Comprehensive settlements to disputes in this area supervised by the courts [106] and the federal Office of Civil Rights [150] provide models of good practice. *Inter alia,* they require health care facilities to develop policies for nondiscriminatory admission of patients with HIV disease; to protect patient confidentiality; and to comply with CDC guidelines by providing education, training, and necessary equipment for rigorous infection control.

The courts have found that persons infected with HIV, even if asymptomatic, cannot be discriminated against in the receipt of health care services [84]. Most courts have decided that private medical or dental offices as well as clinics, hospitals, and dispensaries are "public accommodations" and that the medical field is not exempt from the requirement not to discriminate on the basis of handicap [88, 98]. However, one court held that a physician's private office is "unique in character" and should not be regulated as a public accommodation [87].

It is conceivable that courts may be more likely to uphold discriminatory practices in the future where there is the potential for significant exposure to blood. Pending cases that raise this question involve dialysis units [93, 124].

The professional obligation to treat patients who can clearly benefit must extend to all health professionals, whether in private offices or where there may be exposure to blood. To exempt certain professionals from the obligation to provide nondiscriminatory treatment to patients infected with HIV would jeopardize the health of those most in need of medical attention. It would also unfairly shift the burden from physicians who choose to opt out to those dedicated to providing care without prejudice.

ACCESS TO INNOVATIVE TREATMENTS

The HIV epidemic has revitalized a perennial debate about whether there is legal right of access to experimental or innovative treatments for hopelessly ill patients.[20] Traditionally, the law will not provide an enforceable entitlement to particular medical services unless they are necessary in an emergency.[21] The health care provider may not discriminate on the basis of a patient's serological status. But what if the refusal to treat does not involve discrimination but is based on a valid clinical, research, or financial consideration?

Persons with AIDS claim the right to unimpeded access to innovative pharmaceuticals approved by the federal Food and Drug Administration, including the right to adequate financing. AIDS patients have successfully sued both the state [85] and hospitals [86] for rationing their access to AZT and aerosolized pentamidine on the grounds of inadequate resources rather than for clinical reasons. The state of Missouri limited medical coverage for AZT to recipients who have a history of cytologically confirmed *Pneumocystis carinii* pneumonia (PCP) or an absolute T4/helper/inducer lymphocyte count of less than 200, in accordance with the FDA approval statement. A federal court ordered that Medicaid coverage for the drug must be determined by the physician's decision that the drug is medically necessary [85]. A federal district court in Texas prohibited a hospital AIDS clinic from using a waiting list to control access to AZT and pentamidine, because it violated state public policy that no person be denied medical treatment for fiscal reasons [86].

In the treatment of HIV disease, often the most promising pharmaceuticals are as yet unapproved. The only realistic access to such innovative treatments for hopelessly ill patients may be through participation in a clinical trial. There is no established legal right to experimental therapy. Yet patients have bitterly disputed decisions to exclude them from clinical investigations. In some cases the exclusion appeared almost arbitrary. One subject, for instance, was prevented from continuing experimental medication after arriving forty-five minutes late for a clinical trial appointment [95]. Patients have even contested the discontinuation of a clinical investigation because the preliminary results indicated the drug was ineffective. In one such case the patient contended that the drug had stabilized his condition [91].

This search for a promising therapeutic intervention vividly illustrates the human anguish of AIDS patients. The potential conflict between patients' rights of access to unproven pharmaceuticals and valid research goals is powerful. If patients succeed in achieving an ethical or even a legal entitlement to unimpeded access to experimental drugs, the ability of researchers to conduct scientifically sound research could be compromised by a lack of subjects willing to participate in controlled clinical trials.

HIV-INFECTED HEALTH CARE PROFESSIONALS: TESTING
AND LIMITATIONS ON THE RIGHT TO PRACTICE

A strong ethical argument can be made that health care professionals who are infected with HIV should be permitted to continue their normal practice, provided they are capable of doing so.[22] The potential harm to patients is negligible if rigorous infection control procedures are used. The risk of transmission of HIV from health care professional to patient is estimated to be exceedingly low, with no documented case of transmission.[23] The burden on health care professionals if they are denied the right to practice, on the other hand, is considerable.[24] The professional can lose his or her livelihood, and disclosure of information to colleagues and patients can be psychologically harmful.

This relatively straightforward ethical analysis, however, is not reflected in the professional literature or judicial case law. The American Medical Association's ethical position is that a "physician who knows he or she is seropositive should not engage in any activity that creates a risk of transmission of the disease to others." If professionals are infected with HIV, they should consult their physician and employer to determine whether it is safe to continue to practice.

The AMA position, which opposes *any* risk to patients, is exceedingly harsh. That standard could well require hospitals to place some limits on the right of an HIV-infected professional to practice. The guideline to consult the professional's physician and employer begs the question, for it does not specify the circumstances that might warrant limitations on the right to practice. One rational standard, for example, would be to allow the professional to practice normally (with supervision and careful infection control), but to avoid the performance of invasive procedures where blood exchange is possible.

The problem with the AMA's ethical position that any risk must be avoided is that it could be used by the courts to set an enforceable legal standard of care. Failure of hospitals or health care professionals to comply with that standard could result in liability. In fact, in a growing number of cases hospitals, clinics, and group practices are summarily excluding health care professionals infected with HIV, purporting to respond to ethical guidelines [122]. More worrisome is the argument that, since it is ethically wrong for infected professionals to treat patients, there is a correlative duty to screen workers. The courts, moreover, have been inconsistent in resolving disputes between health care facilities and their HIV-infected employees.

The contrasting decisions of the federal courts in *Glover* [113] and *Leckelt* [114] illustrate the dilemma. In *Glover* the Eighth Circuit Court of Appeals found that a decision of a facility for mentally retarded persons to screen its staff who are in direct contact with patients is unconstitutional. The basis for the policy was the hospital's concern about clients who bite or scratch staff and become exposed to their blood. The appellate court upheld the district court's view that the risk to patients was low, "approaching zero." Courts [125] and human rights agencies [128] have also held that a hospital's repeated refusals to allow an HIV-infected nurse to return to work constitute unlawful discrimination. In one case the hospital even refused the nurse's offer to be transferred to working in the supply room [128].

The federal district court in *Leckelt* took a very different view of a clinic's decision to dismiss a nurse after he refused to disclose the results of an HIV test conducted at an anonymous test site. The nurse had been previously treated for syphilis and was a chronic carrier of hepatitis B virus. The court held that the nurse was not discriminated against, because disclosure of the test result was the necessary first step in safeguarding the security of patients.

Health care facilities support their decisions to dismiss, or limit the practice of, infected health care professionals on public health, ethical, and economic grounds. They suggest that the prospect of transmission of HIV during a professional career of performing invasive procedures is a real risk: "gloves cannot prevent penetrating injuries by needles or other sharp instruments," such injuries are common, and the consequences of infection of patients are severe [122]. They also argue that there is an ethical obligation not to permit any known risk of transmitting HIV infection to patients [122]. Some hospitals stress the economic hardship they would suffer if they knowingly continued to employ a professional infected with HIV; the perception is that the public would refuse to be treated in a facility known to have infected professionals on its staff [121].

The impact of hospital policies on HIV-infected health care professionals has been significant. A nurse was subjected to "full isolation procedures," with his colleagues "fully masked, gowned and gloved" while in his presence [119, 126]; a director of anesthesiology was denied contact with patients and was then disciplined when he personally assisted a patient who had vomited and was in immediate danger of aspirating [120]; a gynecologist was forced out of a lucrative medical partnership despite his offer to do no "hands-on" work [123]. Even health care professionals who contracted HIV from occupational exposure have been dismissed or penalized by the hospital where the exposure took place [124, 125].

Thoughtful resolutions of the rights and duties of HIV-infected health care professionals have been ironed out in court-approved settlements. These settlements have characteristically permitted health care professionals to continue to practice but to be limited in the performance of seriously invasive procedures. The settlements also required health care professionals to use rigorous infection control procedures at all times and to submit to regular medical examinations and supervision by their physician and the hospital [125]. Settlements have also required the health care facility to provide special training for the infected professional [116] and education for all personnel [117].

CHANGES AND TRENDS IN THE PATTERN OF DISCRIMINATION

Human rights commissions report that, early in the HIV epidemic, employment discrimination was "systemic," meaning that the problem was "company or industry wide, that a tacit or written policy existed which would adversely affect any person with AIDS who came into contact with the policy" [150]. However, complaints of discrimination and cruel behavior have been significantly reduced when employers have introduced AIDS education programs in the workplace.

The same changing pattern of discrimination is apparent in education, housing, and public accommodations. Traditional forms of discrimination—such as exclusion of children from school, refusal to rent or sell property, or refusal to provide personal services—are declining.

Complaints about discrimination in health care, nursing, and social services have predominated in recent years, and this trend is likely to continue. Major issues to be faced in the coming years will involve admissions of HIV-infected students to medical and dental schools; employment of HIV-infected health care workers, particularly those performing invasive procedures; and access of HIV-infected patients to nursing homes, hospitals, private medical and dental offices, and other health care facilities.

There are many reasons for the changing complexion of discrimination since the beginning of the HIV epidemic. Most important, public opinion surveys show that the overwhelming majority of respondents understand the primary modes of transmission of HIV.[25] Attitudes toward persons at high risk of HIV, while initially hostile,[26] are softening. Educational programs designed to promote greater acceptance and tolerance of persons infected with HIV have achieved a measure of success.[27]

The shifting pattern of discrimination is further explained by the rapid ethnographic changes in the HIV epidemic.[28] As the epidemic moves from the gay community to intravenous drug users, there is a greater likelihood that persons with HIV disease will have impeded access to services. Intravenous drug users have traditionally been underserved in the health care systems because of their socioeconomic class and because of the lack of expertise and willingness among many health care professionals to treat drug abuse.

Often the reason for discriminatory practice is not pure prejudice or even ignorance or irrational fear. Rather, exclusion of HIV-infected persons is intended to eliminate all risk of infection through exposure to blood. That is why health care and emergency services have become the new focal points for discrimination. These service providers should recognize that they cannot expect to eliminate all risk. As long as strict infection control procedures are used, however, occupational risks should remain within acceptable limits.

Discrimination is also fueled by financial concerns. Persons with HIV disease can increase costs by driving up insurance premiums or deterring potential customers. But the very purpose of civil rights law is to get beyond the inequities of a market economy and to set standards of equal opportunity that cannot be compromised.[29]

Nondiscrimination for persons infected with HIV is consistent with the prevailing sense of justice in America. With continued AIDS education, rigorous enforcement of handicap law, and increased tolerance of gays and IV drug users, discrimination can be reduced and, with it, the public health advanced.

NOTES

This article was originally published as the second part in a two-part series in the *Journal of the American Medical Association* 263 (1990): 2086–93, © 1990, American Medical Association, and is reprinted with permission. The AIDS Litigation Project was supported under a contract from the National AIDS Program Office (NAPO), U.S. Public Health Service. I would like to thank Lane Porter, J.D., M.P.H. (American Bar Association); and Hazel Sandomire, J.D. (Columbia Law School); James Allen, M.D., and Iris Gelberg of NAPO; and Richard Riseberg, J.D., Chief Counsel, U.S. Public Health Service.

1. Government reports: Presidential Commission on the Human Immunodeficiency Virus Epidemic, *Report* (Washington, D.C.: U.S. Government Print-

Office, 1988); Centers for Disease Control, *Recommended Additional Guidelines for HIV Antibody Counseling and Testing in the Prevention of HIV Infection* (Washington, D.C.: Public Health Service, 1987). Medical reports: Institute of Medicine and National Academy of Sciences, *Confronting AIDS: Directions for Public Health Care and Research* (Washington, D.C.: National Academy Press, 1986; 1988 update); American Medical Association Board of Trustees, "Prevention and Control of Acquired Immunodeficiency Syndrome: An Interim Report," *Journal of the American Medical Association* 258 (1987): 2097–2103. Public health report: Association of State and Territorial Health Officials, *Guide to Public Health Practice: AIDS Confidentiality and Antidiscrimination Principles: Interim Report* (Washington, D.C.: ASTHO, 1987). Legal reports: American Bar Association, AIDS Coordinating Committee, *AIDS: The Legal Issues* (Washington, D.C.: ABA, 1988); American Bar Association, *Policy on AIDS* (Washington, D.C.: ABA, August 1989).

2. *School Board of Nassau County v. Arline,* 107 S. Ct. 1123 (1987).

3. Centers for Disease Control, "Guidelines for Prophylaxis against *Pneumocystis Carinii* Pneumonia for Persons Infected with HIV," *Morbidity and Mortality Weekly Report* 38, no. S-5 (1989): 1–9.

4. Federal Office of Civil Rights, Department of Health and Human Services, *AIDS* (Washington, D.C.: DHHS, 1987).

5. San Francisco AIDS Referral Panel, *Annual Report* (San Francisco: AIDS Referral Panel, 1989); San Francisco Human Rights Commission, *Report on Sexual Orientation and AIDS* (San Francisco: Human Rights Commission, 1987–88); AIDS Discrimination Cases Handled by the Office of the City Attorney, Los Angeles. Personal communication from David Schulman, January 27, 1989; New York City Commission on Human Rights, *Reports on Discrimination against People with Aids* (New York: Commission on Human Rights, 1983–1987; updates, 1988, 1989).

6. R. J. Steele et al., *Identification and Assessment of State and Local Strategies to Prevent Discrimination* (Silver Spring, Md.: Birch and Davis Associates, 1989); B. Bridgham and M. Rowe, *AIDS Discrimination: A Review of State Laws That Affect HIV Infection, 1983–1988* (Washington, D.C.: Intergovernmental Health Policy Project, 1989).

7. National Gay Rights Advocates, *Protection against Discrimination under State Handicap Laws: A Fifty State Analysis* (San Francisco: NGRA, 1989).

8. L. Gostin, "Public Health Strategies for Confronting AIDS: Legislative and Regulatory Policy in the United States," *Journal of the American Medical Association* 261 (1989): 1621–30.

9. 20 U.S.C. sections 1400 et seq.

10. Centers for Disease Control, "Education and Foster Care of Children Infected with Human T-Lymphotropic Virus Type III/Lymphadenopathy-Associated Virus," *Morbidity and Mortality Weekly Report* 34 (1985): 517–21.

11. Association of American Medical Colleges, *The HIV Epidemic and Medical Education* (Washington, D.C.: AAMC, 1989).

12. Op. Tex. Att. Gen., No. JM-1093; AIDS Lit. Rptr., Oct 13, 1989, p. 3467.

13. Health Insurance Association of America and American Council of Life Insurance, *Survey of Health and Life Insurance Companies Concerning AIDS* (Washington, D.C.: HIAA and ACLI, 1986).

14. D. P. Andrulis, V. B. Weslowski, and L. S. Gage, "The 1987 U.S. Hospital AIDS Survey," *Journal of the American Medical Association* 262 (1989): 784–94.

15. L. Gostin, "Hospitals, Health Care Professionals and AIDS: The 'Right to Know' the Health Status of Professionals and Patients," *Maryland Law Review* 48 (1989): 12–54.

16. Centers for Disease Control, "Recommendations for Prevention of HIV Transmission in Health-Care Settings," *Morbidity and Mortality Weekly Report* 36 (1987): S2–S18.

17. A. Jonsen, "The Duty to Treat Patients with AIDS and HIV Infection," in *AIDS and the Health Care System*, ed. L. Gostin (New Haven, Conn.: Yale University Press, 1990); Council on Ethical and Judicial Affairs, American Medical Association, "Ethical Issues Involved in the Growing AIDS Crisis," *Journal of the American Medical Association* 259 (1988): 1360–61.

18. P. M. Arnow et al., "Orthopedic Surgeons' Attitudes and Practices Concerning Treatment of Patients with HIV Infection," *Public Health Review* 104 (1989): 121–29.

19. *Doe v. Shasta General Hospital, Shasta City,* Cal. Super. Ct. No. 92336 (1988).

20. B. Freedman, "Licensing of New Drugs: The Balance between FDA Regulation and the Hopes of the Terminally Ill," *Hastings Center Report* 19 (1989): 14–20.

21. T. Brennan, "Ensuring Adequate Health Care for the Sick: The Challenge of the Acquired Immunodeficiency Syndrome as an Occupational Disease," *Duke Law Journal* (1988): 29–78.

22. L. Gostin, "HIV-Infected Physicians and the Practice of Seriously Invasive Procedures," *Hastings Center Report* 19 (1989): 32–39.

23. J. R. Allen, "Health Care Workers and the Risk of HIV Transmission," *Hastings Center Report* 18 (1988): S2–S5.

24. L. M. Peterson, "AIDS: The Ethical Dilemma for Surgeons," *Law, Medicine and Health Care* 17 (1989): 139–44.

25. D. A. Dawson, AIDS Knowledge and Attitudes for January–March 1989: Provisional Data from the National Health Interview Survey; Advance Data from *Vital and Health Statistics* 176 (August 15, 1989): 1–12.

26. R. J. Blendon and K. Donelan, "Discrimination against People with AIDS: The Public's Perspective," *New England Journal of Medicine* 319 (1988): 1022–26.

27. P. D. Cleary, "Education and the Prevention of AIDS," *Law, Medicine and Health Care* 16 (1988): 267–73.

28. S. R. Friedman, J. L. Sotheran, and A. Abdul-Quader, "The AIDS Epidemic among Blacks and Hispanics," *Milbank Quarterly* 65, Suppl. 2 (1987): 455–99.

29. *United States v. Pelzer Realty Co.,* 484 F.2d 438, 443 (5th Cr. 1973), *cert. denied,* 416 U.S. 936 (1974).

COMPILATION OF CASES

Many of the cases in the compilation are from primary source material and are not reported elsewhere. Primary sources include the Lambda Legal Defense Fund (a lesbian and gay rights advocacy organization), the Columbia Law School AIDS Clinic, the American Civil Liberties Union, and others. Readers who want a more detailed understanding of the methodology of how the cases were collected and reported and an expanded citation form are directed to L. Gostin, L. Porter, and H. Sandomire, *The AIDS Litigation Project*. 2 vols. (Washington, D.C.: U.S. Government Printing Office, 1990).

EDUCATION

1. *Martinez v. School Board of Hillsborough County, Fla.*, 861 F. 2d 1502 (11th Cir. 1989), *reversing*, 711 F. Supp. 1293 (M.D. Fla. 1988).

2. *Child v. School Board of Fairfax County*, 875 F. 2d 314 (4th Cir. 1989).

3. *Doe v. Dolton Elementary School District No. 148*, 694 F. Supp. 440 (N.D. Ill. 1988).

4. *Robertson v. Granite City Community Unit School District No. 9*, 684 F. Supp. 1002 (S.D. Ill. 1988).

5. *Doe v. Belleville School District No. 118*, 672 F. Supp. 342 (S.D. Ill. 1987).

6. *Parents of Child v. Coker*, 676 F. Supp. 1072 (E.D. Okla. 1987).

7. *Ray v. School District of DeSoto County*, 666 F. Supp. 1524 (M.D. Fla. 1987).

8. *Thomas v. Atascadero Unified School District*, 662 F. Supp. 376 (C.D. Cal. 1986).

9. *Phipps v. Saddleback Valley Unified School District*, 251 Cal. Rptr. 720 Cal. App. 4th 1988).

10. *District 27 Community School Board v. Board of Education*, 502 N.Y.S. 325 (Sup. Ct., Queens County 1986).

11. *Bogard v. White*, Clinton Cir. Ct. No. 86-144, Ind.; ACLU.

12. *Moore v. School Board of Manatee County*, U.S. Dist. Ct., M.D. Fla.; AIDS Lit. Rptr., Jan. 27, 1989, and Dec. 23, 1988.

13. *New York v. Dow*, U.S. Dist. Ct., Conn.; AIDS Lit. Rptr., June 10, 1988.

14. *Child, by Parent v. Spillane and the School Board of Fairfax County, Va.*, U.S. Ct. of Appeals (4th Cir.); Lambda, Apr. 29, 1989.

DISCRIMINATION: EMPLOYMENT

15. *Chalk v. U.S. District Court, C.D. Cal.*, 840 F. 2d 701 (9th Cir. 1988).

16. *Shuttleworth v. Broward County*, 639 F. Supp. 654, 649 F. Supp. 35 (S.D. Fla. 1986).

17. *Evans v. Kornfeld,* Pa. Ct. Common Pleas, Luzerne County, No. 3468-C of 1988; ACLU.

18. *Raytheon v. Fair Employment and Housing Commission, Estate of Chadbourne,* 261 Cal. Rptr. 197 (Cal. App. 2d 1989).

19. *M.A.E., Estate of J.J.E. v. Doe and Roe,* 586 A. 2d 285 (Sup. Ct. N.J., 1989).

20. *Doe v. 315 232 Street Corp.,* No. 17150-1988, N.Y. Sup. Ct., Bronx County, 1988; Colum. AIDS Law Clinic.

21. *Chapoton v. Majestic Caterers and Karageorge,* Cir. Ct., City of Roanoke, Va.; Lambda, Mar. 21, 1988.

22. *Cronan v. New England Telephone,* 41 F.E.P. 1273 (Mass. 1986).

23. *T. v. A Financial Service Company,* N.Y. Sup. Ct., 1988; Colum. AIDS Law Clinic.

24. *Brunner v. al Attar,* Dist. Ct., Harris County, Tex., 295th Jud. Dist. No. 86-42628; ACLU.

25. *Nieto v. Clark, Thomas, Winters and Newton,* Tex. Dist. Ct., Travis County; AIDS Lit. Rptr., Aug. 12, 1988, and Mar. 10, 1989.

26. *Illinois Department of Human Rights v. Fossett Corp.,* Cir. Ct., Cook County, Ill.; AIDS Lit. Rptr., Feb. 26, 1988.

27. *Wolfe v. Tidewater Pizza,* Va. Sup. Ct., Jan. 1988.

28. *Trueman v. Camden,* Mich. Cir. Ct., Wayne County, May 16, 1984.

29. *Garner v. Rainbow Lodge,* U.S. Dist. Ct., S.D. Tex., Houston Div. H-88-1705 (1989); Lambda.

30. *Cain v. Hyatt,* 1989, West Law 17511 (E.D. Pa. 1989).

31. *Crowley v. Idelman Telemarketing,* U.S. Dist. Ct., E.D. Va.; AIDS Lit. Rptr., Feb. 12, 1988.

32. *Severino v. North Fort Myers Fire Control District,* U.S. Dist. Ct., M.D. Fla.; AIDS Lit. Rptr., Nov. 11, 1988.

33. *Houseknecht v. White,* U.S. Dist. Ct., E.D. Pa., Civ. Act No. 88-9586; ACLU, Dec. 16, 1988.

34. *Chinchilla v. Social Service Agency of Orange County,* U.S. Dist. Ct., C.D. Cal., Case No. 8704811, FFF(Kx); ACLU, July 16, 1987.

35. *Rice v. Bloomer,* U.S. Dist. Ct., E.D. Va., No. 87-162-A; ACLU, Feb. 18, 1987.

36. *McCormick v. Hechnier,* U.S. Dist. Ct., Md.; Lambda.

37. *Little v. Bryce and Randall's Food Market,* 733 S.W. 2d 937 (Tex. App. 1987).

38. *Doe v. Sinicola and Sons Excavating,* Oakland County Cir. Ct., Mich., No. 86-320825NZ; ACLU, Apr. 8, 1987.

39. *Griffin v. Tri-Met,* Ore. Cir. Ct., Multnomah County; AIDS Lit. Rptr., Mar. 10, 1989.

40. *Foulks v. Sup. Provision,* Mich. Cir. Ct., Wayne Country, Nov. 17, 1988.

41. *Farris v. Marriott Corp.,* Cal. Sup. Ct., Riverside County; AIDS Lit. Rptr., Feb. 12, 1988.

42. *Burgess v. Your House of Raleigh,* 380 S.E. 2d 769 (N.C. 1989).

43. *Shawn v. Legs Co. Partnership,* Sup. Ct. N.Y.; AIDS Lit. Rptr., Mar. 10, 1989.

44. *Doe v. Independent Office Machines*, Ct. of Common Pleas, Montgomery County, Pa.; AIDS Lit. Rptr., Nov. 29, 1988.

45. *Mosby v. Joe's Westlake Restaurant*, Cal. Sup. Ct., San Francisco County, No. 865045; ACLU.

46. *Herrera v. Eastman Kodak*, Cal. Sup. Ct., Los Angeles County; ACLU.

47. *Doe v. Dept. of Health and Human Services*, Admin. complaint of employment discrimination filed with DHSS in Ala. June 9, 1986; ACLU.

48. *Shannon v. Charter Real Hospital*, Admin. complaint, Dallas, Apr. 28, 1986; ACLU.

49. *Doe v. Beaverton Nissan*, Equal Employment Opportunity Commission and Ore. Civil Rights Case No. ST-EM-HP-870108-1353.

50. *Rohloff v. New York State Division for Youth*, N.Y.S. Division of Human Rights; Colum. AIDS Law Clinic, 1988.

51. *Iacono v. Town of Huntington Security Division*, N.Y.S. Div. of Human Rights; Colum. AIDS Law Clinic, 1989.

52. *Doe v. New York National Guard*, N.Y.S. Div. of Human Rights, Mar. 9, 1989; AIDS Lit. Rptr., Mar. 24, 1989.

53. *Butler v. Southland Corp., 7–11 Stores*, Cir. Ct., Baltimore, Md., Sup. Ct., Jan. 27, 1989.

54. *Isbell v. Poor Richard's*, W. Va. Human Rights Commission; AIDS Lit. Rptr., Sept. 23, 1988.

55. *Bernabei v. Del Cars*, Ill. Human Rights Commission; ACLU.

56. *Sweetland v. Telecheck*, Kan. Commission on Civil Rights; AIDS Lit. Rptr., Dec. 23, 1988.

57. *Bowers v. Baker & McKenzie*, N.Y.S. Human Rights Commission 1B-E-D-86-115824; National Law Journal, Sept. 14, 1987.

58. *Racine Education Association v. Racine Unified School District*, 385 N.W. 2d 510 (Wis. 1988).

59. *Scott Eckholdt v. Perkins School for the Blind*, Mass. Committee against Discrimination, Case No. 87-BEM-1194, filed Nov. 11, 1987; ACLU.

60. *B. v. A Construction Co.*, N.Y.C. Commission on Human Rights; Colum. AIDS Law Clinic, 1988.

61. *N. v. A Restaurant*, N.Y.C. Commission on Human Rights; Colum. AIDS Law Clinic, 1989.

62. Note: *Employment Discrimination Cases Handled by the San Francisco AIDS Legal Referral Panel*, Annual Rpts. 1987, 1988.

DISCRIMINATION: HOUSING AND PROPERTY

63. *Baxter v. Belleville*, U.S. Dist. Ct., S.D. Ill., Lexis 10298 (1989).

64. *Poff v. Caro*, 549 A. 2d 900 (N.J. Super. 1987).

65. *Kleinfeld v. McNally Real Estate*, N.Y. County Sup. Ct.; Lambda, July 15, 1988.

66. *Braschi v. Stahl Associates*, 543 N.E. 2d 49 (N.Y. Ct. App. 1989).

67. *Marbru and Berkeley Association v. Berg*, Civ. Ct. N.Y. County; Lambda.

68. *Clover Court Realty v. Lombardi*, N.Y. County Civ. Ct., May 9, 1988.

69. *Whitman Walker Clinic and Thomas v. Sibay,* Cir. Ct. Arlington County, Va.; Lambda.

70. *People v. 49 West 12 Tenants Corp.,* Sup. Ct. N.Y. County, No. 43604/83, Aug. 1984; NGRA.

71. *West 22nd St. Association v. Thomas and Thomas,* 144 Misc. 2d 292 (N.Y. Sup. Ct. 1989).

72. *C. v. A Landlord,* N.Y.S. Division of Human Rights; Colum. AIDS Law Clinic, 1988.

73. *Weingarten v. Gruenberg,* N.Y.C. Commission on Human Rights; AIDS Lit. Rptr., July 15, 1988.

74. *Note: Housing Discrimination Cases Handled by the San Francisco AIDS Legal Referral Panel,* Annual Rpts. 1987, 1988.

DISCRIMINATION: PUBLIC ACCOMMODATIONS AND COMMERCIAL ESTABLISHMENTS

75. *Jasperson v. Jessica's Nail Clinic,* 1989 WL 154205 (Cal. App. 2d).

76. *Dimicelli & Sons Funeral Homes v. New York City Commission on Human Rights,* N.Y. County Sup. Ct., Jan. 9, 1987.

77. *People v. Vartoughian,* Beverly Hills Municipal Ct.; AIDS Lit. Rptr., Apr. 14, 1989.

78. *Gittleson v. Jacumba Foundation,* Cal. Super. Ct., Los Angeles County, Mar. 8, 1989; AIDS Lit. Rptr., Mar. 24, 1989.

79. *Townsend v. Post-Newsweek Station,* Mich. Cir. Ct., Wayne County. Oct. 4, 1985.

80. *Doe v. Lacarenza Funeral Home,* Conn. Sup. Ct., Stamford, No. CV87-0090916S; ACLU Nov. 9, 1987.

81. *Cooper, Commissioner v. Northwest Airlines,* Human Rights Dept., Minn.; NGRA, Sept. 16, 1987.

82. *Tema S. Luft v. Nail Gallery;* Md. Commission on Human Rights.

83. *Tama S. Luft v. All That Glitters;* Md. Commission on Human Rights.

DISCRIMINATION: HEALTH CARE

Failure to Treat HIV-Infected Patients

84. *Doe v. Centinela Hospital,* 57 U.S.L.W. 2034 (C.D. Cal. 1988).

85. *Weaver v. Reagen,* 886 F. 2d 194 (8th Cir. 1989), *affirming,* 701 F. Supp. 717 (W.D. Mo. 1988).

86. *Dallas Gay Alliance v. Dallas County Hospital District,* 719 F. Supp. 1380 (N.D. Tex. 1989).

87. *Elstein v. State Division of Human Rights,* Sup. Ct., Onondaga County (N.Y.); AIDS Lit. Rptr., Sept. 9, 1988.

88. *Hurwitz v. New York City Commission on Human Rights,* 142 Misc. 2d 214 (N.Y. Sup. Ct. 1988).

89. *Stepp v. Review Board of the Indiana Employment Security Division,* 521 N.E. 2d 350 (Ind. App. 4th 1988).

90. *Mair v. Barton*, 705 F. Supp. 520 (D. Kan. 1987).
91. *DeVito v. H.E.M.*, 705 F. Supp. 1076 (M.D. Pa. 1988).
92. *Doe v. Lankenau Hospital*, U.S. Dist. Ct., E.D. Pa.; AIDS Lit. Rptr., Nov. 29, 1988.
93. *Roe v. Cumberland County Hospital System*, U.S. Dist. Ct., E.D.N.C., Case No. 88-62-CIV-3, June 10, 1988; ACLU.
94. *Doe v. Howard University Hospital*, complaint filed.
95. *Bleyenberg v. Gustafson and Miller*, Dist. Ct., Harris County, Tex.; AIDS Lit. Rptr., Apr. 29, 1988.
96. *Beardon v. Sutter Place Dental Group*, Cal. Super. Ct., San Francisco; AIDS Lit. Rptr., Dec. 9, 1988, and Feb. 24, 1989.
97. *Johnson v. District of Columbia*, D.C. Super. Ct., Civ. Div.; AIDS Lit. Rptr., Apr. 29, 1989.
98. *Walsh v. Cicmanec*, Cal. Super. Ct., San Diego, Jan. 31, 1989; AIDS Lit. Rptr., Mar. 10, 1989.
99. *Brogan v. Kimberly Services*, Cal. Super. Ct., San Francisco; AIDS Lit. Rptr., Sept. 23, 1988.
100. *McKenany v. Four Seasons Nursing Center*, Dist. Ct., Travis County, Tex., Dec. 2, 1986; ACLU.
101. *Vermont v. Lunt*, Dept. of Health; AIDS Lit. Rptr., Mar. 25, 1988.
102. *G.S. v. Karim Baksh, D.D.S.*, Ill. Human Rights Commission, No. 1987CPO113, Sept. 26, 1988; NGRA.
103. *Frazier v. Marcus Garvey Nursing Home*, N.Y.S. Division of Human Rights, No. 9K-B-D-88-132002; Colum. AIDS Law Clinic, 1988.
104. *Doe v. St. Francis Hospital*, N.Y.S. Division of Human Rights, No. 3-P-D-87-123301; Colum. AIDS Law Clinic, 1987.
105. *B. v. A Dentist*, N.Y.C. Commission on Human Rights; Colum. AIDS Law Clinic, 1989.
106. *Levert v. SSEU Local 371*, N.Y.C. Commission on Human Rights, No. 10286460-PA, Apr. 27, 1988; N.Y.C. Dept. of Health.
107. *Whittacre v. Northern Dispensary*, N.Y.C. Commission on Human Rights, Nos. AU-00015021387, GA-0023030687-DN; ACLU, Feb. 1988.
108. *F.R. v. M.G.H.*, Mass. Commission on Human Rights, Doc. No. 007-85-SO, Sept. 28, 1987.

Refusal to Provide Premises to Health Care Professionals

109. *Whitman Walker Clinic v. C. J. Coakley*, Cir. Ct. Arlington County, Va.; Lambda; AIDS Lit. Rptr., Jan. 12, 1989.
110. *Seitzman v. Hudson River Association*, 513 N.Y.S. 2d 148 (App. Div. 1987).
111. *Barton v. New York City Commission on Human Rights*, 531 N.Y.S. 2d 979 (Sup. Ct. 1988), *affirmed*, 542 N.Y.S. 2d 176 (1989).
112. *Action AIDS v. Dirot Del and U.S. Realty*, Philadelphia Commission on Human Relations; AIDS Lit. Rptr., Sept. 23, 1988.

HIV-Infected Health Care Professionals

113. *Glover v. Eastern Nebraska Office of Retardation*, 867 F. 2d 461 (8th Cir. 1989), *cert. denied*, 110 S. Ct. 321 (1989).

114. *Leckelt v. Board of Commissioners of Hospital District 1,* 714 F. Supp. 1377 (E.D. La. 1989).

115. *Doe, M.D. v. Cook County,* U.S. Dist. Ct., N.D. Ill., Mar. 11, 1988.

116. *Doe v. National Education Center and Strayer,* U.S. Dist. Ct., E.D. Pa.; AIDS Lit. Rptr., Nov. 29, 1988, and Apr. 29, 1989.

117. *Galiher v. Los Angeles County,* U.S. Dist. Ct., C.D. Cal.; AIDS Lit. Rptr., Jan 13, 1989.

118. *Doe v. U.S. Attorney General,* 723 F. Supp. 452 (N.D. Cal. 1989).

119. *Rhodes v. Charter Hospital,* U.S. Dist. Ct., S.D. Miss.; AIDS Lit. Rptr., Mar. 10, 1989.

120. *Mark Bible v. Mother Francis Hospital,* U.S. Dist. Ct., E.D. Tex.; ACLU, 1987.

121. *Laredo v. Southwest Community Health Services,* U.S. Dist. Ct., N.M., Aug. 1987; Lambda.

122. *Doe v. Washington University Dental School,* Mo. Cir. Ct., St. Louis County; AIDS Lit. Rptr., Dec. 23, 1988, and Feb. 10, 1989.

123. *Gordon v. Blanchard,* Cal. Sup. Ct., Los Angeles County; AIDS Lit. Rptr., May 13, 1988.

124. *Hartford Hospital Nurses v. Hartford Hospital,* Conn. Sup. Ct., Hartford, June 19, 1987; ACLU.

125. *Dept. of Health and Human Services v. Charlotte Memorial Hospital,* DHHS No. 04-84-3096, Aug. 5, 1986, Charlotte, N.C.; ACLU.

126. *J. v. A Medical Center,* N.Y.S. Division of Human Rights; Colum. AIDS Law Clinic, 1988.

127. *Doe, R.N., v. New York Hospital,* N.Y.C. Commission on Human Rights; AIDS Lit. Rptr., Oct. 28, 1988.

128. *Dade County Fair Housing and Employment Appeals Board,* No. E-1097; ACLU, Aug. 1987.

129. *Note: Health Care Discrimination Cases Handled by the San Francisco AIDS Legal Referral Panel,* Annual Rpts. 1987, 1988.

DISCRIMINATION: INSURANCE

130. *Kentucky Central Life Insurance v. Webster,* 651 F. Supp. 935 (N.D. Ala. 1986), 841 F. 2d 397 (11th Cir. 1988).

131. *American Council of Life Insurance v. District of Columbia,* 645 F. Supp. 84 (D.D.C. 1986).

132. *Lilley v. Protective Life Insurance,* 1989 West Law 8831 (E.D. La. 1989).

133. *Zachary Trading v. Northwest Mutual Life Insurance,* 668 F. Supp. 343 (S.D.N.Y. 1987).

134. *Cheney v. Bell National Life Insurance,* 527 A. 2d 331 (1987).

135. *Life Insurance Association of Massachusetts v. Commissioner of Insurance,* 403 Mass. 410 (1988).

136. *Health Insurance Association of America v. Corcoran,* 140 Misc. 2d 255 (N.Y. Sup. Ct. 1988).

137. *People v. Health America,* Cal. Sup. Ct., San Francisco; AIDS Lit. Rptr., Nov. 29, 1988.

138. *Horner v. Great Republic Insurance,* Cal. Sup. Ct., San Francisco, No. 852522, Jan. 31, 1985; ACLU.

139. *Northwest Mutual Life Insurance v. Barth,* U.S. Dist. Ct., S.D.N.Y., 85 Civ. 8360, GLG; ACLU.

140. *Frantz v. Coastal Insurance,* Cal. Sup. Ct., San Francisco; AIDS Lit. Rptr., Jan. 13, 1989.

141. *National Gay Rights Advocates and David Hurlibert v. Great Republic Insurance,* Cal. Sup. Ct., San Francisco; AIDS Lit. Rptr., Oct. 18, 1988.

142. *Charon v. First Columbia Life Insurance,* Ill. Cir. Ct., Cook County, Chancery Div., June 7, 1988; ACLU.

143. *Murphy v. State Farm Insurance,* Cal. Sup. Ct., Alameda County; AIDS Lit. Rptr., June 10, 1988.

144. *Kraemer v. Time Insurance,* Ill. Cir. Ct., Cook County, Ch. 87CHO7208, July 23, 1987; ACLU.

145. *Pinney v. Aetna Life Insurance,* Sup. Ct., N.Y. County, No. 2828, Mar. 1986; ACLU.

146. *Doe v. Connecticut Mutual Life Insurance,* Mass. Sup. Ct., Suffolk County, No. 88-6453-C; Lambda.

147. *Starkey v. Arvida Corp.,* Fla. Commission on Human Rights; AIDS Lit. Rptr., Mar. 11, 1988.

148. *National Gay Rights Advocates v. Health America,* Cal. Dept. of Corporations, Nov. 7, 1986.

149. *Note: Insurance Discrimination Cases Handled by the San Francisco AIDS Legal Referral Panel,* Annual Rpts. 1987, 1988.

150. Discrimination: Cases from four civil rights agencies
Federal Office of Civil Rights, Department of Health and Human Services
San Francisco Human Rights Commission
Los Angeles Office of the City Attorney
New York City Human Rights Commission

The History of Transfusion AIDS: Practice and Policy Alternatives

Harvey M. Sapolsky and
Stephen L. Boswell

The relatively small threat of contracting AIDS through blood transfusions in the United States has led to significant improvements in the overall quality of American blood services, nearly all of which could have been achieved without the existence of this new health menace. Nonautologous exposures to blood are always hazardous. Transfusions save lives, but they can also transmit life-threatening diseases. Transfusion recipients are not alone in being endangered. Health care personnel are placed at risk through accidental blood spills and needlesticks. However, as blood-banking service expanded in the 1960s and 1970s, the handling and use of blood became incautious. Convenience rather than safety often guided behavior. But fear of AIDS is now so great that attention has focused on efforts to reduce risk, forcing long-needed changes in medical practice.

The number of transfusions, previously increasing in the United States, has leveled off in recent years as greater care is being taken in prescribing blood. New tests for rare as well as common hazards are being applied to blood. Autologous donations, the safest kind, are up sharply. Research on blood substitutes has expanded. The handling of blood is more carefully audited. Appropriately, health care personnel worry about their exposures to blood. Witness the increased use of gloves and masks whenever contact with blood is possible.[1]

These and other precautions have reduced the risk of disease transmission, including the transmission of AIDS, but they have not eliminated it. The tests are not perfect; medical mistakes and accidents still happen. The risk of contracting AIDS through transfusion may grow if the disease spreads, as some still predict, from the current high-risk groups to the general population, further contaminating the pool of available blood donors.

Irrespective of the actual risk, the search for increased safety caused by the fear of AIDS alone may be sufficient to alter drastically the structure of blood banking. In the United States, and nearly everywhere else, the provision of blood for transfusions is largely a community responsibility. Voluntary donors give blood for those in need without personal knowledge of the recipient and without direct monetary reward. But several of the remaining ways in which the safety of transfusions can be enhanced would require the breaking of these bonds of community, improving chances for some recipients while perhaps harming those for others. Individual gain at the potential expense of the community is not uncommon in society. In this instance, however, the gains and losses are measured in lives.

AIDS IN THE BLOOD SUPPLY: DIFFERING PERCEPTIONS OF RISK

The first case of immune deficiency linked to blood products was reported in a Florida hemophiliac in January 1982.[2] Although the man's death precluded the elimination of other possible causes of his immune deficiency, and made his exclusion from known risk groups problematic, it nonetheless generated great concern, especially among the epidemiologists at the Centers for Disease Control (CDC). By July two more cases had been documented: the first in a Denver hemophiliac; the second in a hemophiliac living in Ohio.[3] That same month the *Morbidity and Mortality Weekly Report,* a weekly publication of the CDC, reported the case histories of these three hemophiliacs.[4] What until that time had been viewed as a problem of sexually active gay and bisexual men, intravenous drug users, and Haitians had suddenly also become an important problem for those who received blood products.

It was not long thereafter that the first transfusion-related AIDS case was reported in an infant. The infant was transfused at the University of California at San Francisco for Rh incompatibility at two weeks of age and had died of profound immune suppression at twenty months. One of the units of blood that the child received was from a donor who at the time of his donation was well but who died of AIDS eighteen months later. A second transfusion case was discovered three days after the announcement of the first.[5] The donor, a man with a history of intravenous drug use, had given blood during a blood drive conducted by the New York Blood Center.

What was becoming clear by the end of 1982 was that AIDS was caused by a transmissible agent that behaved very similarly to hepatitis B. It could be sexually transmitted, and it was endemic in many of the same groups as was the hepatitis virus, especially gay men and intravenous drug users. As with hepatitis B, the agent appeared to have a carrier state in which individuals were unaware of their infection or the potential danger their donation represented to others. Individuals so infected appeared well, and thus were able to donate blood and plasma without remonstration. In fact, because bacteria and protozoa can be easily separated from blood products during their preparation, it seemed increasingly likely that the cause of AIDS was a virus, the only organism small enough to pass through the filters used in preparing many blood products, as hepatitis viruses had already clearly demonstrated.

Weighing this evidence, the CDC epidemiologists began warning representatives of the several blood-banking organizations that the blood supply was possibly being contaminated with AIDS. These discussions culminated in a meeting in Atlanta in early January 1983, at which proposals were presented to screen out from the blood donor pool members of high-risk groups. Since the AIDS antibody test was then not available, members of high-risk groups would have to self-identify through questionnaires and/or interviews.[6]

Blood banking in the United States is divided into two distinct sectors, and so too was the response to the screening proposals. The plasma sector, which is controlled by a handful of large pharmaceutical firms and which pays its blood donors, indicated its intention to adopt screening protocols that included direct questioning of potential donors about sexual preferences, AIDS symptoms, and contact with individuals diagnosed with AIDS.[7] In fact, Alpha Therapeutics Corporation, a major plasma collector, had already stopped procuring plasma in Los Angeles, New York, and San Francisco—major epicenters of the AIDS epidemic—in late 1982; and two weeks before the meeting, it had begun interrogating donors at all other collection sites about their membership in high-risk groups.[8] One of the main uses of plasma is for the production of fractions, which are vital in the treatment of hemophilia. The American Hemophilia Association, which was also represented at the meeting, had already declared its desire that protective measures be implemented immediately. Well that it did, because hemophiliacs were

soon devastated by the AIDS virus. Clotting factors for hemophiliacs
are made from pooled plasma lots composed of as many as 5,000 donations and can be contaminated by a single AIDS virus carrier. Nearly
half of the 15,000 hemophiliacs in the United States are now infected.
Among those with the most severe form of hemophilia, who necessarily
have the greatest exposure to the clotting factor, the infection rate is
estimated to be 70 to 90 percent.[9] The effects of the contamination are
worldwide, because the United States has been the major international
supplier of plasma products.[10] With the recognition that AIDS is caused
by a virus, it has been possible to protect the hemophiliac population
from further risk by the use of a heat treatment to kill the virus in the
processing of plasma fractions.[11]

The other blood-banking sector collects and processes whole-blood
donations for transfusions and is almost entirely composed of nonprofit
regional blood centers and local hospital blood banks that do not pay
donors. Nationally, this sector is represented by three organizations with
somewhat overlapping memberships: the American Red Cross (ARC),
the American Association of Blood Banks (AABB), and the Council of
Community Blood Centers (CCBC).[12] Their representatives opposed the
screening proposal at the January 1983 meeting, arguing that evidence
was not sufficient to exclude gay men from the donor lists or to implement the use of surrogate tests such as the test for hepatitis B core antibody, which had also been proposed. The words one representative
used are often cited to show the concern expressed about disrupting
established routines: "We are contemplating all these wide-ranging
measures because one baby got AIDS after a transfusion from a person
who later came down with AIDS and there may be a few other cases."[13]
The whole-blood collectors feared that a linkage between AIDS and the
blood supply would significantly reduce both blood donations and blood
transfusions. Moreover, they were annoyed by the intrusion of risk-
averse epidemiologists into their professional domain. The opposition
of the whole-blood collectors delayed governmental action intended to
reduce the risks of AIDS transmission through transfusions. It was not
until March 1983 that the Centers for Disease Control made public the
recommendations for widespread screening.[14] This public announcement forced the banks to begin excluding high-risk donors.

Structural differences help explain the inconsistent responses to AIDS
within blood banking. The whole-blood sector relies on voluntary donors. Women and minorities give less frequently than do young white
males. In several cities the gay community provided a readily accessible,

often organized population of young white males to solicit for donations. Through repeated campaigns the blood banks had built good relations with the gay community and found it to be a convenient source
of donations. Many gays regarded the call for screening as scapegoating
and saw in it a threat to their recently won civil liberty gains.[15] Sensitive
to the concerns of the gay community, some influential blood bankers
were reluctant to force the exclusion of gays and doubted the effectiveness of direct questioning of donors to achieve that exclusion. In contrast, plasma collectors pay their donors. If one group of donors were
excluded, another would be found quickly to maintain the supply. Their
relationship with donors was simply a financial one, with no attempt to
build long-term trust or mutual support.

The plasma sector is also highly competitive; its products are inter-
changeable among manufacturers and are marketed internationally. The
buyers of these products are knowledgeable about quality differences,
some being government medical agencies and other individuals who
must be in constant contact with medical specialists because of their
illness. The firm with a demonstrably safer product would rapidly gain
business.[16] Once donor screening was suggested as a possibility for reducing the risk of transmitting AIDS, plasma collectors had no choice
but to adopt it on the fear that one of them would.

The whole-blood sector lacks many of these characteristics. It is
dominated by nonprofit blood-collecting agencies that are local monopolists, supplying all or nearly all of the blood transfused within a given
region. Blood quality in transfusions is more the responsibility of the
supplier than it is of the purchasing hospitals. Nationally, the Red Cross,
the AABB, and the CCBC coordinate policies, effectively cartelizing the
whole-blood sector by refraining from competing with one another. A
hospital seeking an alternative to its local blood center would have difficulty obtaining services from an extraregional supplier. Although hospitals can be licensed to draw their own supply, there have been economic and professional obstacles that limit this option for most hospitals.

The structure of blood banking in the United States was altered in
the early 1970s, when—at the urging of the nonprofit collectors—the
federal government adopted policies favoring voluntary blood donations in collections for transfusions.[17] Richard Titmuss, the English sociologist, had just published a widely praised comparative analysis of
the American and British blood-banking systems, which helped focus
public attention on the risks of transfusion-related hepatitis.[18] In a devastating critique of the American system, Titmuss argued that payment

for donations significantly increased the hepatitis hazard for transfusion recipients. In Britain, where the most a donor could get for his donation was a cup of tea or a glass of stout, hepatitis was not a problem; but in the United States, where payment was permitted, the gift of life was often something else, he claimed. The nonprofit collectors, under pressure to improve the safety of transfusions, promoted this view, inaccurate though it was; they sought the elimination of commercial collectors, as well as the elimination of payment for donors from the whole-blood sector.

The critique was quite misleading, because transfusion hepatitis rates do not correlate well with donor payment. Sweden pays all its donors but has a low hepatitis rate. Japan switched in the 1960s from a largely paid donor system to an exclusively voluntary one without greatly altering its high hepatitis rate. The low rate that Titmuss observed in Britain probably had more to do with the fact that British blood is transfused there than the fact that British donors are unpaid. Incredibly, Titmuss failed to mention the extra precautions that the British transfusion service took to keep the hepatitis rates down. It has avoided collections in areas with large concentrations of immigrants from Third World countries, where hepatitis is endemic. It also has labeled blood donations by race and did not transfuse the blood donated by Pakistani, African, and other immigrants. In addition, Titmuss ignored the fact that some of the leading medical institutions in the United States, the Mayo Clinic and the Massachusetts General Hospital among them, paid donors but had low hepatitis transfusion rates as a result of careful donor-screening practices.[19]

Ironically, paid donations were not a major factor in American blood collections by the early 1970s because the commercial collectors, which did most of the paying, had already shifted their attention to the plasma market, which was rapidly growing due to the discovery of important plasma products. Plasma donations are more demanding in terms of donor time, and usually require compensation. Federal policies encouraging voluntary donations for transfusion merely assured the nonprofits that competition from commercial collectors would remain limited. The nonprofits attempted to consolidate their position further through a cooperative program of regionalization that certified dominant collectors as monopoly suppliers in designated areas.[20]

Not surprisingly, these actions had little effect on the national hepatitis rate. Like AIDS, hepatitis is a complex scientific problem that has eluded a quick solution.[21] Research on control techniques continued during the 1970s, but the nonprofits devoted much energy to reducing their responsibility for the continuing presence of hepatitis in the blood supply. They persuaded the federal government and some state governments to require the labeling of blood by donor source, either paid or volunteer, with the implication that the transfusion of paid donor blood held a special legal liability for the transfusing agent. At the same time, they obtained legislation in nearly all states designating blood a service rather than a product, thus exempting themselves from liability other than for negligence when hepatitis or any other disease is transmitted via transfusion. Because they set their own practice standards, through professional organizations with relatively little governmental supervision, negligence itself becomes difficult to prove.[22]

The nonprofit blood banks hold a unique position in American medicine. They are protected from commercial competition, exempt from most consumer suits, and free to divide geographical markets among themselves. As economists often remind us, monopolists prefer the quiet life free from public scrutiny. When the AIDS crisis appeared, the blood bankers' inclination was essentially to deny that it was a major threat to blood safety. A week after the Atlanta meeting, the ARC, the AABB, and the CCBC issued a joint statement arguing that the evidence regarding the transmissibility of AIDS via transfusions was "inconclusive" and "incomplete."[23] The only screening they advocated was much less intense than that employed by the plasma sector. Specifically, potential donors would be given brochures describing AIDS symptoms and would be asked to sign forms indicating that people with AIDS or in contact with AIDS victims should not donate, but they would not be directly questioned about their sexual preferences. And when the AIDS antibody test was developed in 1985, the associations jointly proclaimed it to be entirely sufficient to protect the blood supply. There was no longer a need to worry about getting AIDS through transfusions, they implied. Unlike many in the society who have sought to exploit public fears about AIDS, the nonprofit blood bankers have continually offered reassurance that all was safe despite AIDS.[24]

THE SEARCH FOR SAFER TRANSFUSIONS

Despite the reassurance offered by the national associations, some professionals recognized that the blood supply would be increasingly contaminated unless immediate action was taken. The screening of donors alone would not protect transfusion recipients. A screening test for blood was needed. Until a direct test for the AIDS virus was developed, a surrogate test was required. Dr. E. Engleman, medical director of the Stanford University Blood Bank, was the first to try such a test. A research hematologist whose interest focused on a type of blood cell known as a lymphocyte, Engleman stood apart from the pathologists-turned-administrators who were usually in charge of blood banks in the United States. He noted that people with AIDS and many individuals in high-risk groups who appeared well had abnormalities in their T cells, a subset of lymphocytes. Aware of the growing evidence of a long incubation for AIDS, Engleman proposed using a T-cell test to screen donations for AIDS-infected units. His attempts to gain support for the T-cell test among fellow blood bankers were frustrated, the argument being that the benefits of costly surrogate testing could not be proven—as indeed they could not be until an actual test for the virus was developed.

Engleman nevertheless instituted the test at Stanford. In one dramatic incident the Stanford bank discarded a unit from a person who had donated thirteen times in the San Francisco Bay area before being diagnosed as having AIDS. The T-cell test had rejected the unit given at Stanford, but the other dozen units were transfused elsewhere. When the AIDS antibody test finally became available, it was learned that 5 percent of blood discarded at Stanford was HIV positive, whereas only 0.01 percent of blood donated by individuals with normal T cells was positive. Thus, HIV-positive donors were 500 times more frequent in the group with T-cell abnormalities than in those with no abnormalities.[25]

Admittedly, the T-cell test was difficult to administer and relatively expensive. Other surrogate tests were also suggested for use in screening the blood supply to prevent transfusion-related AIDS. Unlike the T-cell test, which discriminated among units of blood on the basis of abnormalities closely associated with AIDS or the preclinical stages of the disease, these tests sought evidence of past infections, which occurred frequently in those at risk for AIDS. Chief among them was the hepatitis B core antibody test, which utilized equipment already available at most blood banks and was not especially costly.

The Food and Drug Administration's Blood Products Advisory Committee studied the issues pertaining to screening the blood supply in early 1984, concluding that surrogate testing, and most specifically the hepatitis B core antibody test, was not appropriate as a means of identifying those at high risk for developing AIDS because it screened out too much of the blood supply. The incidence of hepatitis in the United

States was much higher than the perceived incidence of HIV infection (AIDS) in 1984. To exclude large numbers of individuals because these individuals are at higher risk of transmitting AIDS, it was argued, would add significantly to the cost of blood and blood products. The blood banks not only would incur the cost of this testing but also would be faced with the added cost of recruiting more donors and processing additional blood to replace the discarded units. Irwin Memorial Blood Bank in San Francisco estimated that the use of the test for antibodies to the hepatitis B core antigen would result in a 5 to 7 percent increase in deferrals.[26]

The committee did recommend that small-scale experiments be conducted with another test, beta-2 microglobulin, a cell surface glycoprotein present on certain human immune cells and found in elevated concentration among patients with AIDS. This test, it concluded, seemed to be more specific for blood that might transmit AIDS. Very much aware of costs, the committee sought a test that would incorrectly exclude as few units of blood as possible. Less attention was given to the issue of test sensitivity—the ability to identify as many of the infectious units as possible.

The flaw in this thinking is that high-risk, asymptomatic individuals who would later develop AIDS could still donate blood. It was known at the time that beta-2 microglobulin seemed to be elevated with increased frequency in those with AIDS. However, little was known about the test's behavior in those who were asymptomatic but at high risk. If, as many suspected, there is a long latent period before the onset of symptoms, and if beta-2 microglobulin is elevated only in the later stages of AIDS, then large numbers of potentially infectious individuals might be missed. The committee seemed to be arguing that in the tradeoff between sensitivity and specificity, which always occurs when screening tests are employed, test specificity is of greater importance. Put another way, if surrogate tests were going to be employed, the committee desired that the added costs of those tests be borne by those who receive the blood rather than those who process it. These added costs would be measured in lives lost rather than in dollars spent.

In spite of the committee's recommendations, some nonprofit blood banks and several plasma companies began to employ surrogate tests for AIDS. In large part these decisions were made because of growing public pressure on the blood industry to take aggressive steps to protect the blood supply, but other factors also played a role in these decisions. The concern over the growing threat of lawsuits arising from transfusion-associated AIDS contributed greatly to the increase in surrogate testing. As was pointed out earlier, competition among the various companies in the plasma sector also added to the use of surrogate tests. In fact, in at least one case, competition among nonprofit blood banks may have contributed to the wider adoption of surrogate testing. San Francisco's Irwin Memorial Blood Bank adopted the hepatitis B core antibody test, in part, because of perceived differences in quality between the blood in its possession and blood from nearby Stanford University Blood Bank, where the T-cell test was being used.[27]

The pressure to employ surrogate testing was largely mitigated when the Department of Health and Human Services announced on April 23, 1984, that the cause of AIDS had been identified. With the identification of the offending agent, a virus, came a promise that a blood test would be "widely available within about six months," which should "identify AIDS victims with essentially 100 percent certainty."[28] One year later, in March 1985, the Food and Drug Administration licensed antibody kits that were able to identify those exposed to the AIDS virus with 93 to 99 percent certainty.

Surrogate testing was not the only issue around which controversy centered. Early in the epidemic calls for directed donation were often heard. The calls emanated from patients and their families, and in some locations led to the development of "blood clubs."[29] "Directed donation" means that the potential recipient of blood designates those who will be allowed to donate on his or her behalf. By its very nature, directed donation cannot be employed in every situation where a transfusion is necessary. For example, virtually all situations where the need for blood cannot be anticipated are not amenable to this kind of donation. However, with proper planning many transfusions could be accomplished within the framework of directed donations.

Many nonprofit blood bankers opposed the widespread use of directed donations. In opposing it, they cited four points. First, they argued that there was no reason to expect that directed donation was any safer than the traditional anonymous system. But this contention was incorrect, and the blood bankers knew it. Many obvious criteria could be used to decrease one's risk of being transfused with HIV-positive blood. One obvious criterion, for example, might be to select women as donors, since women were far less likely to have been exposed to HIV than were men. Further, at the time the argument that directed donations were no safer than regular donations was being made, a prominent East Coast blood banker had on the wall of his office a map displaying the relative risk of various blood-transmitted diseases by zip code of the donor's residence. There were wide and predictable variations based on this criterion. Clearly, there were ways to affect one's risk of receiving HIV-tainted blood, and most of them were readily available to those who wished to utilize a directed donor program.

Second, those who opposed directed donations argued that patients would place great pressure on those they selected to donate on their behalf, and that this pressure would cause donors to be untruthful about their ability to meet donor requirements. What the blood bankers did not acknowledge was that this problem already existed in the anonymous system. Many of the techniques developed by blood bankers a decade earlier to increase the supply of blood facilitated this kind of pressure. Blood drives at schools, work, and other social gatherings were far more successful because of the peer pressure created within these social contexts. In fact, many blood bankers had already recognized the adverse effect such peer pressure might have on donor behavior and in early 1984 began to establish twenty-four-hour telephone lines so that donors who deemed themselves at higher risk of HIV infection and later regretted having donated could confidentially ask that their blood not be used for transfusion.[30] Further, most blood banks that employed directed donation did not allow the recipient of the donation to know whose blood was actually used. Thus, the patient would never know that a high-risk individual whom he had solicited as a directed donor had excluded his blood from human use.

Third, the blood bankers argued that directed donation would be more costly than the anonymous system already in place. Costs, however, depend on one's perspective. The costs of concern to the blood banker are not the costs perceived by society as a whole or by the individual who receives a unit of HIV-positive blood. Even when viewed from the perspective of the blood banker, however, a system of directed donation would not necessarily be more costly. In 1984 an article published in the *New England Journal of Medicine* cast doubt on the blood bankers' assertion when Thomas Jefferson University's blood bank analyzed its nascent directed donor program—a program initiated largely at the insistence of cardiac surgeons who feared the migration of patients if directed donation were not available. Contrary to the arguments put forth in the communiqué from the AABB, the ARC, and the CCBC, the researchers who analyzed the program found that it "resulted in savings to the institution of $4,142 in four months. The annual figure is $12,426—a substantial reduction in operating expenditures."[31] These savings, in part a result of decreased recruitment costs, run counter to the argument put forth by the nonprofit blood bankers and suggest that, in addition to improving the quality of the blood supply, directed donation might decrease its costs as well.

Fourth, the blood bankers contended that directed donation would result in de facto discrimination against those who are socially isolated. In particular, they argued that the poor and the elderly would be adversely affected in a two-tiered blood supply. That is, the use of directed donors would undermine the ability of blood banks to find anonymous donors, and the resulting burdens would fall disproportionately on those who found it difficult to locate directed donors. This contention assumes that directed donation will adversely affect the anonymous donor pool, which is not necessarily the case. Although it is undoubtedly true that some participants in a directed donor program would have previously been anonymous donors, it is incorrect to assume that all directed donors would have previously donated. To the extent that directed donors have not participated in the anonymous pool, the blood they donate represents additional blood that would not have been available without a directed donor program. And to the extent that the blood donated in this fashion is safer than anonymously donated blood, the overall quality of the blood supply improves. There are three possible scenarios.

The first scenario is one in which the individual who donates in a directed donor program has never been an anonymous donor. The overall effect of this individual's donation will be to increase the availability of blood within the anonymous system. In the second, the donor has previously been an anonymous donor and the directed donation withdraws blood from the anonymous pool temporarily. In this situation the donation would have no net impact on the overall supply of blood. However, the additional blood donated by those who were not previously blood donors would increase the available blood within the anonymous pool. In the final scenario the donor has previously been an anonymous donor but, in order to remain eligible to give blood should an emergency arise for a friend or family member, he or she elects to refrain from anonymous donation permanently. The extent to which this is a realistic concern is uncertain. In order for it to have an adverse effect on overall blood availability, however, the loss of blood as a consequence of this phenomenon would have to outweigh the amount of blood gained from those who did not previously participate in the anonymous donor system.

Regardless of the comparative safety of blood obtained by directed
donation vis-à-vis blood that is anonymously donated, a strong directed
donation program would not a priori result in additional costs to the
blood banker, as the Thomas Jefferson University's blood bank was
quick to realize. Further, the actual risk of contracting AIDS from a
blood transfusion may be only one factor in the patient's well-being.
Los Angeles' Cedars-Sinai Hospital concluded that "we function with a
philosophy that incorporates a concern for the patient's psychological
responses to illness, as well as his need for blood. . . . [B]y providing
these very frightened patients with knowledge that the blood to be received is from their chosen donors . . . we enhance their general well-
being and eventual recovery."[32]

As time has passed, pressure in favor of directed donation has grown.
Legislators in several states—Florida and Georgia were two early examples—have introduced bills requiring blood banks to accept the
practice. Irwin Memorial Blood Bank, located in San Francisco, one of
the metropolitan areas hardest hit by the AIDS epidemic, adopted such
a program in June 1984.[33] Its variation reflected the disdain the blood
bank harbored for the concept. Irwin advised patients "that blood from
directed (family and friend) donors is at best no safer than blood from
other volunteer donors [and] there is actually a danger that direct donations may be less safe."[34] Patients desiring directed donation were
required to have their physicians place the request for blood at least one
week prior to the anticipated transfusion. An additional charge of $15
was assessed against each directed donor. The actual donation had to
occur on a second visit, thus making it more inconvenient for the directed donor.

In contrast to the controversy surrounding directed donation, one
source of blood was recognized as inarguably safer than blood obtained
from other individuals—either through directed donation or anonymous donation. A rarity prior to AIDS, autologous transfusions—
achieved through either the predeposit of blood or its intraoperative
salvage—now account for as much as 2 percent of blood usage and are
growing in popularity.[35] Blood banks had not encouraged the practice,
despite the safety advantages offered patients who can anticipate their
need for blood and who are healthy enough to provide the donation.
Autologous collections cause inventory complications for blood banks
and contradict their donor recruitment message that blood is a community responsibility. But the fear of AIDS among patients and sur-

geons has left the banks with little choice other than to advocate the maximum possible use of autologous donations.

RISKS REMAIN

About 3 percent of the AIDS cases recorded in the United States are attributed to the therapeutic exchange of blood. The AIDS toll is certain to grow, but not likely the transfusion-related share of that toll. The AIDS antibody test provides an important, although imperfect, defense against the spread of the disease through blood services. So, too, do improvements in medical practice.

The number of units of whole blood and red cells transfused annually in the United States, which peaked at approximately 12 million units in 1986 after years of steady growth, is now declining.[36] In the absence of a national blood data system, precise figures are not available; but estimates are that in 1987, the most recent year for which there are complete data, the rate of red cell transfusion was 15 percent lower than could have been expected if the historic growth in transfusion rates had been sustained.[37] The growing tendency in many medical centers is to avoid transfusion unless defined need criteria are met. It is becoming less common for a physician to order a unit of blood to put the blush back into the cheeks of a patient about to be discharged from a hospital. And physicians and patients think harder than they once did about the risks of transfusions when considering surgery.

Ultimately, it is the AIDS test that guards transfusions. Not all uses of blood can be avoided, nor can all recipients provide for themselves. When someone else's blood is to be transfused, safety depends on the effectiveness of the screen. In AIDS testing, as in testing for many other diseases, the screen is less than perfect. Some infected units will get through.[38]

The most commonly used screening test for AIDS is the enzyme-linked immunosorbent assay (ELISA). Blood bank procedures require each donated unit to be screened by the ELISA test immediately after collection. Positive units are often rescreened. If the rescreening test is also positive, the unit is usually considered unusable and not transfused. (Many, but not all, blood centers discard initially reactive units, even though this status is not predictive of the disease.) A confirming test, usually the Western blot, is performed before the donor is notified of a positive status. Most ELISA positives turn out to be false positives.[39] The ELISA screen is purposely set low so as to eliminate as many dangerous units as possible. The intent of this process, however, is that some blood pass the screen in order that there will be blood for transfusions. A perfect screen for a low-incidence population, such as blood donors under current conditions, would mean substantially reduced blood availability. As it is, nearly 1 percent of donated blood is discarded on the chance that it might be HIV infected.[40]

For the potential recipient the issue is not how many units are discarded but how many infected units are passed into inventory and transfused. As a result of technican error, faulty test batches, or mishandled units, some HIV-infected units will get through. More significantly, the AIDS screen as an antibody test has inherent limitations. One problem is that infected individuals do not immediately produce antibodies to HIV. Several weeks will pass before antibodies begin appearing in the blood of a virus carrier. Those in the terminal stage of the disease may also be antibody free. There are also reports of a few victims who do not produce detectable antibodies in the middle stages of the disease.[41] Absent the use of a test for the HIV viral antigen, which is under consideration, there will always be some false negatives as long as infected individuals donate blood. And some potentially infected individuals will continue to donate, if only because blood banks unintentionally provide a convenient and confidential way to discover one's antibody status. The question then becomes: How many infected units pass into the blood supply and cause AIDS?

Several factors complicate the calculation of the blood-related AIDS transmission rate. Not all collected blood is transfused; upward of 10 percent of the units are discarded because they are outdated. Transfusion recipients are often severely ill; as many as half die immediately or shortly after the transfusion because of their underlying condition. Not every infection necessarily will produce a defined AIDS case; AIDS-related complex, milder infirmity, or no disease may result. And the incubation period for AIDS may be longer than ten years; consequently, not all cases contracted since the antibody screen was implemented have yet been identified.

Blood bankers, concerned about the impact that fear of AIDS was having on public confidence in the safety of the blood supply, were overenthusiastic about the effectiveness of the antibody test and proclaimed its arrival as ensuring the total elimination of HIV infection risk from blood use.[42] Since then they have had to acknowledge the test's inherent limitations and to revise their estimates of the continuing AIDS risk in transfusions. At first the rate was cited as 1 in a million. Then it was 1 in 300,000. Still later it was 1 in 100,000.[43] Currently it is listed as between 1 in 10,000 and 1 in 100,000, although some researchers claim it is as high as 1 in 5,000.[44] Given approximately three and a half million transfusions, that means there are between 35 and 700 new cases each year still being transmitted through the blood supply.

AIDS, of course, is not the only hazard of transfusions. Several thousand transfusion hepatitis cases, most of the elusive type C, are transmitted each year, with a significant fatality rate. HIV-2, a virus related to the AIDS agent, has been detected in blood, although not yet in great frequency. The human T-cell leukemia/lymphoma virus, HTLV-1, has also been found in the United States blood supply, with a transmission rate that is much greater than that of HIV-2. A screening test for HTLV-1 was instituted in early 1989. A test for hepatitis C became available in 1990. Other screening tests are in development, but their efficaciousness has not been determined.[45] Not surprisingly, there is still much public fear about the safety of the blood supply, a fear that affects potential donors even though they are not at all threatened directly by these transfusion dangers.[46] Donations are down by about 6 percent, and in some regions a supply crisis has been averted only because usage has also declined.

Science can make transfusions safer. Better tests and the development of vaccines will help, but the significant gains will be in the introduction of blood substitutes, artificially produced substances that can duplicate the life-sustaining traits of blood components. Helpful, too, will be the use of recombinant human growth factors to stimulate the endogenous production of various blood cell lines.[47] Chief among these new hormones is erythropoietin, which can stimulate the production of red blood cells in certain individuals.[48] Much work along these lines is under way, enhanced by the accumulating progress being recorded in biotechnology. When they occur, the advances may alter the structure of blood banking and eliminate the need for recruiting and screening blood donors. Given its emphasis on research, Genentech or some other biotechnology firm is more likely to be the supplier of the substitutes than are the American Red Cross and the other traditional blood collectors.

SEEKING GREATER SAFETY

Even without a breakthrough in synthetic blood research, the structure of blood banking seems certain to change. The fear of AIDS, disproportional though it may be to the actual risk, is sufficient among transfusion recipients and medical staffs to force a continuing search for alternatives to the random draw from the community blood donor pool. Provision of autologous donations, however, is likely to satisfy no more than 10 percent of the demand for blood, because of the unpredictability of individual need and because of the frailty of many recipients. The search then will be for safer homologous sources. At least three exist, each of which threatens blood banking as it is currently structured.

One is directed donations, in which donors provide blood to designated recipients, usually friends or relatives, who actively solicit their contributions. As was mentioned, blood bankers have generally opposed this form of donation because it undermines the basic ideology of the blood system: that blood banks serve the community rather than individuals, operating like a community charity rather than a bank with individual accounts. But—as demonstrated in insurance, schools, and other social systems—individuals and groups often have much to gain by withdrawing from community pools. This should be especially true for achieving isolation from a disease focused in defined groups that are separated from most of the rest of the population.[49]

A second alternative is to obtain blood for transfusions from locations that have a very low AIDS incidence. This already occurs to some extent in the United States, because high-donating rural areas subsidize low-donating urban areas in most regions. It is also the unintended by-product of a little-publicized program that imports red cells from Switzerland and Germany to New York City, where a chronic blood shortage exists because of inadequate donor recruitment. The Swiss and German Red Crosses overbleed their populations to obtain sufficient supplies of plasma for domestic processing. As a result, they produce a surplus of several hundred thousand red cell units, which they ship to the New York Blood Center in exchange for blood-processing equipment, deftly avoiding the embarrassment that a transfer of cash would involve.[50] Further extension of such programs would increase the safety of the blood supply in many American cities but would require recognition that the concept of community responsibility for blood is inadequate or at least requires substantial expansion.

A third alternative is to expand donor exclusion so that other high-risk groups will be prevented from contributing to the blood supply. Such an expansion of donor exclusion criteria was recently proposed by the Food and Drug Administration when it suggested that Haitians be banned from donating blood. The reasons for the FDA's proposal were straightforward. First, the Haitian community has a much higher prevalence of HIV infection than the United States population as a whole.[51] The FDA argues that, since the blood test for HIV is not 100 percent accurate, a disproportionate fraction of HIV-infected Haitian blood will enter the blood supply. Second, the FDA argues that adequate screening of Haitian donors is not possible, because heterosexual intercourse is believed to be the primary mode of transmission among Haitians.[52] Fearing the loss of large numbers of potentially safe donors, blood banks do not currently screen people who have multiple heterosexual partners.

The proposal to eliminate Haitian blood donors created great controversy and led to numerous protests around the country, including a march by more than 100,000 people in New York City. Although the Haitian donor ban may decrease the risk of transfusion AIDS in the United States, the decrease comes with a price. The price of such a plan is borne disproportionately by the communities affected. There is, of course, a precedent. The gay community, one of the first groups recognized to be at increased risk of HIV infection, is largely excluded as well. The net effect of expanding the donor exclusion criteria is to further diminish the notion of community responsibility for blood.

Paying donors is yet another option that is likely to be considered in order to reduce the risk of AIDS transmission in transfusions. The use of direct financial incentives, of course, would reverse federal policies favoring voluntary—that is, noncash—donations established in the 1970s and strongly supported by the nonprofit collectors. But, as was previously mentioned, several of the nation's leading medical institutions once used cash payments to create panels of frequently tested and monitored blood donors to protect against transfusion hepatitis. Today the same procedures could be used to recruit more women, middle-aged donors, or other donors who are less likely to harbor HIV or to engage in high-risk behavior.

Paying blood donors is an anathema to nonprofit collectors, who argue that money is a corrupting force in blood banking, tempting both the collector and the donor to conceal the truth about the quality of the blood they supply. Ignored is the fact that some voluntary donors currently receive substantial cash-equivalent rewards in the form of extra vacation days and time off from work and that blood banks sell blood and other products to hospitals for cash. Confusing blood bankers' arguments against payments, directed donations, and increased imports

are their concerns about the future of blood banking. Each of the reform proposals holds potential for increased competition from hospitals and commercial blood collectors, which are likely to be responsive
to the real or imagined fears of transfusion recipients and medical staffs
about the safety of blood. But there is a more compelling public policy
question: How will attempts to reduce the risks of transfusions affect
those who may not be able to take advantage of the additional protections made possible by implementing the proposals and who therefore
must rely on the community supply of blood?

Titmuss claimed that blood-banking systems are symbolic of the relationships favored within a society. Voluntary systems, he believed,
encourage altruism and strengthen the bonds of community, because
these systems are based on the giving by one stranger to save another.
Payment systems, he thought, destroy community by creating a market
in the gift of life. Titmuss did not discuss directed donations, but he
would undoubtedly view them as divisive and dangerous, replacing trust
among strangers with tribal and family-defined selfishness.

However, the problem we face today is that disease can spread by
either altruistic or selfish acts. Not every carrier is aware of his or her
exposure to the virus. Tests provide no guarantee that the uncompen-
sated gift from a stranger is safer than the compensated gift from a
stranger. The random draw from the community blood pool can be
quite hazardous, depending on the pool's composition. Titmuss was
mistaken in believing that voluntary donations would eliminate the
hepatitis problem. We have no assurance that voluntary blood donations will protect absolutely against AIDS.

Frightened people will seek to protect themselves. Better public understanding of AIDS will surely reduce fears, but it will not eliminate
them. Small risks as well as large risks encourage avoidance. Physicians,
entrepreneurs, and policy analysts are certain to inform us how that
avoidance can be achieved. The reality is that neither the fear nor the
risk of transfusion-transmitted AIDS will disappear.

Some cannot fend for themselves when fending is required. The elderly, the poor, and the friendless are most vulnerable in systems that
permit payment and directed donations. But donor payments may actually decrease blood collection costs by reducing recruitment expenditures and blood wastage. Much, although not all, blood use is financed
through insurance and public benefit programs. Increased costs, if there
are any, can be absorbed by adjusting reimbursement levels or through
charity drives. More difficult, if this blood collection method becomes
common, is the identification of directed donors for those in society

who are alone or in high-risk groups. Here churches, fraternal orders, clubs, and other voluntary organizations may be willing to provide donors for those in need. It is not clear that altruism disappears when alternative donation systems exist. Those who donate for friends and relatives may be quite ready to step forward for others as well.

The more people withdraw from the community pool by making private arrangements to protect themselves, the more likely it is that the shrinking pool will become increasingly disadvantageous for those who must continue to use it. This is the result in too many institutions, urban public schools being but the most dramatic example. A cartel of nonprofit organizations is not sufficient to manage this problem, because they tend to deny the risks and fears that drive people from the community-based arrangement. Blood banking needs to be made more responsive to the public's concerns if it is to retain broad support.

One possibility would be to remove the exemption from strict liability standards that blood banks have obtained in most jurisdictions. The purveyors of nearly all other products in the United States are held strictly liable for faults that cause illness or death independent of any negligent acts in product preparation or distribution. With the burden of liability shifted back to the blood banks, they would soon adopt one or more of the methods previously described that would reduce the hazards of transfusions. Protections that are certain to be available for some could be made available for all.

Another possibility would be for the federal government to encourage interregional and international transfers of blood. In a focused epidemic some areas suffer more than others. The task then is to even the risks of transfusion transmissions among locations. Surgical candidates in New York, Newark, or San Francisco need not suffer greater risks of contracting AIDS simply because New York, Newark, and San Francisco are especially burdened by AIDS. Like other disaster victims, they should expect government-directed assistance from those who are spared or at least less threatened.

The measure of community is not the sharing of risks but the effective management of hazards that may or may not be evenly distributed within a population. There are opportunities to reduce anxiety and risk for all, but we cannot realize these opportunities by denying the existence of dangers or ignoring the possibility of risk avoidance. Instead, to seize these opportunities we must acknowledge and use the many motivations that guide behavior in society, altruism being only one of them.

The justification in the United States for favoring community responsibility for blood has been that it was safer. But that is not the case in at least some locations. What is necessary is to make blood use safer for all, for the friend as well as for the stranger. Protecting organizations that hold small empires and convenient ideologies does not reduce the risks of transfusions or build community. Finding ways to give reassurance to those who must be transfused is the more responsive and more responsible course to serve the community.

NOTES

An earlier version of this essay, with the title "AIDS, Blood Banking and the Bonds of Community" by Harvey M. Sapolsky, appeared in *Daedalus* 118 (Spring 1989) and in Stephen R. Graubard, *Living with AIDS* (Cambridge: MIT Press, 1990), 297–308, and is reprinted with permission.

1. The precautions needed to limit exposures go beyond gloves and masks and are described in Centers for Disease Control, "Recommendations for Prevention of HIV Transmission in Health-Care Settings," *Morbidity and Mortality Weekly Report* 36, Suppl. 2S (August 21, 1987).
2. Randy Shilts, *And the Band Played On: Politics, People, and the AIDS Epidemic* (New York: St. Martin's Press, 1987).
3. Ibid.
4. *Morbidity and Mortality Weekly Report* 31 (December 10, 1982): 644–46.
5. Shilts, *And the Band Played On.*
6. William A. Clark, "Preventing AIDS Transmission: Should Blood Donors Be Screened?" *Journal of the American Medical Association* 249, no. 5 (February 4, 1983): 567–70; Andrea Rock, "Inside the Billion-Dollar Business of Blood," *Money,* March 1986, pp. 140–51; Shilts, *And the Band Played On;* Ross D. Eckert, "AIDS and the Blood Bankers," *Regulation,* September–October 1986, pp. 15–24, 54.
7. Clark, "Preventing AIDS Transmission," p. 569; "ABRA Releases Recommendation on AIDS and Plasma Donors," *CCBC Newsletter,* February 4, 1983, p. 1.
8. Alpha Therapeutics Corporation, "Press Information: Alpha Therapeutics Acts to Protect Hemophiliacs from AIDS Epidemic," January 12, 1983; D. J. Gury, "AIDS and the Paid Donor," *Lancet* 2 (1983): 575.
9. Gina Kolata, "Hemophilia and AIDS: Silent Suffering," *New York Times,* May 16, 1988, p. 1.
10. The international plasma business is discussed in Piet J. Hagen, ed., *Blood: Gift or Merchandise* (New York: Alan R. Liss, 1982).
11. Centers for Disease Control, "Safety of Therapeutic Products Used for Hemophilia Patients," *Morbidity and Mortality Weekly Report* 37 (July 29, 1988): 441–44; Margaret W. Hilgartner, "AIDS and Hemophilia," *New England Journal of Medicine* 317, no. 18 (October 29, 1987): 1153–54.
12. Alvin Drake, Stan Finkelstein, and Harvey M. Sapolsky, *The American Blood Supply* (Cambridge, Mass.: MIT Press, 1982), especially chap. 4.

13. Clark, "Preventing AIDS Transmission," p. 568.

14. Office of Biologics, U.S. Food and Drug Administration, *Recommendations to Decrease the Risk of Transmitting Acquired Immune Deficiency Syndrome (AIDS) from Blood Donors* (Washington, D.C.: FDA, March 24, 1983); Centers for Disease Control, "Prevention of Acquired Immune Deficiency Syndrome (AIDS) Report of Inter-Agency Recommendations," *Morbidity and Mortality Weekly Report* 32 (March 4, 1983): 101–3.

15. Clark, "Preventing AIDS Transmission," p. 569. See also Shilts, *And the Band Played On.*

16. Reuben A. Kessel, "Transfused Blood, Serum Hepatitis, and the Coase Theorem," *Journal of Law and Economics* 17, no. 2 (October 1974): 265–89.

17. For a more detailed analysis of the structure and performance of blood banking in the United States, see Drake et al., *American Blood Supply.*

18. Richard M. Titmuss, *The Gift Relationship: From Human Blood to Social Policy* (New York: Pantheon Books, 1971).

19. Harvey M. Sapolsky and Stan Finkelstein, "Blood Policy Revisited," *Public Interest* 46 (Winter 1977): 15–27; Comptroller General of the United States, *Hepatitis from Blood Transfusions: Evaluation of Methods to Reduce the Problem* (Washington, D.C.: General Accounting Office, February 13, 1976).

20. "As GAO Investigates, Blood Commission Seeks Regionalization," *American Medical News,* April 14, 1978, p. 1.

21. Harold M. Schmeck, Jr., "Scientists Seek Ways to Limit Lasting Harm of Hepatitis Infection," *New York Times,* May 19, 1988, p. B15; Janice Hopkins Tanne, "The Other Plague," *New York Magazine,* July 11, 1988, pp. 34–40.

22. Gilbert M. Clark, ed., *Legal Issues in Transfusion Medicine* (Arlington, Va.: American Association of Blood Banks, 1986); Lynn Shodahl, "Liability for Transfusion-Transmitted Disease," *William Mitchell Law Review* 14 (1988): 141–67; David A. Roling, "Transfusion-Associated Acquired Immunodeficiency Syndrome (AIDS): Blood Bank Liability?" *Baltimore Law Review* 16 (1986): 81–116; Stan N. Finkelstein and Harvey M. Sapolsky, "Controlling Post-Transfusion Hepatitis: A Proposal to Publicize Hepatitis Rates of Transfusion Facilities," *American Journal of Law and Medicine* 5, no. 1 (Spring 1979): 1–9; "Blood Bank Is Cleared in Colorado AIDS Case," *New York Times,* June 5, 1988, p. 29; Beth Rabkin and Michael Scott Rabkin, "Individual and Institutional Liability for Transfusion-Acquired Diseases," *Journal of the American Medical Association* 256, no. 16 (October 24, 1986): 2242–43; Patti J. Miller et al., "Potential Liability for Transfusion-Associated AIDS," *Journal of the American Medical Association* 253, no. 23 (June 21, 1985): 3419–24. On recent developments see Stuart Wasserman, "Nation's Blood Supply on Trial," *Boston Globe,* January 3, 1989, p. 1.

23. American Association of Blood Banks, American Red Cross, and Council of Community Blood Centers, Joint Statement on Acquired Immune Deficiency Syndrome (AIDS) Related to Transfusion, January 13, 1983.

24. Harvey M. Sapolsky, "AIDS and the Blood Supply: Is Honesty the Best Policy?" in *AIDS: Public Policy Dimensions* (New York: United Hospital Fund, 1987), pp. 107–14.

25. E. Engleman, "AIDS and the Blood Supply: A Report to the Presidential Commission on the Human Immunodeficiency Virus Epidemic," May 9, 1988.

26. E. J. Power, *AIDS and the San Francisco Blood Supply*, contract No. 433-4520.0 (Washington, D.C.: U.S. Congress, Office of Technology Assessment, April 1984).

27. Ibid.

28. M. Heckler, Secretary, U.S. Department of Health and Human Services, Statement announcing the discovery of the possible etiological agent for AIDS, Washington, D.C., April 23, 1984.

29. "As AIDS Scare Hits Nation's Blood Supply," *U.S. News and World Report*, July 25, 1983, p. 72.

30. "Blood Bank Opens AIDS-Risk Hotline," *Santa Ana Register*, January 10, 1984.

31. S. K. Ballas et al., "Designated Blood Donations," *New England Journal of Medicine* 310 (1984): 124.

32. L. Pura et al., "Directed Donor Program: A Three-Fold Benefit," paper presented at the 36th annual meeting of the American Association of Blood Banks, New York, November 1983.

33. "Irwin Initiates Directed Donation Program," *AABB News Briefs*, July 1984, p. 4.

34. *Blood Policy and Technology*, OTA-H-260 (Washington, D.C.: U.S. Congress, Office of Technology Assessment, January 1985).

35. D. M. Surgenor, "The Patient's Blood Is the Safest Blood," *New England Journal of Medicine* 316, no. 9 (1987): 542–44; Pearl T. C. Y. Toy et al., "Predeposited Autologous Blood for Elective Surgery," *New England Journal of Medicine* 316, no 9 (1987): 517–20; Johanna Pindyck et al., "Blood Donations by the Elderly," *Journal of the American Medical Association* 257, no. 9 (1987): 1186–88; Lawrence K. Altman, "The Safest Blood: One's Own," *New York Times*, December 2, 1986, p. C1; B. U. Anderson and P. A. Tomasulo, "Current Autologous Transfusion Practices: Implications for the Future," *Transfusion* 28, no. 4 (1988): 394–96; "Autologous Blood Transfusions: Principles, Policies and Practices," *Forum Focus* (Spring 1988): entire issue. Note also "Contact Lasers Reduce Pain, Blood Loss in Mastectomies," *Modern Healthcare*, November 1988, p. 90.

36. D. M. Surgenor et al., "Collection and Transfusion of Blood in the United States, 1982–1988," *New England Journal of Medicine* 322 (1990): 1646–51.

37. The figure for the Massachusetts General Hospital is a 25 percent reduction. See "AIDS: Out of Tragedy Comes Good," *MGH News* 46, no. 8 (November 1987): 2.

38. Don Dagani, "The Problem of Diagnostic Tests," *Chemical and Engineering News*, November 23, 1987, pp. 35–40; Deborah M. Barnes, "Keeping the AIDS Virus Out of the Blood Supply," *Science* 233 (August 1, 1986): 514–15; Philip P. Mortimer, "Serological Tests," in *Blood, Blood Products and AIDS*, ed. R. Madhok, D. D. Forbes, and B. L. Evatt (Baltimore: Johns Hopkins University Press, 1987), pp. 125–42.

39. Thomas F. Zuck, "Human T-Cell Lymphotropic Virus, Type III, Antibody Testing in the United States: Experience of the First Year," in *AIDS: The*

Safety of Blood and Blood Products, ed. J. C. Petricciani et al. (New York: Wiley, 1987), p. 221.

40. Personal communication with Michael Barry, 1989.

41. H. A. Kessler et al., "Diagnosis of Human Immunodeficient Virus Infection in Seronegative Homosexuals Presenting with an Acute Viral Syndrome," *Journal of the American Medical Association* 258 (September 4, 1987): 1196–99.

42. Lawrence K. Altman, "Blood Supply Called Free of AIDS," *New York Times,* August 1, 1985, p. 1.

43. Gerald H. Friedland and Robert S. Klein, "Transmission of the Human Immunodeficiency Virus," *New England Journal of Medicine* 317, no. 18 (October 29, 1987): 1126.

44. "AIDS Risk Cited in Donated Blood," *Boston Globe,* August 25, 1988, p. 8; J. R. Bove, "Transfusion-Associated Hepatitis and AIDS: What Is the Risk?" *New England Journal of Medicine* 317 (1987): 242–45; Philip M. Boffey, "Federal Panel Calls for Improved AIDS Test," *New York Times,* July 16, 1986, p. A20; Gina Kolata, "New Blood Test Raises Thorny Issues," *Science* 233 (July 11, 1986): 149–50.

45. "Testing for HTLV-1 Infection Should Begin among Blood Donors, Yale Researcher Tells NHLBI Panel," *The Blue Sheet* 30, no. 44 (November 4, 1987): 2; "Red Cross Plans Blood Test for Cancer Virus in Donors," *New York Times,* April 29, 1988, p. A1.

46. "AABB Public Opinion Poll Reveals Surprising Views," *AABB News Briefs* 11, no. 6 (July 1988): 1; see also "AIDS: A Multicountry Assessment," *Public Opinion* 11 (May–June 1988): 36–39.

47. J. E. Groopman, J. M. Molina, and D. T. Scaddem, "Hematopoietic Growth Factors: Biology and Clinical Applications," *New England Journal of Medicine* 321 (November 23, 1989): 1449.

48. J. W. Ischbach et al., "Recombinant Human Erythropoietin in Anemic Patients with End-Stage Renal Disease: Results of a Phase III Multicenter Clinical Trial," *Annals of Internal Medicine* 111 (1989): 992–1000.

49. The insurance analogy is discussed in two articles by Harvey M. Sapolsky: "Prospective Payment in Perspective," in *Health Policy in Transition,* ed. Laurence Brown (Durham, N.C.: Duke University Press, 1987); and "An Evaluation of the New Jersey DRG Hospital Payment System," *New Jersey Medicine* 85 (January 1988): 32–37.

50. See Drake et al., *American Blood Supply,* chap. 7, for a discussion of the "Euroblood" program. There is currently discussion of extending the program to Atlanta, which is said also to experience chronic supply problems. According to the American Blood Commission, overall blood imports are up, accounting for perhaps as much as 5 percent of the 12 million units used in the United States each year.

51. "FDA Defends Plan as Based on HIV Data but Might Re-examine," *American Medical News,* June 15, 1990, p. 3.

52. Collaborative Study Group of AIDS in Haitian-Americans, "Risk Factors for AIDS Among Haitians Residing in the United States: Evidence of Heterosexual Transmission," *Journal of the American Medical Association* 257 (February 6, 1987): 635–39.

Scientific Rigor and Medical Realities: Placebo Trials in Cancer and AIDS Research

David J. Rothman and Harold Edgar

In the recent debates on the ethics of placebo-based trials in the evaluation of new drugs to combat AIDS, a sharp line is often drawn between the need to satisfy the principles of "sound science" and the readiness to satisfy "humanitarian impulses." The proponents of sound science contend that the only procedure that will demonstrate the efficacy of a new agent is a placebo trial in a population that is randomly selected; in such a trial both the subjects and the investigators must be ignorant, or blinded, as to who is receiving the active agent and who the inert substance. Although half the subjects will receive an inactive ingredient, proponents believe that the long-term good of establishing knowledge outweighs all other considerations. Those opposed to placebo trials contend that, although the new substance is of unknown efficacy, it may work, and therefore may give persons with AIDS an opportunity, both psychological and pharmacological, to extend their lives. But an evaluation of the ethics of placebo trials in the AIDS era does not require us to pursue an either/or approach, a rigid opposition of scientific progress and compassion, with no ground between these two extremes. In fact, the choices are not so stark, mostly because the principles of sound science are not so rigid and immutable as many of its advocates insist. The placebo-based random clinical trial does not have the hegemony in drug development that its proponents suggest—and the departures from the standard have not come at the price of ignorance or malfeasance. The evidence for this proposition comes most powerfully from cancer research. The way cancer researchers have pursued drug development casts a very different light on the AIDS controversies and deserves sustained analysis.

Long before the AIDS crisis, the issue of scientific rigor and patient needs was confronted in the cancer research field, surfacing most notably in the disputes that marked the relationship of the National Cancer Institute (NCI) and the federal Food and Drug Administration (FDA). The NCI, a government-funded research organization, actively develops and tests new drugs. In formal terms it has the same relationship to the FDA that any other drug manufacturer has; that is, the drugs it develops must be licensed by the FDA before distribution. But in reality the FDA-NCI relationship is far more complicated, and the NCI generally follows special procedures that depart from FDA requirements. Probably the most important difference between the two organizations is on the matter of demonstrating drug efficacy, in effect, on the kinds of clinical trials appropriate to demonstrating efficacy.

A 1982 congressional hearing clarified these differences. The hearings were occasioned by a series of articles in the *Washington Post,* describing protocols in which cancer patients were ostensibly used as guinea pigs in research. These patients, the article contended, were receiving drugs that investigators knew were too toxic, or ineffective, and the FDA was failing to supervise or regulate their work. (Even as late as 1981, the predominant fear among outsiders was not that patients were unable to enroll in protocols but that patients would be misused by researchers.) The cancer investigators, for their part, insisted that the patients were fully informed about the risks and benefits, that drugs ineffective against one type of tumor might be effective against another type, and that high drug toxicity was unavoidable in light of the present state of knowledge. But what emerged most vividly in the course of the hearings was the shared commitment among cancer researchers to doing something, anything, for the terminally ill cancer patient. When death was the alternative, they were ready to try new and admittedly dangerous drugs on patients who wanted a shot, even a long shot, at a remission or cure, and if this commitment brought them into conflict with the FDA, or with the gold standard of random clinical trials (RCTs), so be it. The first loyalty was to the patient.

Vincent DeVita, director of the NCI, explicated this position fully. "The most serious toxicity of all," he declared in his testimony, "is the unnecessary death from cancer. . . . Any system of drug distribution we develop that denies any cancer patient access to these resources is wrong."[1] The NCI arrangements aimed to maximize distribution with-

out sacrificing oversight. New cancer drugs (all cytoxic—that is, by definition injurious to normal cells) were designated A, B, or C, with a
rough but not complete analogue to Phase I, II, III categories. Drugs in
category A were tested first on patients with advanced disease by oncologists in ten designated institutions; should any of the drugs appear
promising (by evidence of tumor shrinkage or improved quality of life),
they moved to category B, to be tested by a larger group of selected
clinical investigators on a wider range of patients. The drugs that demonstrated effectiveness were then promoted to category C, to be distributed to a still wider network of designated practicing physicians (those
sponsored by NCI grants or contracts). This distribution was akin to
the FDA's "compassionate use" procedure but was much more extensive and systematic.

Several aspects of this system made clear the extent to which cancer
drug development was treatment oriented. First, this considerable distribution of drugs took place *before* the FDA actually licensed them.
Second, drugs were moved into category A without extensive animal
tests (since they were known to be toxic). Again and again cancer researchers made the point that the true toxicity was cancer. As Dr. James
Holland of New York City's Mt. Sinai Hospital put it: "Can it be more
ethical to deny the possible good effects to most, by avoiding all toxicity
in order to do no harm to one? The unmitigated disease must be calculated as a toxic cost of cancer. Underdosing, in an attempt to avoid
toxicity, is far more deadly."[2] Third, no one at NCI disputed that
"leakage" occurred; that is, physicians who received drugs in A or B
category and did not exhaust their supply sent the remainder on to still
other physicians for use with their patients. DeVita was not very apol-
ogetic about the leakage, insisting that "sometimes patients benefit."[3]
Finally, and perhaps most important, and we will return to explore this
point in more detail later, the trials with cytoxic drugs against advanced
cancers were almost always single armed—that is, not controlled and
not placebo based.

The cancer investigators in their testimony made no secret of their
disdain for the FDA regulatory apparatus. "Innovation and regulation
are constantly in conflict," argued Dr. Emil Freireich, of the University
of Texas System Cancer Center, and formerly at the NCI. "In our country we have gone extremely to the side of regulation, much to the detriment of innovative creative science. . . . It is truly ironic that the mechanisms designed for protection create serious harm to thousands of
individuals with cancer without any potential for benefit. . . . Speaking

as a physician-scientist . . . there is continuous frustration resulting from excessive regulation. . . . It is clear that any new knowledge requires additional risk."[4] Indeed, these researchers were impatient not only with the FDA but with the idea of government paternalism, and if some of this attitude may have been the product of professionals wanting to maintain ample discretion, it also reflected a deep concern for the desperately ill patient. When Dr. John Ultmann, director of the Cancer Research Center at the University of Chicago, was asked whether in category A or Phase I studies the researchers might be sacrificing patient welfare for scientific knowledge, he insisted that "throughout this process, above all else we are doctors."[5] And when California congressman Henry Waxman invoked the need for the government "to protect the public from drugs that are going to kill them, poison them, maim them," Dr. Holland reminded him that with cancer drugs the injunction to "do no harm" was meaningless, for "all the patients who would have benefitted will be undertreated."[6]

In the immediate aftermath of the 1981 hearing, the NCI and the FDA established a joint task force. Its report, aptly titled *Anticancer Drugs: The NCI's Development and the FDA's Regulation,* spelled out further differences between the more patient-centered risk-taking procedures at the NCI and the more paternalistic and "sound science" oversight at the FDA.[7] For one, the cancer researchers were so committed to patient care that they were unwilling to continue to test a new drug against all types of tumors when the drug had shown little efficacy in its initial tumor screens. Conceding that some drugs had proven effective only against one or two types of tumors (and if the screening had not been complete, this efficacy would have been missed), the researchers were nevertheless "reluctant to enroll patients with a given tumor in a study of a drug already shown ineffective in several other tumors; they prefer, instead, to try a drug with which there is little prior experience."[8]

For another, the FDA required that, before any drug could be licensed to be used in combination therapies (together with other drugs), its own individual efficacy had to be established. By the gold standard, drug X should not be added to drugs Y and Z unless drug X had independently demonstrated its efficacy. The cancer researchers took a contrary position; they were ready to go with what worked, regardless of testing requirements. Thus, in Phase III studies the NCI focused on the patient and the disease, not on the drug. "Most research oncologists are convinced that they will obtain the best therapeutic results with drug combinations, so that the design at this stage that will clearly illustrate the value of a drug may appear unethical." The FDA staff accused the NCI of being unwilling to do proper testing; the NCI responded that over the past decade, as a result of its testing methods, a number of drugs had found "secure places in the practice of clinical oncology and . . . overall survival of cancer patients has improved."[9]

The task force also had to address the issue that the *Washington Post* had raised about the appropriateness of using cancer patients in Phase I, or NCI category A, tests for toxicity. Here, too, it concluded that patients should be permitted to make their own determinations of risk and that the FDA should not decide what risks were or were not allowable. "While the Task Force recognized that people do not have an absolute right to harm themselves consciously, neither should they be absolutely precluded from seeking treatment which holds out hope of benefit." Even an overall response rate of 9.5 percent (the average response rate to Phase I drugs) was reason enough to let the patient make the choice.[10]

The task force then confronted two especially controversial aspects of NCI procedures. First was the NCI's unwillingness, and the general unwillingness of cancer researchers, to adhere to the placebo trials. Although it acknowledged the widespread perception that "NCI protocols are not scientifically adequate; they are biostatistically flawed," the task force unapologetically defended the NCI procedures in language that is well worth scrutinizing: "There are difficulties in creating ethical controlled trials in a uniformly fatal disease, and there are restrictions on the number of patients to be studied because of the known drug toxicity. *Ideal experimental design must be compromised to achieve the best possible patient care.* As a result, many Phase II studies have used historical controls, and Phase III studies [have used] combination therapies. Thus they may not be compared with experiments that can be performed in other kinds of illnesses."[11] In other words, the need to treat desperately ill patients ruled out the use of placebos or the testing for efficacy of the individual drugs that went into combination therapies.

This same rationale supported the distribution of the drugs in group C testing. Although the efficacy of these drugs had not been proved by FDA standards, and although the drugs were being distributed to hundreds of physicians, the task force defended the procedure. First, it noted that the drugs were distributed only to a selected group of qualified physicians; second: "The Task Force believes that Group C status is an appropriate method for bringing important medications to patients who need them."[12] Once again the needs of patients took first priority.

The task force's endorsement of the practice of distributing cytoxic drugs whose efficacy had not been established in placebo-based clinical trials was only the latest entry in a decade-long debate on the standards that should be satisfied before drugs were made available. This same controversy erupted, with even more heat, around the release of AIDS drugs. Were the new agents to undergo placebo trials? Should the active agent be given to all subjects, and its efficacy measured against past knowledge of the course of the disease?

The FDA, in fact, does not insist on placebo-controlled studies or rule out the use of historical controls. Its 1985 regulations defining "adequate and well-controlled studies" (section 314.126) open with the statement: "The purpose of conducting clinical investigations of a drug is to distinguish the effect of a drug from other influences, such as spontaneous change in the course of the disease, placebo effect, or biased observation." It then lists five types of controls that are "recognized." The first is placebo concurrent control; the others include a "no treatment concurrent control," or control through comparison with another active agent. Fifth—and by no coincidence last on the list—is the historical control: "The results of treatment with the test drug are compared with experience historically derived from the adequately documented natural history of the disease . . . in comparable patients or populations. Because historical control populations usually cannot be as well assessed with respect to pertinent variables . . . historical control designs are usually reserved for special circumstances. *Examples include studies of diseases with high and predictable mortality (for example, certain malignancies)*" (italics added). Hence, the FDA does accept historical controls as a type of control in clinical trials, in contradistinction to the reliance on "isolated case reports" or "random experience."

Many investigators object to this position, insisting that historical controls are never an adequate base for measuring the efficacy of a drug. One of the most persistent critics has been Thomas Chalmers, who was dismayed to report, on the basis of a survey of abstracts presented to the 1971 meeting of the American Association for Cancer Research, that only 21 percent of the protocols had used clinical trials. He found it "surprising that this crucial concept has not caught on to a greater extent" and marshaled arguments for its use. Noting that "many clinical investigators believe that they cannot deprive their patients of the opportunity to receive a new drug," he countered that "the experience with every new cancer drug, when it is introduced into man, is such that either the risk of drug toxicity and mortality is greatest during its early use, or impotent doses are used at first to avoid unknown toxic effects. In either case little benefit to the first patients treated with the new agent can be anticipated." Moreover, Chalmers continued, if a drug shows some signs of early efficacy, investigators will then not undertake randomized trials but will accept the pilot test results as definitive. From Chalmers's perspective, the only way to avoid the predicament is to randomize from the first patient; otherwise, a state of ignorance is certain to prevail.[13]

Franz Ingelfinger, then editor of the *New England Journal of Medicine,* ran an accompanying editorial to the Chalmers article, supporting his insistence on the randomized clinical trial. Noting the "ethical and emotional" objections to the trials, Ingelfinger declared: "It is an investigator of strong moral and intellectual fiber who would resist the urge to 'do something' for a fatally sick patient . . . who would use 'cold science' when the pressures are all on the side of warm hope." But researchers must rise to the challenge: "Ethical, as well as scientific, considerations require that medicine depend on the most reliable and best controlled data available—the kind of data that is sought by the randomized clinical trial."[14]

The types of arguments that Chalmers and Ingelfinger raised in defense of the RCT are familiar and have been often repeated. What is more needed is a full explication of the counterposition, one that goes beyond "warm hope" for the subject or the weak fiber of the researcher-clinician. At its core is the proposition, conceded by the FDA but ignored by Chalmers and the others, that placebo-based trials are ethically inappropriate in the case of a "uniformly fatal disease." In the standard medical text on cancer, a chapter on the design of clinical trials declares: "To determine whether a new treatment cures any patients with a disease that is uniformly and rapidly fatal, history is a satisfactory control. . . . Are randomized trials necessary for identifying major advances in treatment? No. There are many examples of therapeutic breakthroughs that were recognized without randomized trials. For the most part, however, these occurred in diseases where the prognosis was 100% predictable before the advent of the new therapy, and hence there was no possibility of bias with regard to patient selection."[15]

This position was also advanced by David Byar, of the NCI's Clinical and Diagnostic Trials Section, in an essay on the "Necessity and Justification of Randomized Clinical Trials." Byer listed six difficulties with historical controls (from missing data to failure to convince others of the results), presented another six arguments in favor of randomized trials (bias is avoided, time trends are no problem, fewer patients need to be treated to get a convincing answer), and comfortably declared that the ethical dilemmas in RCTs were resolved because "there is always some cost in learning something." But Byar was also prepared to support nonrandomized studies "when a new treatment appears that is markedly effective for a disease which before that time was virtually incurable." Those situations, he cautioned, might be rare, but when they arose, "it would be difficult or impossible to justify a randomized study . . . from an ethical point of view." [16]

Some cancer researchers were even prepared to go further in undercutting an exclusive reliance on RCTs. Drs. Edmund Gehan and Emil Freireich, of the M. D. Anderson Hospital and Tumor Institute, writing in 1974, insisted: "A clinical investigator has an ethical responsibility for his patients when they are involved in a clinical trial . . . to administer . . . the treatment that gives him the highest probability of a successful outcome. . . . If preliminary clinical studies suggest that a new treatment is significantly more effective than a standard . . . the physician would not be fulfilling his ethical responsibility if he planned a randomized comparative trial." Hence, the authors concluded: "In clinical trials it is unwise to assign patients to treatments by any single method. In the field of cancer chemotherapy, effective new therapies have been detected, confirmed, and applied widely in practice as a result of prospective and quantitative clinical trials that have not used random allocation of patients. . . . The widespread acceptance of the randomized comparative trial seems based . . . more on the intuitive attractiveness of the technique than on any objective scientific evaluation of the methodology." [17]

Thus, for a number of reasons, the placebo-based RCT is not the gold standard in cancer research, not in principle and not in fact, when the disease is uniformly fatal or virtually incurable. Cancer researchers have openly made the case against the monopoly of RCTs in trial design and in practice have prepared to avoid them, even at the risk of not satisfying FDA procedures. As Dr. Robert Wittes of the NCI concluded: "The placebo or no-treatment control has always had a very limited role in the evaluation of cytoxic therapy in advanced cancer. . . . Clinical oncologists in the United States have been generally unwilling to randomize a patient with advanced progressive cancer to placebo or observation alone." Instead, "the clearest demonstration of a beneficial effect on survival might only come from a comparison with a carefully selected and characterized historical control group.[18] And by 1989 at least, the FDA was on the whole ready to accept the position. In a "Talk Paper" on "Approval of New Cancer Drugs," issued March 3, 1989, as part of a series of papers "to guide FDA personnel in responding with consistency and accuracy to questions from the public on subjects of current interest," the FDA declared that in decisions to approve new drugs "neither safety nor effectiveness is absolute, but must be weighed in particular cases" and that "although randomized clinical trials . . . are the preferable means of evaluation, other study designs may be acceptable, especially for refractory diseases (those malignancies which do not respond to standard therapy), where a clear response may be apparent even without a randomized control."

With the cancer research model to mind, let us now examine the controversies around research design and AIDS drugs, focusing first on the AIDS Drug Development hearings conducted in July 1986 by Congressman Ted Weiss, and then on the ethical dimensions of the decision to make the first large-scale AZT trial placebo based.

The Weiss hearings confronted directly the issue of placebo-based trials, and the testimony split along the lines that we have been tracing. Proponents of the classic-style RCT came predominantly from the realms of infectious diseases, the FDA, and the drug companies (whose products, after all, must pass FDA review). Their model was not the cancer model; the research in AIDS was not to follow on the designs for research in cancer. "We have learned," declared Harvard professor of medicine and infectious disease specialist Martin Hirsch, "in clinical trials of antiviral agents against other fatal diseases . . . that placebo controls are mandatory until an effective agent is found. The same procedures must be followed in HIV infections, or we will pay the price in unnecessary delays and unwarranted deaths. . . . Until you have some evidence of efficacy of a drug you are still justified in doing placebo-controlled trials even in a fatal condition, such as AIDS, because you may do harm with any of these drugs."[19]

Anthony Fauci, director of the National Institute of Allergy and Infectious Diseases, and Dr. Harry Meyer from the FDA both tried to differentiate AIDS from intractable cancer. "Although one can project that within a five-year period most of the patients will succumb to disease," argued Fauci, "in fact, to those of us who see AIDS patients every day, it becomes very clear that the natural history is quite variable. One of the great problems that we could create for ourselves would result from using a control that is not an adequate control and feeling that an agent was helpful when it really was not."[20] This position was also defended by Dr. David Barry, vice-president of research, Burroughs Wellcome (the manufacturer of AZT): Stating unequivocally that AIDS was unlike cancer, he argued that "because of the waxing and waning of some of the clinical manifestations of AIDS, we could not do an uncontrolled study."[21]

Dr. Mathilde Krim, herself a cancer researcher before she established the American Foundation for AIDS Research, most explicitly made the case for having AIDS research follow on the cancer model. (Surprisingly, she remains one of the very few commentators in this debate to do so—the "plague-like" quality of AIDS apparently made the cancer model seem as irrelevant in the laboratory as in the design of the delivery of care.) Her arguments drew on the traditions in cancer research. Noting that "ethically and scientifically satisfying alternatives to placebo-controlled trials have been devised for the study of experimental drugs in cancer patients," she asked why they were not being used in AIDS. Observing, as well, that experimental (group C) drugs were made available to cancer patients before FDA licensing, she wondered why AIDS patients were not coming under the same policy. After all, "AIDS is presently more surely lethal, within a shorter time, than most cancers. There is no known accepted treatment."[22]

The differences that emerged at the Weiss hearing were anything but academic. At that very moment, the first large-scale trial on the new drug AZT was being conducted, and the trial was placebo based. AZT had been first tested on 19 patients with AIDS and ARC; and the highly promising findings from this six-week trial, in which all patients received the drug, were published in March 1986 in *Lancet*. To review some of the highlights: the patients generally tolerated the drug well, 15 of the 19 had increases in helper T cells, 13 patients had a weight gain of 2 kilograms or more, and 6 patients noted cessation of fever or night sweats and an improvement in their sense of well-being. The published report of the study concluded that the trial did not demonstrate whether immunological improvements would be sustained, whether AZT could be tolerated over a long time, whether viral drug resistance would develop, or whether AZT would affect disease progression or survival. "These are issues which can be resolved only by appropriately controlled long-term studies."[23]

On the basis of these findings, a multicenter, placebo-based trial was undertaken in 282 patients; 145 subjects received AZT, and 137 received placebo. Of the patients with AIDS, all had experienced a first episode of *Pneumocystis carinii* pneumonia (PCP) within 120 days; patients with ARC had notable weight loss or other symptoms, such as herpes zoster or lymphadenopathy. The multicenter study was terminated after twenty-four weeks because the first results demonstrated the efficacy of the drug: over this period, 19 subjects in the placebo group but only 1 in the AZT group died. More generally, in 1986, patients with AIDS and PCP had a median survival of twelve and a half months, and after twenty-two months three-quarters of these patients were dead.

Was the design of this trial ethically proper? Should 137 patients have received placebo? This question was actually the subtext of the testimony at the Weiss hearing. Dr. Krim, in effect, said no, asking why "any AIDS patient should be forced to accept cornstarch pills. . . . This practice has long been abandoned in the experimental treatment of patients with advanced cancer."[24] From her perspective, a median survival of twelve and a half months made AIDS an intractable and uniformly fatal disease, and historical controls would have been sufficient to establish efficacy. On the other side, the remarks by Drs. Fauci and Meyer about the standards for research and the variability of the disease patterns in AIDS were clearly intended to defend the protocol's design.

Whatever the nature of the dispute, it is apparent that were AZT an anticancer drug, the trial would not have been placebo based. Had 19 patients with advanced cancer and no known therapeutic agent done as well as the first 19 patients on AZT, the next trials would have given the drug to all subjects. The goals of treatment would have taken first precedence. Put another way, that the AZT trials were placebo based testifies to the fact that the treatment of AIDS was based not on the cancer model but on a more generalized medicine model, really an infectious disease model.

This formulation has several implications that merit notice. First, in light of the initial definitions of what constituted the AIDS crisis, it is not surprising that the research design followed an infectious disease model. AIDS was a plague, an infection, the result of a viral agent, not a chronic illness of cellular origin. And those working in infectious diseases, unlike those in cancer research, generally had considerably less day-to-day contact, and less intense contact, with terminally ill patients than their counterparts in oncology. Most of the research in infectious diseases, although certainly not all, did not involve desperately ill patients willing to take high risks for the slimmest possibility of a gain. Inevitably, in the realm of infectious diseases, the commitment to placebo-based random trials did not have to come up against agonizing questions.

By the same token, the FDA staff, driven for a variety of reasons to maximize safety and minimize risk, were also committed to rigorous RCTs; and the group that stood out against this orientation, the cancer researchers, had over the years been able to insulate their operations, through the NCI, from systematic FDA oversight.[25] Hence, it was the infectious disease–FDA model, not the cancer model, that structured the design of the AZT tests.

A recognition of this process has a direct relevance to deliberations on the ethics of clinical trials, for it makes apparent that science comes in a variety of models, and the process by which one or another subsumes a particular area of medicine is determined not by immutable canons of research but by historical and social contingencies, or, if you will, by metaphors. Since the first designation of AIDS was of a plague, not a chronic disease, the models of infectious disease, not cancer, took hold. Put another way, a committee charged to analyze the ethics of trials is confronting a choice not between science and compassion but between which model of science is most appropriate to AIDS.

NOTES

The authors would like to acknowledge research support from the American Foundation for AIDS Research.

1. *National Cancer Institute's Therapy Program,* Joint Hearing before the Subcommittee on Health and the Environment of the Committee on Energy and Commerce (House of Representatives) and the Subcommittee on Investigations and Oversight of the Committee on Science and Technology, 97th Cong., 1st sess., October 27, 1981 (Washington, D.C.: U.S. Government Printing Office, 1981) p. 154.
2. Ibid., p. 256.
3. Ibid., p. 218.
4. Ibid., pp. 261, 264, 265, 268.
5. Ibid., p. 272.
6. Ibid., pp. 279, 283.

7. Joint Task Force, National Cancer Institute and U.S. Food and Drug Administration, *Anticancer Drugs: The NCI's Development and the FDA's Regulation* (Washington, D.C.: U.S. Department of Health and Human Services, January 28, 1982).

8. Ibid., p. 33.

9. Ibid., p. 36.

10. Ibid., p. 69.

11. Ibid., pp. 90–91 (italics added).

12. Ibid., pp. 101–2.

13. Thomas C. Chalmers, Jerome Block, and Stephanie Lee, "Controlled Studies in Clinical Cancer Research," *New England Journal of Medicine* 287 (July 13, 1972): 75–78.

14. Franz Ingelfinger, "The Randomized Clinical Trial," *New England Journal of Medicine* 287 (July 13, 1972): 100–101.

15. Richard Simon, "Design and Conduct of Clinical Trials," in *Cancer: Principles and Practice of Oncology*, 2nd ed., ed. V. DeVita, S. Hellman, and S. Rosenberg (New York: Lippincott, 1985), pp. 332–33.

16. David Byar, "The Necessity and Justification of Randomized Clinical Trials," in *Controversies in Cancer*, ed. H. Tagnon and M. Staquet (New York: Masson Publishing, 1979), chap. 10.

17. Edmund A. Gehan and Emil J. Freireich, "Non-randomized Controls in Clinical Trials," *New England Journal of Medicine* 290 (January 24, 1974): 198–203 (quotations from pp. 202–3).

18. Robert E. Wittes, "Antineoplastic Agents and FDA Regulations: Square Pegs for Round Holes?" *Cancer Treatment Reports* 71 (1987): 795–806, at pp. 799, 804.

19. *AIDS Drug Development and Related Issues*, Hearing before a Subcommittee of the Committee on Government Operations (House of Representatives), 99th Cong., 2d Sess., July 1, 1986 (Washington, D.C.: U.S. Government Printing Office, 1986), pp. 52, 69.

20. Ibid., p. 104.

21. Ibid., pp. 115–16.

22. Ibid., pp. 23, 38–39.

23. Robert Yarchoan et al., "Administration of [AZT] to Patients with AIDS or AIDS-Related Complex," *Lancet* 1 (March 15, 1986): 575–80.

24. Ibid., p. 39.

25. For an overview of the tension between FDA regulation and AIDS activism, see our article: "New Rules for New Drugs: The Challenge of AIDS to the Regulatory Process," *Milbank Quarterly*, 68, Suppl. 1 (1990): 111–42.

Entering the Second Decade: The Politics of Prevention, the Politics of Neglect

Ronald Bayer

In 1991 the AIDS epidemic in the United States entered its second decade. More than 200,000 people have been diagnosed with AIDS; 140,000 are dead. It is a time of great promise but also of great risk. Remarkable advances have been made in the biomedical realm, and public policies have been designed to limit the spread of HIV infection and protect the rights of those who are infected or at risk of infection. These are singular accomplishments—all the more so since they have come as a consequence of intense political conflict, spurred by the demands of those who have borne the burden of disease and their allies. But these achievements also set the stage for new controversies in public health. The central political and ethical question of privacy, which was debated in the epidemic's first phase, has now been joined, although not displaced, by the question of equity. How America responds to the new issues concerning access to potentially life-prolonging therapies will have a profound impact on the shape and course of the epidemic in the next years. The situation will be far different in the Third World, where, because of the international maldistribution of professional and economic resources, access to new therapeutic regimes will be all but beyond reach. A single virus may thus create two very different epidemic patterns: one that permits increasingly effective clinical responses; another where men, women, and children continue to succumb, with an enormous toll in human suffering and social dislocation.

Inevitably, public policy will be affected by changing perceptions of the dimensions of the epidemic. Estimates of the number of infected individuals made in 1986 were, it is now clear, too high. Indeed, figures presented in late 1989 suggest that no more and perhaps fewer Americans were infected at that time than were assumed to be infected three years earlier.[1] Equally important, epidemiological trends first noticed in the last years of the 1980s made it clear that, although heterosexual transmission of HIV continues to occur, the spread of infection has remained largely confined to those groups first identified as being at increased risk. The prospect of a rapid spread of HIV among the general population, which served as a specter haunting public policy and which fueled public anxieties, is not currently considered likely. Gay and bisexual men, intravenous drug users, their typically female sexual partners, and their offspring will continue to bear the epidemic's greatest burden of disease, suffering, and death. Sexual orientation and the lines of social cleavage that tend to limit sexual contact between the poor, urban underclass and the broader society have served thus far to contain the epidemic.

Because the epidemic of HIV infection appeared less threatening than was previously thought, many people feared that only limited resources would be allocated to it—at a time when major infusions of funds for care would be needed. It is in that light that Michael Fumento's *Myth of Heterosexual AIDS* must be read; its polemical thrust is directed at those who appealed for resources to meet the challenge of AIDS.[2] The angry reaction from gay groups such as the Gay Men's Health Crisis and especially ACT UP, in the summer of 1988, when the New York City Health Department revised downward by 50 percent the estimated number of infected New Yorkers, must also be understood in that light.[3] At the same time, the increasing association of AIDS with the underclass may fundamentally weaken the political alliance that underlay the voluntarist consensus which dominated public discourse about prevention policies in the epidemic's first decade.

Even more critical to an understanding of the evolving political debates about AIDS and the public health are recent clinical developments. The therapeutic impotence of the early years of the epidemic has begun to give way to a sober yet more optimistic perspective. Progress has been made not only in meeting the challenge posed by opportunistic infections but also in slowing the progression of disease in those who are infected but still asymptomatic. Although it is still too soon to speak of AIDS itself as a chronic disease, HIV infection will increasingly require the kind of long-term clinical management associated with such conditions. As a consequence, public health officials are no longer intent solely on preventing the further spread of infection; rather, they face the task of creating the necessary medical infrastructure to ensure that the million or more infected Americans are provided with appropriate clinical supervision. It is within this changed context that screening, reporting, and partner notification—issues that figured prominently in the early days of AIDS prevention—have taken on new significance and have provoked fresh debates about the appropriate role of the state. The traditional approaches of public health officials to epidemic disease, approaches that were vigorously challenged in the early and mid-1980s, have found new support from those who had previously found them inadequate or ethically unacceptable.

No issue has consumed more attention in the debates over public policy and AIDS than the use of the antibody test to identify those infected with HIV. In the period following the test's development, controversy centered on the role of testing in supporting the radical modifications of behavior that were universally deemed critical to altering the epidemic's course. Out of these debates emerged a broad consensus, often codified in state statutes, that testing should be conducted only with the informed voluntary and specific consent of individuals. Despite that standard, and the carefully defined, though always contested, exceptions to its scope, many clinicians and hospitals undertook surreptitious testing of patients, justifying their practices by the belief that the protection of health care workers and sound diagnostic work required such screening.[4] In Illinois organized medicine went further, successfully pressing the governor and legislature, despite opposition from the state's chief health official, to permit testing at the discretion of the clinician.[5] In New York State four medical societies, including the New York Medical Society, unsuccessfully brought the commissioner of health to court because of his failure to designate AIDS a sexually transmitted disease, a determination that would have permitted testing without consent.[6]

With the announcement in mid-1989 that clinical trials had revealed the efficacy of early therapeutic intervention in slowing the course of illness in asymptomatic but infected persons and in preventing the occurrence of *Pneumocystis carinii* pneumonia, the political debate about testing underwent a fundamental change. Gay groups such as Project Inform in San Francisco and the Gay Men's Health Crisis in New York, which had formerly opposed testing, now began to encourage people in high-risk groups to determine whether or not they were infected.[7] Physicians pressed more vigorously for the "return of AIDS to the medical mainstream," so that testing might be routinely done under conditions of presumed consent.[8] Public health officials—most notably in New York and New Jersey, which had borne much of the burden of AIDS—launched aggressive testing campaigns.

Although physicians and public health officials have typically avoided the language of compulsion, stressing instead routine testing, the threat of coercion loomed before gay activists, their liberal political allies, and proponents of civil liberties. So, too, did the risk of increased stigmatization and discrimination.

With the promise of early therapeutic intervention came the unraveling of the alliances that had been forged in the first phase of the epidemic. A powerful movement emerged, supported by obstetricians and pediatricians, for the routine screening of pregnant women who could transmit HIV to their offspring and the mandatory screening of infants at high risk for infection. The public health practice of testing for syphilis and hepatitis B served as a model for the testing of pregnant women; the widescale and broadly accepted tradition of screening for congenital conditions such as phenylketonuria (PKU) served as the standard for the screening of infants. The promise—with little evidentiary base—that early intervention might protect the fetus or at least enhance the life prospects of babies at risk for HIV infection had begun to override ethical concerns about the coercive identification of infected women, most of whom were black or Hispanic, as well as about the potential burdens of exclusion from housing, social services, and health care itself that might be imposed on those so identified.

The erosion of the alliance that had resisted the application of traditional public health practices could be seen also in the shifting trends on the issue of reporting the names of those infected with HIV to confidential public health department registries. Such reporting requirements had been fiercely resisted by gay groups and their allies because of concerns about privacy and confidentiality. The requirements also had been opposed by public health officials in areas with large numbers of AIDS cases because of the potential impact on the willingness of individuals voluntarily to seek HIV testing and counseling. As a consequence, the reporting requirements had become policy in only a handful of states. It was thus a great setback for those who opposed reporting that the Presidential Commission on the Human Immunodeficiency Epidemic—appointed by President Reagan and skillfully chaired by Admiral James D. Watkins—urged in its mid-1988 final report the universal adoption of a policy first chosen by Colorado three years earlier.[9]

That decision was all the more distressing since much of the commission's final report contained proposals broadly applauded by liberal critics of the Reagan administration's failure to commit either sufficient resources or political leadership to the struggle against AIDS.

Ultimately more significant were the fissures that had begun to appear in the alliance opposing named reporting in those states where the prevalence of HIV infection was high and where gay communities were well organized. In New York, for example, the same suit brought by the medical societies that sought to compel the commissioner of health to declare AIDS a sexually transmitted disease demanded that HIV infection be made a reportable condition.[10] What made the (ultimately unsuccessful) suit so remarkable was the posture of the opposing sides. Historically, clinicians had resisted efforts by public health officials to require the reporting by name of individuals with infectious diseases, arguing that such policies represented an intrusion upon the doctor-patient relationship. In this instance the representatives of clinical medicine were asserting that reporting was critical to the public health while the state's chief health official resisted such a perspective. That apparent paradox can be explained only by the unique political alliances that had been created early in the epidemic between gay organizations, civil liberties groups, and public health officials.

But by June 1989, even that feature of the political landscape of public health had begun to change. In an address that was met with cries of protest, Stephen Joseph, commissioner of health in New York City, told the Fifth International Conference on AIDS that the prospect of early clinical intervention necessitated a "shift toward a disease control approach to HIV infection along the lines of classic tuberculosis practices."[11] A central feature of such an approach would be the "reporting of seropositives" to ensure effective clinical follow-up and the initiation of "more aggressive contact tracing." Joseph's proposals opened a debate that was only temporarily settled by the defeat of New York's mayor, Edward Koch, in his bid for reelection. When the newly elected mayor, David Dinkins, selected Woodrow Myers, formerly commissioner of health in Indiana, to replace Joseph, his appointment was almost aborted, in part because he had supported named reporting.[12] The festering debate was ended only by a political decision on the part of the mayor, who had drawn heavily on support within the gay community, to stand by his appointment while promising that there would be no named reporting in New York.

In New Jersey, which shared with New York a relatively high level of HIV infection, the commissioner of health also supported named reporting, but in that case the politics surrounding the issue were very different. There both houses of the state legislature endorsed without dissent a confidentiality statute that included named reporting of cases of HIV infection.[13] New Jersey simply exemplified a national trend. For, although only nine states at the end of 1989 required named reporting without any provision for anonymity, states increasingly were adopting policies that required reporting in at least some circumstances.[14] Finally, in late 1990 the House of Delegates of the American Medical Association went on record as supporting named reporting. So, too, did the CDC, if in a somewhat circumspect fashion.[15] And always the arguments were the same. New therapeutic possibilities provided the warrant for reestablishing a standard of traditional public health practice.

Ironically, pressure to extend the provision of Medicaid coverage for early treatment and to expand government-funded clinics to treat those with HIV infection will inevitably result in the creation of records on growing numbers of infected individuals regardless of whether states adopt mandatory reporting requirements. The move toward early clinical intervention is, then, incompatible with the preservation of anonymity. As a result, creating and enforcing regimes to protect the rights of infected persons from acts of discrimination will assume greater importance than in the epidemic's first years. In this context state-level protections for individuals with HIV infection will be crucial. But even more important will be the enforcement of the Americans with Disabilities Act by the Congress, legislation that provides those with HIV infection rights extended to those with other impairments.

The move toward reporting was linked only in part to the argument that state health departments needed the names of individuals to ensure adequate clinical follow-up. Also important was the assertion from public health officials that effective contact tracing, now more critical than ever because of the need for early clinical intervention, could be undertaken only if those with HIV infection, but not yet diagnosed as having AIDS, could be interviewed. Despite its central and well-established role in venereal disease control, the notification of the sexual and needle-sharing partners in the context of AIDS had been a source of ongoing conflict between gay groups and civil liberties organizations, on the one hand, and public health officials who had proposed such a strategy in the early years of the epidemic, on the other. This standard disease control measure had always been predicated on the willingness of those with sexually transmitted diseases to provide public health workers with the names of their partners in exchange for a promise of anonymity. AIDS activists had viewed contact tracing as a threat to confidentiality and as a potentially coercive intervention. Indeed, opponents of contact tracing typically denounced it as "mandatory."

With time and a better understanding of how contact tracing functions in the context of sexually transmitted diseases, some of the most vocal opponents of tracing yielded their principled opposition, at least in private meetings and discussions, and instead centered their concerns on the cost of so labor-intensive an intervention. Support for voluntary contact tracing was ultimately to come from the Institute of Medicine and the National Academy of Sciences, the Presidential Commission on the HIV Epidemic, the American Bar Association, and the American Medical Association.[16] Indeed, it was the AMA's support for tracing— justified by its executive director, James Sammons, as having "the potential in the heterosexual society to substantially reduce the proliferation and spread of AIDS"—that provided the grounds for the group's support for mandatory HIV reporting.[17]

Most important in pressing for the adoption of contact-tracing programs at the state level, where all such programs are organized and funded, has been the Centers for Disease Control.[18] Critically involved in the training of workers in SDS clinics and in the funding of local venereal disease programs, the CDC had from the outset urged the adoption of this standard public health approach to AIDS and HIV infection. In February of 1988 the federal agency took on a more aggressive posture, making the adoption of partner notification by the states a condition for the receipt of funds from its HIV Prevention Program.[19] Despite such pressure the response on the part of the states was variable. Those most heavily burdened by AIDS continued to favor programs that encouraged infected individuals to notify their own partners. Of the states that stressed the role of professional public health workers—the "provider referral" model—most tended to have relatively modest AIDS case counts.[20] Thus, local epidemiological factors as well as political forces continued to influence the course of public health policy. But the trend was unmistakable, and in 1991 a New York City Health Department panel was constituted to examine the issue of partner notification. The panel—which included representatives of community-based organizations such as the Gay Men's Health Crisis, as well as experts in medical ethics—gave its support, in principle, to an expanded program of partner notification.

In part, both the early and the lingering resistance to partner notification can be explained by the conflation of the standard public health approach to sexually transmitted disease control with policies and practices that are rooted in a very different tradition, entailing a "duty to warn" or protect those who might be threatened by individuals with communicable conditions. In the early part of this century, courts and legislatures adopted legal norms that imposed on those with infectious diseases a duty to inform those whom they might place at risk through contact. Physicians who knew that their patients could place family members or neighbors in danger could be held civilly liable for failure to warn those at risk.[21] With the decline of infectious disease as a social threat, this legal tradition fell into disuse. It was given new life, however, with the 1976 case of *Tarasoff v. Regents of California,* in which the court held that psychotherapists have a duty to protect the identifiable potential victims of their patients' violent acts. While some state courts have rejected *Tarasoff,* others have handed down rulings that placed limits on the principle of the inviolability of physician-patient communications, holding that clinicians have a duty to protect or warn identifiable individuals who might be harmed by those under their treatment.[22] That line of cases set the stage for the debate over whether physicians could be held liable for failing to warn the partners of those who, though infected with HIV, planned to act in a way that posed a risk of viral transmission.

The early and strict confidentiality rules surrounding HIV screening and medical records all but precluded physicians from assuming their *Tarasoff*-like duties, especially in New York and California. In recent years the recognition that such limitations placed physicians in a position that sometimes violated professional ethical norms, the realization that some patients could pose a grave threat to unsuspecting partners, and the increasing importance of early therapeutic intervention have led to modifications of early confidentiality restrictions. Such modifications are often opposed on principled grounds by those who believe that physician-patient communications should never be violated and by those who argue that such breaches of confidentiality would have the counterproductive consequence of reducing patient candor, thus limiting the capacity of clinicians to effectively counsel and persuade individuals who might harm their partners. At the same time, the modifications in the standard of strict confidentiality have been given strong support in a number of state legislatures, and by the American Medical Association and the Association of State and Territorial Health Officials.[23]

As of 1990 no state had imposed on physicians a duty to warn un-suspecting partners. But about a dozen had adopted legislation granting physicians a "privilege to warn or inform," thus freeing physicians from liability for either warning or not warning those at risk.[24] Reflecting profound concerns about the centrality of confidentiality to the struggle against AIDS, New York's 1989 confidentiality statute went further and, borrowing from the tradition of contact tracing, stipulated that the identity of the threatening party not be revealed to those being warned.[25] To those—the American Bar Association, for example[26]—who believed that adequate warnings require the identification of the infected party to the individuals placed at risk, such compromises represented an un-due limitation imposed by a mistaken interpretation of the ethics of confidentiality.

The question of how to respond to individuals whose behavior rep-resents a threat to unknowing partners inevitably provoked continued discussion of the public health tradition of imposing restrictions on lib-erty in the name of communal welfare. The specter of quarantine has haunted all such discussions, not because there was any serious consid-eration in the United States of the Cuban approach to AIDS—which mandates the isolation of all persons infected with HIV[27]—but because of fears that even a more limited recognition of the authority to quar-antine would lead to egregious intrusions on privacy and invidiously imposed deprivations of freedom.

In spite of fierce opposition to all such efforts, between 1987 and 1990 more than a dozen states had brought AIDS within the scope of their quarantine statutes. At the same time, many of these states mod-ernized their disease control laws to reflect contemporary constitutional standards detailing procedural guarantees, and to require that restric-tions on freedom represent the "least restrictive alternative" available to achieve a "compelling state interest."[28]

Soon after he resigned as commissioner of health in New York City at the end of 1989, Stephen Joseph bluntly made the case for the careful exercise of the power of quarantine. He did so on the occasion of the continuing uproar surrounding the appointment of Woodrow Myers as his successor. Gay and civil liberties groups opposed Myers, in part, because he had supported quarantine legislation in Indiana and had reportedly exercised the authority then granted him under state law. They demanded that such policies never be pursued in New York. No such pledge could or should be made, stated Joseph in an editorial writ-ten for the *New York Times*.[29] Among his last formal acts had been the signing of a detention order for a woman with infectious tuberculosis because of her repeated unwillingness to take the medication that would render her noninfectious. "It is virtually certain that at some point, a New York City Health Commissioner will be faced with an analogous situation concerning the transmission of the AIDS virus. When all lesser remedies have failed, can anyone doubt what would be the proper course of action for the Commissioner to take, faced with . . . an infected individual who knowingly and repeatedly sold his blood for transfusion?" When and if a treatment became available that would render HIV-infected persons less infectious, "would there not then be a clear obligation to take all reasonable measures to ensure that the infected take their medication, thus protecting others?" In characteristically vigorous form— but in language emboldened by the freedom to speak without the constraints of office—Joseph reasserted the traditional claims of public health. His boldness was reinforced by his belief that with advances in therapy AIDS and its control would follow the model established by earlier infectious diseases.

With the exception of the few notable cases that have received press attention, there is no well-documented review of the extent to which newly revised quarantine statutes have been applied to the AIDS epidemic. There are, however, data to suggest that the power vested in public health officials by such laws has been used more often to warn those whose behavior has posed a risk of HIV transmission than to incarcerate. But in any case the numbers have been small. It is clear, therefore, that the enactment of revised quarantine laws has been responsive to political pressures and the belief in the efficacy of symbolic bulwarks.

The enactment of statutes criminalizing behaviors linked to the spread of AIDS has paralleled the political receptivity to laws extending the authority of public health officials to control individuals whose behavior poses a risk of HIV transmission. Such use of the criminal law, broadly endorsed by the Presidential Commission on the HIV Epidemic, called upon a tradition of state enactments that made the knowing transmission of venereal disease a crime.[30] Though they almost never were enforced, the existence of these older laws served as a rationale for new legislative initiatives. Between 1987 and 1989 twenty states enacted such statutes, the vast majority of which defined the proscribed acts as felonies despite the fact that older statutes typically treated knowing transmission as a misdemeanor.[31] Moreover, aggressive prosecutors have relied on laws defining assaultive behavior and attempted murder to bring indictments even in the absence of AIDS-specific legislation.

Any effort to determine the extent to which prosecutions for HIV-related acts have occurred must confront the difficulty of monitoring the activity of local courts when there is neither a guilty verdict nor an appeal to a higher state tribunal. One survey, relying on newspaper accounts as well as official court reports, estimated that between fifty and one hundred prosecutions had been initiated involving acts as diverse as spitting, biting, blood splattering, blood donation, and sexual intercourse with an unsuspecting partner.[32] Though small in number, these cases have drawn great attention. In the vast majority either the defendant was acquitted or the prosecution was dropped. In the small number of cases that produced guilty verdicts, however, there have been some unusually harsh sentences. In Nevada, where prostitution is both legal and regulated, a woman was sentenced to twenty years' imprisonment in 1989 under a statute that made solicitation by those who tested positive for HIV a felony. In the same year, an Indiana appeals court upheld a conviction for attempted murder against an individual who had splattered blood on emergency workers seeking to prevent him from committing suicide.[33]

Whatever the allure of such measures and of the rediscovery of traditional public health approaches in the effort to combat the spread of HIV infection, it has remained clear that the AIDS epidemic will be stemmed only when radical voluntary changes in behavior are made and sustained. Educational campaigns and counseling programs, most effectively undertaken by groups linked to the populations at risk, have remained the centerpiece of that preventive effort. Such efforts are still limited by moralistic trends in American society, and especially by those reflecting the abhorrence of homosexuality. The most striking failure in the preventive realm, however, is rooted in the unwillingness to commit the resources necessary for the provision of drug abuse treatment.

The dimensions of that failure were underscored in the 1988 preliminary report of the Presidential Commission on the HIV Epidemic.[34] A vast expansion in government efforts was needed. One and a half billion dollars a year would be necessary for drug abuse treatment and education. Only such an investment could make possible the provision of immediate treatment to all drug users who might seek such help. For the Reagan administration, which had placed its emphasis on a moral appeal to abstinence and which had entertained the idea of a return to harsh street-level enforcement of drug use and possession statutes, the call for the massive funding of drug abuse treatment programs must have seemed the siren call of a discredited liberalism. For those who were all too familiar with the inadequacy of available services, and the difficulties that would follow even if there were a commitment of resources, the commission's declaration provided some reason for hope.

The call for greater attention to the problem of drug abuse in the light of the AIDS epidemic was repeated by the Institute of Medicine and the National Academy of Sciences. In the 1988 update to its earlier report, *Confronting AIDS,* the IOM-NAS painted a bleak picture linking intravenous drug use, heterosexual transmission, and the birth of infants with HIV infection. "The Committee believes that the gross inadequacy of federal efforts to reduce HIV transmission among IV drug users, when considered in relation to the scope and implications of such transmission, is now the most serious deficiency in current efforts to control HIV infection in the United States."[35] Relying on the report of the Presidential Commission, the IOM-NAS also called for an annual expenditure of $1.5 billion. But despite these appeals, little has been done. In its first report to President George Bush, issued in December 1989, the National Commission on Acquired Immune Deficiency Syndrome lamented the failure of the White House National Drug Control Strategy to give appropriate attention to AIDS. Like its predecessor, the National Commission—chaired by June Osborn, a well-known critic of federal AIDS policy, and vice-chaired by David Rogers, a persistent voice for increased federal support to the cities most severely affected by the epidemic—called for the availability of treatment "on request" for all drug users.[36]

Concern about budgetary deficits, ten years of ideological opposition to welfare state–like programs by conservative national administrations, and the absence of a strong political constituency capable of effectively clamoring for the needs of the underclass have resulted in the politics of neglect. This context helps to explain why black and Hispanic community leaders are opposed to the halfway measures of needle exchange and education about the use of bleach to cleanse drug injection equipment.[37] In the absence of a strong commitment to treatment, such measures appear to write off the needs of the poor. Thus, there has emerged the tragic alliance of the moralistic right and those who speak in the name of the dispossessed. It was the first black commissioner of health in New York City, acting at the behest of the city's first black mayor, who terminated a small and politically hobbled needle exchange program soon after assuming office.[38] More stunning, the commissioner sought to cancel a municipal contract that funded a community-based group to provide drug users with bleach and education about how to sterilize injection equipment.[39]

The failure to fund drug abuse services was but a portion of a much deeper problem: the failure of the federal government to plan for and assist those localities that were compelled to bear the burden of providing care for large numbers of patients with AIDS. And such patients were but a fraction of those who would increasingly be defined as in need of care. In mid-1989 the Public Health Service announced that chemoprophylaxis could dramatically affect the likelihood of developing *Pneumocystis carinii* pneumonia.[40] Soon thereafter, clinical investigators announced that the use of AZT could retard the onset of disease in asymptomatic individuals whose immune systems had already begun to show the impact of HIV infection.[41] Writing in the *Journal of the American Medical Association*, researchers predicted that "rather than a fulminant disease treated primarily inside the hospital, the disease will become a largely chronic condition requiring years of outpatient monitoring and pharmacologic intervention."[42] To meet the challenge of chronic HIV infection, it would be necessary to create and fund an infrastructure capable of providing ongoing clinical services to more than half of those with HIV infection. Some predicted that such care soon would be necessary for a million individuals.

Here, then, was a paradox not new to the American health care system. Extraordinary advances in medicine must inevitably confront the social reality of the most inequitable system of medical care among advanced democratic societies. Thirty to forty million Americans have no health insurance at all. Of those who are insured, many are inadequately protected. Virtually the whole cost of prescription drugs must be borne by those for whom they are prescribed. Could such a health care system meet the challenge of providing between five hundred thousand and one million persons, many of whom are impoverished, with the outpatient clinical services they would need and with the expensive drugs they would require? Would it be possible for a health care system so fundamentally unjust to fashion a just response to those infected with HIV? Before these questions the earlier important debates about discrimination by private medical insurers paled.

Emergency federal programs to assist the states in paying the cost of AZT for those without insurance, Medicaid reimbursement policies, and a host of patchwork programs in the states provided some relief but were clearly inadequate.[43] In its December 1989 report to the president, the National Commission on Acquired Immune Deficiency Syndrome warned that medical breakthroughs would "mean little unless the health care system can incorporate them and make them accessible to people in need."[44] The existence of a medically disenfranchised class meant that, for many, access to care was almost solely through the "emergency room door of one of the few hospitals in the community that treats people with HIV infection and AIDS." Hardly the foundation for the kind of care HIV infection would require in the 1990s.

These were the conditions under which ACT UP, which had rejected conventional political styles of protest for the methods of direct action reminiscent of the 1960s, turned its attention to the shape of the American health care system, going beyond its earlier bold challenge to the bureaucratic structure of new drug development. It was the context in which President George Bush's first address on AIDS, in the spring of 1990, was greeted as hollow by many AIDS activists. No longer was it enough to declare that those who are ill have a right to be treated with "dignity, compassion, care and confidentiality and without discrimination."[45] Federal exclusionary policies in the military, the Foreign Service, and the Job Corps, as well as restrictions on the rights of foreign travelers with HIV infection, made such a declaration seem less than honest. But equally as important was the failure to guarantee that those with HIV infection would have access to the full range of needed clinical and social services.

The situation that prevailed in New York, the epicenter of the American AIDS epidemic, was extreme because of the existence of a number of concurrent sociomedical and economic crises, including drug abuse, homelessness, and dire fiscal conditions. Nevertheless, it revealed that a failure to commit sufficient resources, itself a consequence of federal default, could have catastrophic results—not only for those with HIV-related disorders and the poor, who are dependent on publicly provided medical services, but for the system of health care more generally.

As early as the spring of 1988, investigators writing in the *Bulletin of the New York Academy of Medicine* could assert that "to ignore the possibilities inherent in the empirical evidence available is to create a social calamity even greater than the one already perceived. . . . One can imagine bitter competition for hospital beds. . . . The AIDS epidemic threatens not only individual lives but the city's health care, education and research environment as well. The time is short, the need is great, and is likely to grow rapidly."[46] Within a year three separate reports by public- or voluntary-sector groups detailed how far New York was from being able to meet the demands of the epidemic.[47] Community-based organizations, typically within the gay community, had provided an extraordinary range of services to those with HIV infection and AIDS. They could not, however, meet the needs that public bodies and large private-sector agencies were responsible for meeting. Volunteerism was no substitute for the institutional response that was demanded. Three to five hundred new acute care hospital beds would be needed each year for five years in order to meet requirements of those who became ill. In addition, hundreds of nursing home beds and special housing units would be needed for those requiring less intensive medical care. The capital costs alone for meeting these demands would be over $700 million. And if only half of those who could benefit from ambulatory care for HIV infection were to seek it, the city's already overburdened clinic system would have to absorb an additional 800,000 visits a year. Commenting on the care and attention to detail revealed in each of the report projections, Kenneth Raske, president of the Greater New York Hospital Association, said, "This is the biggest amount of planning for an epidemic with the least amount of action to go along with it."[48]

It was not too soon to start thinking of worst-case scenarios.[49] Middle-class patients together with their physicians might increasingly flee the city in search of medical care in the suburbs. If they remained, and were able to protect their own interests by insulating themselves from the critical shortage of hospital beds, those institutions forced to bear the burden of caring for the poor would be compelled to restrict even further access to inpatient care for "elective" procedures. While middle-class patients would continue to receive increasingly effective outpatient care from their overworked physicians, the poor would face growing delays and waiting lists as they sought out the benefits of early therapeutic intervention. Many, discouraged, would simply not seek care at all.

Shortages would impose the need for rationing, and in the political economy of a city such as New York competition among the desperate would ensue. In what Bruce Vladek, president of the United Hospital Fund, termed the "calculus of misery," it would become increasingly necessary to choose between AIDS cases and the frail elderly for admission to nursing homes; between single adults with AIDS and homeless families with young children for access to newly renovated apartments;

between children and homeless persons dying of AIDS for access to transitional shelter; between HIV-infected pregnant women and women not yet infected for admission to drug abuse treatment programs.

The looming crisis in health care for those with HIV disease set the stage for congressional action that could scarcely have been imagined a short time earlier. Such action was the fruit of dogged efforts on the part of AIDS activists, their allies, and some political leaders from the cities and states that had borne the disproportionate share of AIDS cases. In the winter of 1990 Senator Edward Kennedy, the exemplar of Democratic party liberalism, and Senator Orrin Hatch, a Republican whose stance on abortion often cast him in the role of a conservative, jointly sponsored legislation—the Comprehensive AIDS Resource Emergency Act of 1990—that would provide a major infusion of federal assistance to those localities most severely burdened by AIDS. As the government had responded to natural disasters, the Kennedy-Hatch Bill asked it to respond to the medical disaster of AIDS. "The Human Immunodeficiency Virus constitutes a crisis as devastating as an earthquake, flood or drought. Indeed, the death toll of the unfolding AIDS tragedy is already a hundredfold greater than any natural disaster to strike our nation in this century."[50]

As remarkable as the joint sponsorship of this legislation, which promised to provide $2.9 billion over five years in a complex political formula to the cities and states most severely struck by AIDS, was the overwhelming support the legislation received in the Senate, where the vote was 95–4.[51] When similar legislation, with even greater resource commitments, was voted on by the House of Representatives, the vote was 408–14.[52]

However late in coming, this legislation represented on both symbolic and practical levels an important act of national solidarity. But the hopes of early summer were dashed by the fall, when the Congress, confronted with a severe budgetary crisis, slashed funds for the now-renamed Ryan White Act. What allocations will be made in successive years cannot be foretold. It is certain, however, that such an emergency act cannot be a substitute for fundamental changes in the organization and financing of health care—changes that will be required by the chronic management of the medical and social needs of all HIV-infected persons at a moment when many other medical needs of the nation's poor remain unmet.

With the rapid development of therapies for HIV-related disease, the link between the provision of care and the strategy of prevention has

assumed critical importance.[53] Public health officials have used the occasion of new therapeutic prospects as a justification for rethinking policies adopted in the epidemic's first years. But the prospect of new therapies is not enough. If lives are to be prolonged, and if the public health
goal of preventing the further spread of HIV infection is to be achieved,
these therapies must be available to those who need them. If those with
HIV infection can receive ongoing clinical care, behavioral changes can
be encouraged, supported, and sustained. A failure to provide care and
counseling—especially to the poor, among whom intravenous drug use
plays a critical role in HIV transmission—will entail not only a sentence
of needlessly foreshortened life but a lost opportunity to intervene in
the epidemic's epidemiological course.

New therapeutic possibilities made possible by scientific advances
create the conditions for establishing a moral standard against which to
judge the responses of the American polity to AIDS in the second decade. Unlike the Third World, where absolute scarcity imposes limits
on what can be done to meet the challenge of HIV infection, in the
United States restrictions on governmental efforts will be the consequence of social decisions. History will judge us by the choices we make
at this moment, when the possibilities are greater than at any point
since HIV first made its appearance.

NOTES

Reprinted with permission from *Private Acts, Social Consequences: AIDS and
the Politics of Public Health* (New Brunswick, N.J.: Rutgers University Press,
1991).

1. Centers for Disease Control, "CDC Estimates of HIV Prevalence and
Projected AIDS Cases: Summary of a Workshop, Oct 31–Nov 1, 1989," *Morbidity and Mortality Weekly Report* 39 (February 23, 1990): 110–19.
2. Michael Fumento, *The Myth of Heterosexual AIDS* (New York: Basic
Books, 1990).
3. Expert Panel on HIV Seroprevalence Estimates and AIDS Cases Projection Methodologies, *Report* (New York: City Health Department, February 15,
1989); Richard Dunne, letter to Stephen Joseph, August 18, 1988.
4. *New York Times,* February 17, 1990, p. 1.
5. *Windy City Times,* September 8, 1988, p. 1.
6. *New York State Society of Surgeons, New York State Society of Ortho-
paedic Surgeons, New York State Society of Obstetricians and Gynecologists,
and the Medical Society of New York v. David Axelrod,* New York State Court
of Appeals, May 2, 1991.

7. *PI Perspective,* April 1988, p. 7; *New York Times,* August 16, 1989, p 1.

8. Frank S. Rhame and Dennis A. Maki, "The Case for Wider Use of Testing for HIV Infection," *New England Journal of Medicine* 320 (May 11, 1989): 1248–54.

9. Presidential Commission on the Human Immunodeficiency Virus Epidemic, *Report* (Washington, D.C.: U.S. Government Printing Office, 1988), p. 76.

10. *Society of Surgeons et al. v. Axelrod.*

11. Stephen C. Joseph, "Remarks at the Fifth International Conference on AIDS," Montreal, June 5, 1989, mimeo.

12. *New York Times,* January 19, 1990, p. B1.

13. *Newark Star Ledger,* January 5, 1990.

14. Intergovernmental Health Policy Project, "HIV Reporting in the States," *Intergovernmental AIDS Reports,* November–December 1989.

15. CDC, "Update: Public Health Suveillance for HIV Infection—United States, 1989 and 1990," *Morbidity and Mortality Weekly Report* 39 (1990): 860.

16. Institute of Medicine and National Academy of Sciences, *Confronting AIDS: Update 1988* (Washington, D.C.: National Academy Press, 1988), p. 82; Presidential Commission, *Report,* p. 76; American Bar Association, AIDS Coordinating Committee, *Policy on AIDS* (Washington, D.C.: American Bar Association, 1989); *American Medical News,* July 8–15, 1988, p. 4.

17. *American Medical News,* July 8–15, 1988, p. 4.

18. Kathleen Toomey and Willard Cates, "Partner Notification for the Prevention of HIV Infection," *AIDS,* 39, Suppl. 1 (1989): 557–62.

19. *Federal Register* 53, no. 24 (February 1988): 3554.

20. Kathleen Toomey, "Partner Notification for HIV Prevention: Current State Programs and Policies in the United States," paper presented at the Fifth International AIDS Conference, Montreal, June 7, 1989.

21. Donald H. J. Hernann, "AIDS: Malpractice and Transmission Liability," *University of Colorado Law Review* 58 (1986–87): 63–107.

22. Vanessa Merton, "Confidentiality and the 'Dangerous' Patient: Implications of *Tarasoff* for Psychiatrists and Lawyers," *Emory Law Journal* 31 (Spring 1982): 263–343.

23. Board of Trustees, American Medical Association, December 1989; Association of State and Territorial Health Officials, National Association of County Health Officials, and U.S. Conference of Local Health Officers, *Guide to Public Health Practice: HIV Partner Notification Strategies* (Washington, D.C.: Public Health Foundation, 1988).

24. Intergovernmental Health Policy Project, "1989 Legislative Overview," *Intergovernmental AIDS Reports* 2 (January 1990): 1–3.

25. New York State, Public Health Law, Article 27-F.

26. American Bar Association, House of Delegates, *Report No. 124* (Washington, D.C.: American Bar Association, February 12–13, 1990).

27. Ronald Bayer and Cheryl Healton, "Controlling AIDS in Cuba," *New England Journal of Medicine* 320 (April 13, 1985): 1022–24.

28. This conclusion is based on a review of all AIDS-related legislation in the files of the Intergovernmental Health Policy Project, Washington, D.C.

29. *New York Times,* February 10, 1990, p. 25.

30. Presidential Commission, *Report,* pp. 130–31.

31. This information is derived from a review of all AIDS-related legislation in the files of the Intergovernmental Health Policy Project, Washington, D.C. See, generally, Martha A. Field and Kathleen M. Sullivan, "AIDS and the Criminal Law," *Law, Medicine and Health Care* 15 (Summer 1987): 46–60.

32. Lawrence O. Gostin, "The AIDS Litigation Project: A National Review of Court and Human Rights Commission Decisions, Part 1: The Social Impact of AIDS," *Journal of the American Medical Association* 263 (April 11, 1990): 1963.

33. Larry Gostin, "The Politics of AIDS: Compulsory State Powers, Public Health, Civil Liberties," *Ohio State Law Journal* 49 (1989): 1041.

34. *New York Times,* February 25, 1988, p. 1.

35. Institute of Medicine and National Academy of Sciences, *Confronting AIDS: Update 1988,* p. 84.

36. National Commission on Acquired Immune Deficiency Syndrome, *Report Number One* (Washington, D.C.: U.S. Government Printing Office, December 5, 1989), mimeo.

37. Harlan Dalton, "AIDS in Blackface," *Daedalus* 118 (Summer 1989): 205–28.

38. *New York Times,* February 14, 1990, p. B1.

39. *AMA News,* May 25, 1990, p. 5.

40. Public Health Service, "Guidelines for Prophylaxis against *Pneumocystis Carinii Pneumonia* for Persons Infected with Human Immunodeficiency Virus," *Morbidity and Mortality Weekly Report,* Suppl. 5, June 16, 1989.

41. Paul Volberding et al., "Zidovudine in Asymptomatic Human Immunodeficiency Virus Infection: A Controlled Trial in Persons with Fewer Than 500 CDR-Positive Cells per Cubic Millileter,"*New England Journal of Medicine* 332 (April 5, 1990): 941–49.

42. Peter S. Arno et al., "Economic and Policy Implications of Early Intervention in HIV Disease," *Journal of the American Medical Association* 264 (September 15, 1990): 1494.

43. Intergovernmental Health Policy Project, "AZT: Who Will Pay?" *Intergovernmental AIDS Reports* 2 (May–June 1989): 4–5; Intergovernmental Health Policy Project, "State Financing for AIDS: Options and Trends," *Intergovernmental AIDS Reports* 3 (March–April 1990): 1–8, 12.

44. National Commission, *Report Number One.*

45. *New York Newsday,* March 30, 1990, p. 1.

46. Michael Alderman et al., "Predicting the Future of the AIDS Epidemic and Its Consequences for the Health Care System of New York City," *Bulletin of the New York Academy of Medicine* 64 (March 1988): 181.

47. New York City AIDS Task Force, *Report* (New York: AIDS Task Force, July 1989); Citizens Commission on AIDS, *The Crisis in AIDS Care* (New York: Citizens Commission, March 1989); Mayor's Task Force on AIDS, *Assuring*

Care for New York City's AIDS Population (New York: Mayor's Task Force, March 1989).

48. *New York Times,* April 23, 1989, p. E24

49. United Hospital Fund, "Presidents Letter," February 1990.

50. Senator Edward Kennedy, Letter, February 1990, mimeo.

51. *New York Times,* May 17, 1990, p. B10.

52. *New York Times,* June 14, 1990, p. B9.

53. Donald Francis et al., "Targetting AIDS Prevention and Treatment toward HIV-Infected Persons: The Concept of Early Intervention," *Journal of the American Medical Association* 262 (November 10, 1989): 2572–76.

PART III

Affected Populations

Until That Last Breath: Women with AIDS

Ann Meredith

Since March of 1987, I have been photographing and recording the oral histories of women who are HIV-positive, have ARC, or have AIDS. I wanted to bring to light this "hidden population" of the AIDS epidemic. The individuals whose images appear in this essay graciously consented to be photographed and to have the photographs presented to the public. The resulting portraits and the accompanying statements reveal the personal day-to-day struggles, the hopes, the fears, and the dreams of each of these women as they deal with the physical, emotional, and spiritual ramifications of this chronic disease. Proof that AIDS knows no boundaries, the women portrayed here come from a wide range of geographical areas and backgrounds. They are young; they are old. They are mothers, wives, sisters, and daughters. These are women you know.

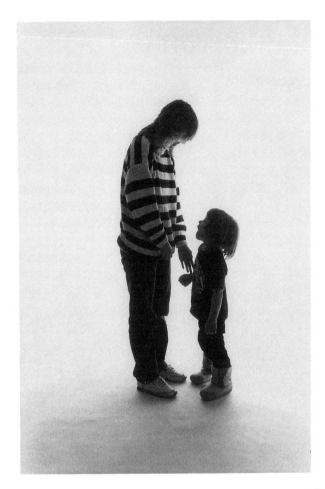

1. Anonymous woman with her five-year-old son (San Francisco, Calif., 1988)
   Age: 30
   Diagnosis: "HIV-positive"
   Sexual preference: Heterosexual (mother of one)
   Transmission: Heterosexual sex with her husband

"I'm thirty. In 1985 my husband died of AIDS. He had a life none of us knew about. I tested HIV-positive in 1985 and believe I got it from sexual contact with my husband. I have a five-year-old son. We got lucky. He's negative. The hardest thing is to keep an emotional balance for him. I have to protect him from the idea of being ostracized because his parent has AIDS. The schools can't keep him out because he's negative, but the kids won't play with him. He'll be considered a leper. What kind of life will he have?"

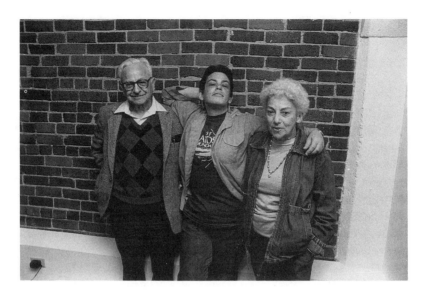

2. Meredith Miller
    Age: 33
    Diagnosis: "AIDS"
    Sexual preference: Heterosexual (mother of two)
    Transmission: Heterosexual sex with her boyfriend
    Died: August 1989

"If I tell you I was diagnosed with a terminal illness, the normal reaction is 'Oh, do you need anything? How are you feeling?' If I say I have AIDS, the first question is 'How did you get it? What have you been doing?' Nobody cares that I am sick, that I hurt, that I'm tired all the time, that each movement is painful. They hear AIDS, and they have a preconceived idea of my life-style and my morality. Hey, nobody told me about AIDS! What is my crime? That I loved somebody too much?"

Meredith

"Don't close the door between you. Offer them every kind of support that you can. Take them in as your friends as well. I think the important thing is to let them know that you love them . . . that the love continues . . . it doesn't stop. Let them know that you love them both verbally and physically.

"How do I feel about Merry being sick? I feel it's just dreadful. Something must be done, there must be a cure. It's just horrible, this disease that is taking so many young people. And to think my daughter is one of the people who is affected by this."

Lillian, Meredith's mother

"Reinhold Niebuhr said the same thing about the Holocaust. When they killed the Jews, we weren't Jews and it didn't bother us. But when they started killing us, then we became concerned. . . . That's what it is now with the heterosexual community."

Al, Meredith's father

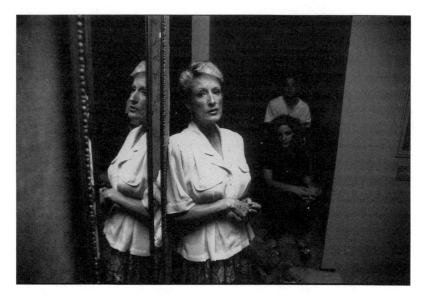

3. Natalie with her daughter, Carolyn, and her son, Doug (Sparks, Nev., 1990)
   Age: 46
   Diagnosis: "I'd prefer not to be labeled."
   Sexual preference: Heterosexual (mother of two)
   Transmission: Heterosexual sex with her husband

"One thing a disease does, especially if it is life threatening, is you don't believe you are immortal anymore. Most people are under an illusion ... I'm not. It adds an edge to life. Life is much more interesting when you live the way people ought to live. I live for today. I don't live in the past, and I don't live in the future. God never promised anybody anything but today."

Natalie

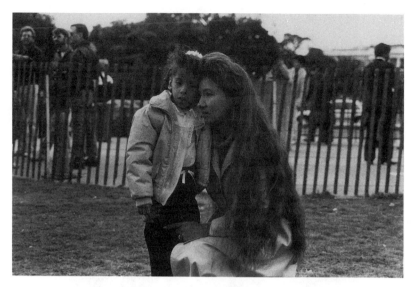

4. Eleana and Rosa (Washington, D.C., 1988)

Eleana is a child with AIDS. Of children affected with the virus, 70 to 80 percent are black, 10 percent are white, and 10 percent are Hispanic (Public Health Hearing on Women and HIV sponsored by the San Francisco Public Health Department; San Francisco, California; June 1987).

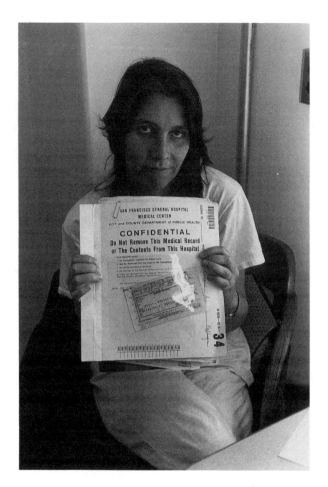

5. Sharon (San Francisco, Calif., 1987)
    Age: 35
    Diagnosis: "AIDS"
    Sexual preference: Lesbian
    Transmission: IV drug use

"Kathy and I have been together for five years. She has stayed with me and
been my friend through this whole thing. Hope is really important. I have
decided to go back home. . . . My family wants me there. I don't know how
much time I have left. I want to be able to enjoy my family. I consider myself
very lucky. I'm a little scared. For once I feel like I am doing the right thing.
Kathy is coming home with me."

                                                                    Sharon

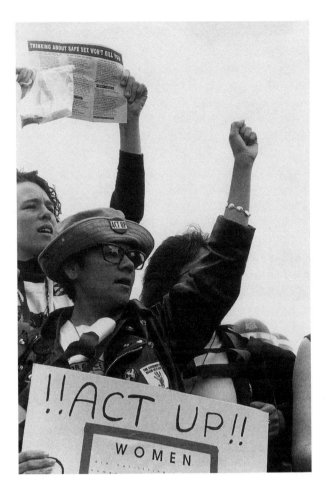

6. ACT UP! WOMEN (San Francisco International Conference on AIDS, June 1990)

Women are the "hidden population" of the AIDS epidemic and comprise the fastest growing segment of AIDS cases. Since 1981 the number of women with AIDS has continued to more than *double* every six months. (Public Health Hearing on Women and HIV sponsored by the San Francisco Public Health Department; San Francisco, California; June 1987).

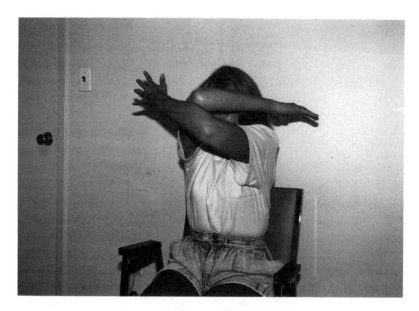

7. "Gertrude" (Long Island, N.Y., 1990)
    Age: 39
    Diagnosis: "HIV-positive"
    Sexual preference: Heterosexual
    Transmission: Heterosexual sex

"I'm one of the 'paranoids' that does things underground. Nobody knows about me because I work, and I don't really trust anybody at all. I'm one of those angry people. I've seen too much in my life. I have chosen not to tell my friends, except two people. There *are* people whose life has to continue. Women more so than men are hated for having this."

"Gertrude"

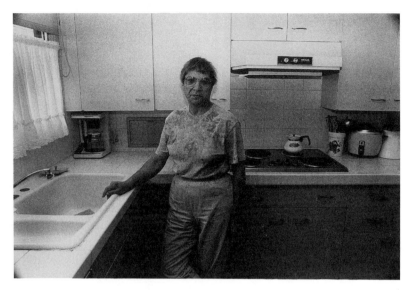

8. Amy (San Francisco, Calif., 1989)
   Age: 58
   Diagnosis: "AIDS"
   Sexual preference: Heterosexual (mother of two)
   Transmission: Blood transfusion

"It's lonely being a woman with AIDS. I don't come in a community. I want people to make it okay. I want the medical profession to recognize the difference between female and male. Women have different problems, both physically and emotionally. I'm an activist, and I'm sorry if I offend anyone, but I'm full of anger and rage. I talk about empowerment and self esteem . . . integrity and women's health issues. I have a lot of things to say!"

Amy

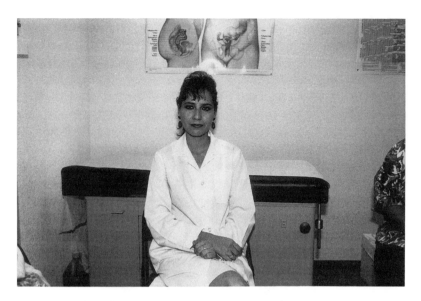

9. Elisa, medical doctor, Compañeros Women's Project (United States–Mexico Border Health Association, Juárez, Mexico, 1990)

"We don't give only medicine and condoms, we give them our time, our dedication, and hopefully an arm to hold on to. We do have limited resources. We work in a very poor country, and we work with people who are very needy. It's hard for people in developing countries to really evaluate and define what need is. What we see . . . the poverty doesn't compare in light of our limited resources. It's a blessing in a way. We have a very important responsibility, and we have to give the best of ourselves."

Rebecca Ramos, project director

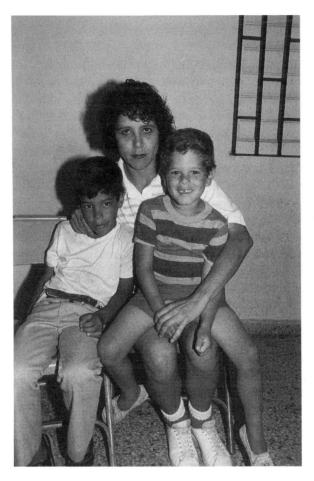

10. Angie with her sons, Xavier and Pedro (Bayamon, Puerto Rico, 1990)
Age: 27
Diagnosis: "HIV-negative, with severe positive symptoms"
Sexual preference: Heterosexual (mother of four)
Transmission: Heterosexual sex

"I have four boys. The oldest is with my mother; the three youngest are with me in my apartment. I had been living with a guy that was a drug user. I don't shoot. I got fearful and got scared, that's why I came to the program. I have been tested the first and second time. Thank God they [the children] have all been negative. I'm worried about it . . . it's a problem for all."

Angie

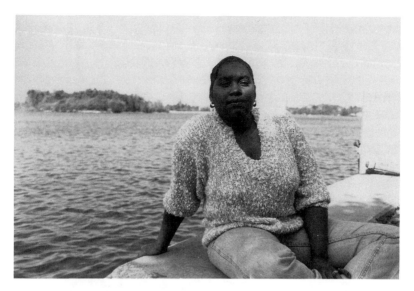

11. Pam (Wilmington, N.C., 1990)
     Age: 27
     Diagnosis: "HIV-positive"
     Sexual preference: Heterosexual (mother of two)
     Transmission: Heterosexual sex

"Me, myself, I'm only positive, and I have energy most of the time. My main concern was for my kids. They're both okay. It's amazing the amount of ignorance there is. It's amazing how little people know about this disease. I am an actual woman that lives and breathes, with kids . . . and I pay bills, too! There's a lot of info about how not to get this disease, but there's nothing that tells you how to live with it once you have it!"

Pam

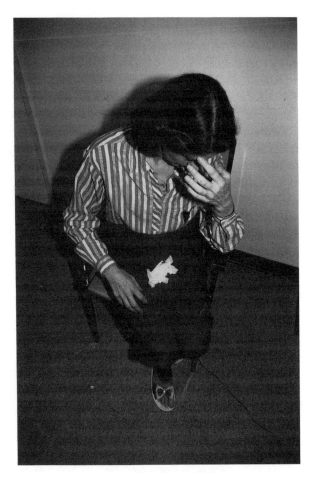

12. Rose, mother of a twenty-two-year-old daughter who died of AIDS (Long Island, N.Y., 1990)
     Daughter: Dawn
     Age: 22
     Diagnosis: "AIDS"
     Sexual preference: Heterosexual
     Transmission: Heterosexual sex
     Died: September 1990

"At the time I questioned everything. It takes a while to accept. Maybe the test is wrong. Maybe the doctor's wrong. . . . But of course, they said 'NO!' There's such a problem with this disease. People will not admit it exists; they think, 'We have no problem on the Island' . . . that it's hyped up by the papers and that it doesn't happen to everybody like you and me. . . .

"Well, we did everything. We did everything that was expected of us, that we were supposed to do. You work hard all your life, make a couple of bucks, get married, you have a family, have a child, and where does it all lead . . . ?"

Rose

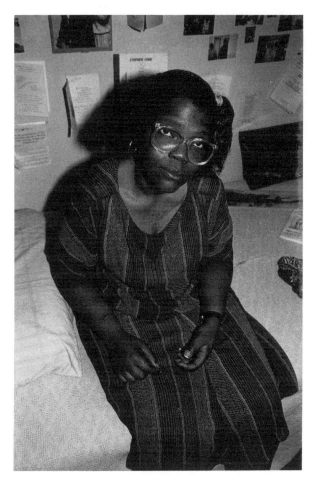

13. Wendi Modesti (Syracuse, N.Y., 1990)
    Age: 37
    Diagnosis: "AIDS"
    Sexual preference: Heterosexual
    Transmission: IV drug use

"What I'm trying to do is put a face on AIDS so that people will begin to associate this disease with human beings. This is a human illness. It's the human element that will take out the fear. I can be anybody's daughter or sister or wife. Stop putting it in the shadows. My name is Wendi Modesti, and I've got AIDS. Let me tell you how I got it so you won't get it."

Wendi

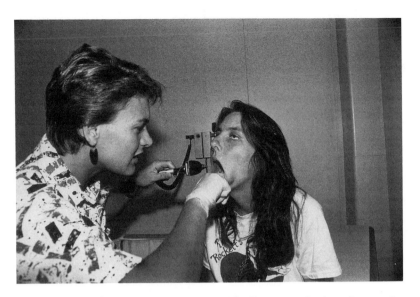

14. Lauren Poole, nurse practitioner with Sharon at Project Aware, San Francisco General Hospital (San Francisco, Calif., 1987)

No personal statement available.

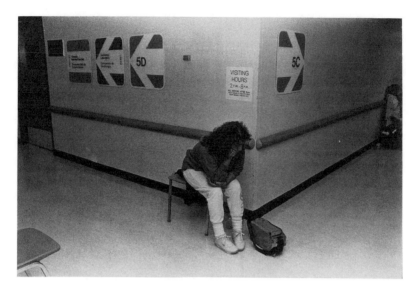

15. A Relative waits, San Francisco General Hospital (San Francisco, Calif., 1987)

No personal statement available.

Riding the Tiger: AIDS and the Gay Community

Robert A. Padgug and
Gerald M. Oppenheimer

He who rides the tiger is afraid to dismount.

Chinese proverb

The dialectic that links gay people, gay men in particular, and AIDS has been central to the entire AIDS crisis. Among Americans gay people have been those most affected by the AIDS epidemic. At the same time, they have been more involved than any other community in both the management of the epidemic and the definition of the discourses our society has devoted to the disease and its sufferers.

These statements are not so uncomplicated as they may at first sight appear. To be sure, many analysts and even casual observers have seen gay people as central to the epidemic, but they have viewed them mainly as either villains or victims, either the cause of the epidemic or merely its foremost sufferers. Such approaches tend to reduce gay reality and experience to the single dimension of disease and, beyond that, to sexual practice. Above all, they prevent a fuller exploration of the complex relationship between AIDS and the gay community in all its richness.

Reductionism of this sort is in many ways the continuation of an old story, one key aspect of which Jean-Paul Sartre underscores in his well-known study of Jean Genet, written more than thirty years ago: "[Genet] never speaks to us *about* the homosexual, *about* the thief, but always *as* a thief and *as* a homosexual. His voice is one of those that we wanted never to hear; it is not meant for analyzing disturbance but for communicating it. . . . He invents the homosexual *subject*."[1] At the heart of Sartre's description is the peculiar position of the homosexual, a position central to his oppression, during the greater part of this century: he (more rarely, she) is the object, never the subject, of public discourse;

245

he is that which is studied, never the student; he is not the actor, the self-conscious creator of his own being, of his own history. He is *silent*. As object of study, therefore, he is the fitting subject of the psychologist and the physician; for the historian he exists only as the individual with a curious "personality defect."

While this situation still exists in large measure for the non-homosexual world, it has effectively come to an end for gay people themselves. In the 1940s and 1950s and then more swiftly during the post-Stonewall 1970s and 1980s, a variety of "homophile" and, later, gay movements laid the groundwork for a gay subjectivity even as they created a gay collectivity.

Gay subjectivity and gay collectivity are intimately connected. For the existentialist Sartre of *Saint Genet,* it is a particular individual of genius who represents the irruption into social consciousness of the homosexual as actor. On the broader stage of history, however, especially in the United States, it has been the collectivity of gay persons, what we shall term here "the gay community," that has been the homosexual actor—as the more Marxist Sartre of the *Critique de la raison dialectique* would doubtless recognize.[2]

It is the dialectical relationship of the gay community to AIDS that we explore here: how AIDS has affected the community and its identity and how the community has affected AIDS. We focus largely on gay men, who are, epidemiologically speaking, the portion of the community most directly affected by the epidemic and whose self-identity and relationships to the non-gay world have been most altered by it.

THE GAY COMMUNITY ON THE EVE OF THE AIDS CRISIS

Homosexual identity emerged as a negative medical, psychological, or biological concept in the late nineteenth and early twentieth centuries.[3] It was only in the post–World War II period that significant numbers of self-identified homosexuals viewed the label in a more positive sense and used it as a basis for common political and social activity that created a real gay community.[4] Like other communities that have their origin in resistance to oppression, the gay community is to a large degree oppositional in nature. It is struggling against the marginalization and stigmatization that homosexuality has traditionally attracted; and, more positively, it is providing the means for self-affirmation for its members. At the same time, the community contains a world of social activities, institutions, and meanings—that is, a living and changing tradition that defines what it means, at any point in time, to be homosexual. Gay institutions are as varied and complicated as those of any similar grouping, without, to be sure, being identical to those found elsewhere. But in addition to its social, political, business, legal, psychological, cultural, and charitable institutions, one of the most notable features of the gay community has always been its profusion of institutions and activities aimed at sexuality.

The sexual institutions of the community have mainly been the product of its male members. Lesbians have certainly developed sexual institutions of their own, and some of them have been similar in type and function to those found among gay men. But lesbians' sexual institutions, besides being fewer in number, have never played as central a role in their lives.[5] Also, except in smaller and less urban areas, gay men's sexual institutions have been quite separate and distinct from those of lesbians. These differences have created numerous tensions within the wider community and have, in most periods, prevented gay men and lesbians from working closely together around issues of sexual practice. In any case it was gay men who mainly created the elaborate world of sexual practices and identities based on sexuality that would be challenged by the AIDS epidemic.

In some ways the sexual institutions of the male gay community— "cruising" streets and areas, pickup bars, bathhouses, movie theaters, "tea rooms" (the polite, and ironic, term for public rest rooms)—are parallel in purpose and nature to those of the heterosexual world. In other, more significant, respects they vary considerably. Part of the variation derives from the historical oppression and persecution of gay sexuality, but the most significant difference lies in the symbolic and social centrality of such institutions to the gay community. For much of this century, and in many places even today, the institutions of gay sexuality represented the only spaces that could be considered truly "homosexual," even taking into account police and community hostility and the need for "discretion" or secrecy.[6] They were the only places where homosexuals could discover each other and begin the process of entering the homosexual world and publicly committing themselves to their homosexuality. It is impossible to separate the sexual aspects of such institutions from their other important social roles.

Whether sexual or not, the institutions of the gay community, those of gay men in particular, appear to be more malleable and adaptable than those of the non-gay world—in part because the gay community is a relatively recent creation and in part because gay institutions have had to live a largely "underground" existence, inhibited by oppression from being linked with, and reinforced by, the older and more permanent institutions of the non-gay world. In much the same way, gay persons have, at least in the past, tended to be more "adaptable" or "theatrical," changing personalities and roles to suit situations and "audiences," especially in circumstances that require hiding one's homosexuality from non-gays (that is, especially, in the need to "pass"). Its malleability would assume a particular importance to the community during the AIDS epidemic.

While all the members of the community have much in common, they also demonstrate significant differences among themselves. These differences tend to cluster around gender, geography, age, race, and ethnicity.

There have traditionally been major differences, as we have already noted, between gay men and lesbians. Lesbians have potential alternative identities in the women's movement or lesbian separatism and differ significantly from gay men in life-style, especially sexual activity. A common "sexual orientation" and a common struggle against oppression have brought gay men and lesbians together, but lesbians have centered their identity far less on sexual acts than their gay male brethren have. Such differences might lead us to conclude that lesbians and gay men do not share enough to form a single community, but this would probably be too strong a statement. Lesbians, like gay men, are quite varied in their politics, sexual style, and other attitudes, and by no means all of them regard feminism as necessarily in opposition to a broad gay identity. In addition, lesbians and gay men have often cooperated around common political agendas and taken part in common social activities, if not always without tensions. To be sure, during the 1970s and early 1980s, the two groups often clashed over sexism and sexual practice, but never so strongly as to break with one another irrevocably.

In terms of geography, the community tends to cluster around large agglomerations of gay people in major urban centers, the so-called gay ghettos, where a wide network of social and political institutions and fairly stable and strong gay identities have been built. In contrast, gay persons in smaller cities or rural areas have tended to be left out of community activities and even gay identity to a substantial degree.[7]

As to age, the "Stonewall" generation (post-1969) was composed, by and large, of younger persons. The community they created—with its emphases on youth, sexuality, and oppositional politics—tended to distance older people, who were, typically, politically and socially more conservative and who often experienced a certain alienation from the community.

Finally, differences of race and ethnicity—differences that by and large mirror similar distinctions, often class based as well, in the wider society—are naturally of major importance, although they have only begun to attract the attention that other distinctions have garnered.[8] This comparative lack of attention is unfortunate, since a large proportion of gay men with HIV-related conditions are from minority groups. It is clear, however, that the gay community is divided by differing ethnic and racial styles, identities, and activities. It also appears that a large proportion of minority-group members engage in homosexual activities without identifying themselves as gay—a fact that is of particular significance in the age of AIDS, when it has become difficult to reach such people through the normal channels of the gay community.

Because of these various internal differences, any particular gay individual will have multiple potential identities, which may, depending on that individual's life history and other circumstances, work together or contradict one another, and will, in any case, modify gay identity in important ways. From the point of view of the gay community itself, the existence of competing behavioral and ideological axes both enriches daily life in countless ways and creates multiple potential areas of conflict and misunderstanding, all of which need to be taken into account in community politics and social life. All this suggests that there is no single gay identity and no single manner of "being" gay but, rather, a multiplicity of gay identities and modes of participation, which, taken together, make up a complex gay community.

Such complexity is apparent in the political history of the community. Although not as much is known in this sphere as we would like, attention to the recent history of the community is essential if we are to comprehend its reaction to AIDS.

The major turning point in gay communal history—the point at which the gay community emerges into history and public consciousness after a long "prehistory" that stretches back at least into the late nineteenth century—is symbolically associated with the extraordinary struggle against police harassment that began at the Stonewall Inn, a gay bar in New York City, in 1969. The struggle sparked by Stonewall, building on decades of slow and difficult community building, led more or less directly to the emergence of a large number of political groups and the politicization of many thousands of hitherto relatively quiescent gay people.[9]

The political groups of the early 1970s, most notably the Gay Liberation Front and the Gay Activists Alliance, were modeled directly on the confrontational street politics of the black and women's movements and the antiwar New Left of the 1960s, and remained closely tied to them in both aims and tactics for some years.[10] Their major public aims were to eliminate discrimination and persecution by the organs of the state, the church, the police, and the medical and psychiatric professions; to remove the stigma associated with homosexuality; and to achieve public recognition of the legitimacy of homosexuality and the homosexual community.[11]

In a more "utopian" and idealistic vein, many of the most self-conscious gay militants asserted not only that gay people had much to teach their non-gay counterparts, especially in the arena of sexuality, but also that the ultimate aim of their political activity was to overcome and eliminate the distinction between gay and straight.

The gay community thus developed a political movement that intersected with the social institutions it had earlier spawned. In the days before Stonewall, collective activity within the community had existed on the very fringes of society and had been essentially unidimensional, taking place largely within institutions oriented toward sexuality—the bars, bathhouses, and "cruising" spaces we have already mentioned. Afterward an entire range of nonsexual political and social institutions—such as political action, legal, and "consciousness-raising" groups, as well as newspapers and journals—emerged, adding significant depth to the community.

At the same time, those institutions based directly on sexuality, although they may have declined in relative importance to the community, expanded immensely in actual number in the 1970s, at least in regions with large and active gay male populations. This profusion of sexual institutions, where sex was freely available or easily arranged, became the most noticeable feature of the gay male community. While there were some tensions between these institutions and those that were political in nature, such tensions remained manageable because the gay political movement itself had as one of its major aims the removal of social obstacles to the expression of gay sexuality.

The politics of the gay male community of the early 1970s, insofar as it was anchored in sexual practice, was, in fact, both potent and divisive. It was potent because it united gay men and provided them with a set of cultural practices that was also a direct challenge to the dominant heterosexual world and around which a strong sense of common identity could be constructed. It was divisive because it fragmented the wider gay community—leading, for example, to tensions between gay men and lesbians and younger and older elements within the community—and tended to prevent strong alliances from being formed with non-gay groups.

However this may be, the deliberate public quality of most of these activities, both sexual and political, is significant. It represents the "coming out" of the gay community, the deliberate desire to tear away the curtain of invisibility that had hitherto enveloped it. To be invisible is to have no public voice and, thus, to be socially powerless, since public speech—public discourse—is central to power in all societies. The addition of a public presence and a public voice to what had been only private—indeed secret—forms of communication between gay persons was thus fundamental for the creation of a viable, self-conscious, and positively identified gay community. Its two sides were the internal consolidation of a gay identity and the external confrontation of all those attitudes, ideologies, and practices in the wider society that had thrust gay people, at least insofar as they were gay, out of society and had forced them to hide in "the closet."

The irruption of the gay community into public discourse and consciousness, with the concomitant building of a positive self-identity, was accompanied by the community's desire to control its own institutions and its own life, free of outside interference. This desire for communal autonomy—another aspect of the desire for communal legitimacy, recognition, and a role in the functioning of the wider society—has become a key characteristic of the gay community, one that has marked it through all successive phases of its existence.

Many of the most important features of this period continued into the later 1970s—above all, the struggle against discrimination, the insistence on a presence in public discourse and consciousness, and the community's need to control its own institutions. But other aspects fell by the wayside as both the external world and the community changed in fundamental ways.

The participatory street politics of the post-Stonewall years was replaced by a politics of membership groups and pressure-group activity. This change is best illustrated by the growth of the National Gay Task Force (later the National Lesbian and Gay Task Force), founded as a membership organization in 1977 and dedicated to lobbying activities,

which soon became the major political organization of the gay community.[12] In addition, the notion that the community was struggling
against oppression as part of a wider fight for human liberation was
replaced by an emphasis on the community as a legitimate "minority"
group—parallel to blacks, Hispanics, and, to some degree, women—
struggling for its own interests. A community that had considered itself
a political *movement* aimed at liberation from oppression was replaced
by a community that emphasized its cultural and social institutions and
its desire to be tolerated—that is, a community that had replaced human liberation with civil rights and equality as its major aims.

This transformation took place in the context of the decline of the
American left wing and the resurgence of a new and more aggressive
right wing. One feature of right-wing ideology was an emphasis on
"moral" issues: sexuality and the family, abortion, women's liberation,
and homosexuality. Homosexuality (like the women's movement and
abortion) was useful to conservative political leaders in creating a new
right-wing ideology and in connecting right-wing religious groups with
right-wing political and economic groups. It was posed as a major challenge to the most fundamental institutions of American society, in particular the family. The homophobia of right-wing groups drew upon
earlier fears and distortions of homosexuality—notably in the sexual
sphere. But these groups also were obsessed with the emergence of a
public gay world and with the establishment of an independent gay
identity and voice. That the right wing specifically called into question
gay civil rights (that is, public recognition of gay legitimacy) and any
public expression of gay sensibility or culture was the natural result of
this obsession. Right-wing confrontation with the gay community was
in many ways a mirror image of the confrontation of the community
with the wider straight society.[13]

The political and public energies of the gay community in the late
1970s were turned to combating this new challenge to its identity and
very existence, best symbolized by the successful efforts of Anita Bryant
and her followers in 1977 to repeal Miami's law prohibiting discrimination against gay people, and by similar campaigns in several other
cities.[14] Such challenges reinforced the minority-group emphasis of the
gay community and its recent discovery of civil rights and pressure-
group methods to achieve its aims.

Such was the gay community on the eve of its confrontation with
AIDS, a complex community with a varied constituency and significant
strengths and weaknesses. The AIDS crisis marks yet another major

turning point in its history—a turning point whose nature was in large measure determined by the prior social and institutional development of the gay community.

AIDS AS A "GAY DISEASE"

The AIDS crisis challenged the most significant elements of the gay community as they had developed in the 1970s. The most obvious challenge was to its sexuality. Early in the epidemic scientists identified AIDS as a sexually transmitted disease, and the exuberant sexuality of the gay male community was implicated in its spread.[15] In addition, the parts of the gay community that were most clearly affected were those that were most central to it; that is, the relatively sophisticated and self-conscious gay "ghettos" of New York, San Francisco, and Los Angeles. Finally, and most significantly for our purposes, the community was challenged in its newfound sense of identity and in its politics, especially the insistence on autonomy, self-determination, and the ending of discrimination against gay people. These and other "internal" problems were intensified through the manner in which AIDS was constructed in the minds of outsiders as a "gay disease."

From the start, in 1981, AIDS was closely connected to homosexuals, since the first patients identified with the syndrome were gay men, and gay men have continued to form the largest single block of persons with AIDS. Early in the epidemic the connection seemed so self-evident that some researchers named the new disease "GRID" or gay-related immunodeficiency syndrome.[16]

The association of gay men with AIDS was, however, never quite so straightforward as it sometimes is made to seem. From the beginning, studies described non-gay persons with AIDS.[17] For example, the first heterosexual patients, including the first women, were reported by the Centers for Disease Control (CDC) as early as August 1981.[18] The first clinical descriptions of immunosuppression in heterosexual intravenous drug users appeared in December 1981. Interestingly, the editorial discussing these findings in the *New England Journal of Medicine,* while acknowledging the existence of heterosexual cases, systematically ignored them in developing a hypothetical causal model of the new syndrome in homosexual men.[19] This example presaged the manner in which the epidemic would largely be handled in the first years: as a problem that mainly affected gay men that would be solved if particular attention was paid to the supposed characteristics of that population.

In these circumstances it was probably inevitable that researchers should initially concentrate on what came to be known in both professional and popular discussion as "the gay life-style" in attempting to comprehend the etiology and epidemiology of the new disease.[20] By "gay life-style," however, they meant the narrow dimension of gay male sexual practice, abstracted from the community in which it took place and from that community's history and the meanings that it imparted to its sexuality.

The identification of homosexuality with AIDS was underscored once scientists publicized the epidemiological concept of high-risk groups. High-risk groups were those whose members were at especially great risk of being infected and of infecting others.[21] The designation of gay men as a high-risk group reinforced the notion that all gay men were diseased or at risk of being so. The effects were mitigated only to a small extent by the designation of additional groups as high risk (IV drug users, hemophiliacs, and Haitians, initially) and by the CDC claim that "each group contains many persons who probably have little risk of acquiring AIDS."[22] Nonetheless, the designation of gay men as a high-risk group reinforced the notion that all gay men were diseased or at risk of being so.

The belief that the gay male community *in toto* formed a risk group lost whatever rationale it had early in the epidemic as it became clear that only certain sexual acts put one at risk for AIDS and that, even in the context of those acts, a large measure of safety was achievable through the use of condoms and other precautions. Nevertheless, the idea that all gay men constituted a risk group was, for all practical purposes, never eliminated, even among professionals, who, as a group at least, had learned the weakness of such a belief and recognized that sexual practice varied among gay men as much as they did among non-gays. The persistence of the identification of the entire gay community as a risk group because of its sexual practices meant that gay sexuality itself was, in effect, identified as the "risky" factor. Scientific medicine thus appeared to support an old idea, largely discredited in the 1970s through the efforts of the gay community, that homosexuality was itself a disease.

Among the groups that were most significant in determining the varying interpretations of AIDS, right-wing ideologists (including leaders of conservative religious movements) were of particular importance. As they extended their anti-gay offensive of the late 1970s, AIDS was a powerful symbol for them, a way of negatively reinserting homosexuality into what one observer has called "a symbolic struggle between purity and pollution."[23] In this type of discourse, punitive messages were central, as was the tendency to identify as the problem not a particular virus but those infected with it—in particular, homosexual men, who had supposedly introduced the virus into the country and served as a reservoir of contamination. These ideas were often echoed by the news media, which either publicized the notion of a "gay plague" during the early years of the epidemic or remained silent about AIDS, except when it appeared to threaten the "general population," implicitly defined as the heterosexual majority.[24]

The isolation felt by the gay community was further intensified by the ambivalent role played by the federal government. Normally a leader in the struggle against disease, and to some extent a mediator among competing groups, the executive branch under President Carter and, to a greater degree, under President Reagan had begun to dismantle institutions aimed at securing the health of the population and was loath to spend additional funds on a new disease that appeared to strike only or mainly at disliked populations.[25] In addition, it was not prepared, at least under Reagan, actively to combat a crisis in such a way as to seem to support the gay community, which it opposed on ideological grounds. Congress, the Public Health Service, and some states and localities were inclined to be more activist in the face of the epidemic, but in general government leadership was notable mainly for its absence.[26]

The gay community thus quickly found itself in a difficult situation. By accepting the identification of gay men and AIDS, it would open itself to the social distancing, hostility, and loss of community empowerment such an identification would entail; by refusing the identification, it would allow AIDS to be ignored and its members to die needlessly. Consequently, the community had to find within itself—in its own institutions, identity, and history—the means to endure the epidemic and to save itself. Just as crucially, it also had to find allies among those groups, mainly heterosexual, that could ally with it for professional, ethical, or philanthropic reasons (such as public health personnel, medical researchers, elements of the political left and center, and representatives of liberal churches).[27] The intertwining of these two themes—internal resources and external alliances or compromises—would come to dominate the entire gay response to AIDS.

THE GAY COMMUNITY'S RESPONSE

The gay community in fact had little choice from the start but to accept one side of the dilemma: it had to identify itself with AIDS in order to provide the necessary care and support to those of its members who had contracted the syndrome. In embracing AIDS as a peculiarly gay problem and reality, however, it would not draw the same connec tions and conclusions from that identification that the non-gay world had drawn. Gay people could hardly accept common metaphors of AIDS that were based on fear and loathing of homosexuality itself. Unlike much of the heterosexual world, the gay community, if it was to survive as such, was incapable of constructing AIDS as a disease of "the other"— the outsider—but was forced to attempt to "normalize" it; that is, to deal directly with the pain, suffering, and social problems it caused without allowing it to abolish gay people and their sexuality in the process.

Paradoxically, in order to deal with AIDS on these terms, the community was forced to strengthen rather than weaken its identification with AIDS: the stronger the identification, the greater the possibility that the community could control the social meaning of the disease, act effectively in dealing with it, and persuade or pressure the heterosexual majority to move in positive ways. It was forced, in other words, to "own" the disease.[28] By owning it, the community could reconstruct both the disease and its relationship to it on its own terms.

The process of identifying the community with AIDS was, of course, never a simple one, nor was it the product of internal community unanimity. Some in the community saw that identification as a trap for gay people, in which the most important achievements of the past would be rolled back in the interest of the heterosexual majority. Many others were quite bewildered by the new epidemic and reacted in panic or disbelief, reactions that inevitably led to an inability to deal with it at all.[29]

Eventually, a small group of gay men, mainly in New York and San Francisco, succeeded in convincing the great majority of the gay community of the need to identify with AIDS in order to combat it. These men alerted other gays to the problem, created new institutions to deal with it, and attacked what they saw as the sluggishness of the community in coming to terms with the new reality.[30] We may take as symbolic of this group the efforts of Larry Kramer, who—in a series of strident but effective articles in the gay press—castigated the community for not acting rapidly enough, and who was instrumental in the founding of New York's Gay Men's Health Crisis.[31]

Even after the community had basically accepted the identification with AIDS and the need to contend with the disease (during 1981 and

1982), there was never perfect agreement regarding the management of the AIDS crisis. The response to AIDS by the gay community was the product of innumerable and only minimally coordinated day-to-day actions, choices, and struggles by particular individuals and groups. That response appears, especially in hindsight, more coherent and rational than it actually was, because it was created within and through gay institutions that already had purpose and meaning and by a community with a relatively firm identity and history of struggle against oppression. By themselves, however, the most determined gay efforts would probably have failed in these and many other areas of the AIDS struggle. What enabled them to succeed as fully as they eventually did was a combination of factors: an American tradition of self-help and voluntarism,[32] the existence of natural allies and sympathizers in the wider non-gay world, and significant resources in community political and social institutions as well as funds, talent, and labor that could be brought to bear on the crisis. In addition, and at least as significant, a peculiar set of historical circumstances existed for the gay community in the first few years of the epidemic. The combination of the relative strength of gay identity and institutions inherited from the 1970s and the widespread avoidance of the crisis by other elements of society provided the gay community with what may be termed a "window of opportunity" through which to claim the major role in the epidemic that it came to play.

Putting this another way, one might say that it was the lack of other claimants to the ownership of AIDS—especially the scientists, physicians, and government officials who normally take control of disease, its meanings, and its treatment in our society—that allowed the gay community in large measure to make good its claim to own the disease and the manner in which it was dealt with. The gay community thus was able to use the power of medicine, medical science, the healing and social professions, and government without granting them nearly as much power over itself as would otherwise doubtless have been the case. In addition, the relative weakness of other so-called groups within the crisis meant that, when they did enter the struggle, they were in large measure forced to negotiate with the gay community over many aspects of the crisis and to rely on it for much of the resources (especially nonmonetary resources) and skills that were necessary to deal with it.

Thus, in embracing AIDS, and in seeing that its own needs and structures were congruent, at least in this arena, with the realities of the wider American health and social spheres, the gay community was able to become the single most powerful force in the struggle against AIDS. But at the same time, in so acting, the community consciously and unconsciously was shifting the site of major elements of its own identity, especially for gay men. As sexuality became a sphere of uncertainty and danger, requiring significant alterations, it was displaced, to a large degree at least, from the center of gay male identity, to be replaced by a new sense of identity built up around the political, cultural, and health care aspects of the AIDS struggle itself.

Like sexuality, however, AIDS has both strengths and weaknesses as a source of gay identity. AIDS provided a powerful and renewed source of strength to gay identity and gay institutions because, at least temporarily, it made any divisions in the community relatively less important, since the common life-and-death struggle took precedence over almost all differences; it formed a set of issues around which all parts of the community, including those excluded by male sexual practice, could work together; and it created a sense of crisis that moved even the most nonpolitical homosexuals and those whose participation in the community had hitherto been marginal to provide their money, labor, and talent for the struggle.

At the same time, the gay community could never embrace AIDS as a source of identity without a profound sense of ambivalence. AIDS could never be truly gay in the same sense that sexuality had been. The disease had become gay in the circumstances of a specific historical conjunction, not because it was gay in any innate sense. AIDS would, thus, always remain tendenciously related to other aspects of gay identity. In addition, not only did non-gays also suffer from AIDS—and they would become increasingly important in the epidemic as time went on—but non-gay institutions also had an interest in the meaning and management of the epidemic, and would have to be dealt with by negotiation and compromise. Finally, a more or less single-minded focus on AIDS could lead to the neglect of other issues important to the community. As a central focus of gay identity, AIDS therefore had serious weaknesses, weaknesses that would emerge more fully in the more recent stages of the epidemic.

Nevertheless, AIDS did become central to gay identity, at least during most of the 1980s, and determined the nature of the gay community and its activities in that period. A number of common, closely intertwined threads run through all the gay responses to the crisis in the period from 1981 to the present. It will be convenient to summarize them at this point, since they form the (sometimes unspoken) context in which gay people confronted AIDS as a disease and as a social reality. In essence, these common threads involve the alteration of the perceived nature of the disease, the reconstitution of the community's institutions and self-identity around the struggle against the disease, and the restructuring of the community's relationship to the non-gay world.

REDEFINITION OF AIDS AND PERSONS WITH AIDS

From the beginning the gay community insisted that AIDS must be viewed as a disease and not as a divine judgment or a revenge of nature. That is, it had to be understood and dealt with in the spheres of medical science, social welfare, and politics rather than those of morality or theology. In short, persons with AIDS must be seen as human beings with a disease rather than as moral outcasts. As such, and as participants in the American "social contract," they deserve to have the full force of society's scientific, healing and caring, and material resources available in their struggle against a deadly pattern of disease.[33] In addition, and crucially, persons with AIDS must be treated not as passive "victims" of a disease but as active participants in the struggle against it, participants who have their own voice and whose viewpoints, knowledge, and skills must be taken into account and respected at all times.

From a gay perspective, therefore, the AIDS crisis must be viewed as a full political and social struggle, in the broadest sense of those terms, and not merely as a medical event. In this perspective gays were, if only implicitly, insisting on the social construction of AIDS as a disease, a social construction whose nature could be contested at every moment.

THE GAY COMMUNITY AS SUBJECT

The gay approach sought to empower not only persons with AIDS but the entire community as well.[34] Here, too, the point has been to avoid the objectification of the community, something it had, as we have seen, struggled against for many years. As a subject, or group of subjects, the community has insisted that there be a gay voice—a public presence—in all aspects of the epidemic and its management. Specifically, gay people have insisted on their need, and right, as those most affected by AIDS, to share power over the crisis: the power to define it, the power to deal with it, the power to negotiate with outsiders over it. This insistence has its roots in prior gay history, but it has been reinforced by the perceived tendency of the non-gay world to ignore gay interests, gay welfare, and gay knowledge and capabilities in defining and confronting the epidemic.

Through its insistence on its right to subjectivity and a voice in the epidemic, the community demanded that it be treated as a community with its own interests, and not merely as a set of individuals who are only loosely connected together by the fact of potential or actual disease. Only the community as a whole could assert the interests of its individual members and combat the tendency of the wider society to exclude gay people as well as people with AIDS. Thus, for example, the community's resources, its legal defense and AIDS advocacy groups, were used in the struggle against HIV antibody testing, quarantine, exclusion from insurance, and the like. Although there was considerable disagreement within the community about the correct approaches to take on each of these issues, there was no debate over the need for gay leadership to defend gay community interests.[35]

TRANSFORMATION OF COMMUNITY INSTITUTIONS

Throughout the crisis the gay community was aware that to meet the challenge of AIDS and survive, it would not only have to confront the outside world, but would, just as significantly, have to restructure its own institutions. This has been a twofold process, involving the creation of new institutions as well as the elimination or alteration of older ones.

With respect to new institutions, the provision of necessary services for those affected by the epidemic has naturally been at the center of the gay response from the earliest days. It is no accident that the first gay institutions that sprang up to deal with AIDS (notably New York's Gay Men's Health Crisis and San Francisco's Shanti Project) were devoted to the care of persons with AIDS and the provision of necessary social welfare services for them, and that the majority of the many hundreds of gay AIDS-oriented institutions that were eventually founded continue to be of this type.[36] The severity of the epidemic, the large numbers of members of the community who have contracted the disease or who are HIV positive, and the unwillingness or inability of major elements of the wider society to provide these services required the gay community to do so.

In addition to such organizations, the community has created a number of more or less formal ways to deal with the grief, pain, and tragedy that AIDS has caused.[37] For example, periodic candlelight vigils and prayer services have been held; and a San Francisco group, whose work has now become national and has been shown in many cities, created a giant quilt containing hundreds of panels in memory of those who have died of AIDS, thus both "individualizing" persons with AIDS and allowing members of the community (and even those not directly connected to it) to share and express their grief and anguish.[38]

The community's attempts to meet the immediate and most urgent needs of people with AIDS through its own efforts have resulted in a partial break with past traditions of gay politics, whose major aims were those of civil liberties and rights rather than health care or the elements of material welfare.[39] Moreover—although the community has continually insisted that society as a whole must deal with the crisis— the community's own efforts, by filling the caregiving void, not only stretched its resources to the limit but may well have allowed the wider society to avoid its responsibilities for a longer period than might otherwise have been the case.[40]

At the same time, some of the most central institutions of the community, those organized around sexual expression, have had to be changed dramatically or, in some cases, simply jettisoned if gay people were to survive at all—HIV is, after all, transmitted, at least in part, through sexual intercourse. What was being abandoned, it is important to stress, were particular *forms* of sexual expression—in particular, those that took place in back-room bars, bathhouses, and other places where sexuality was freely available—rather than gay sexuality itself. In this respect the community acted on the belief that it had to preserve itself during the health crisis without giving up its sexual existence and its control of its own sexuality.

Here again, the major changes that emerged were accompanied by substantial, at times acrimonious, debate within the community over the role of multiple sexual partners and other aspects of gay sexuality as practiced in the 1970s. Some directly implicated "promiscuity" in the spread of AIDS even before HIV had been identified, and many in the community turned to a renewed emphasis on the importance of "monogamy."[41] Others were much more cautious, suspecting that AIDS would be used to attack what they considered the positive features of gay sexuality and gay autonomy, less because of the threat to gay health than because of illegitimate moral and political considerations.[42]

At times the controversies generated were unsolvable within the community, as in the bathhouse controversy in San Francisco and other cities, where certain members of the gay community deliberately used the forces of local and state government to eliminate sexual meeting places that, in their view, were focal points for the spread of HIV infection.[43] Ultimately, as the etiology of AIDS became better known, most activity respecting gay sexuality became focused not on number of partners or site of sexual encounter but on the type of sexuality practiced. Most of the significant changes in sexual behavior that have affected gay men have derived from the safe-sex efforts of the community itself. Safe-sex education was, at least in the early years, considered at least as much a political act as a medical one. Cindy Patton has put the matter well:

> Safe sex organizing efforts before 1985 grew out of the gay community's understanding of the social organization of our own sexuality and from extrapolations of information hidden in epidemiologic studies. Informed by a self-help model taken from the women's health movement and by the gay liberation discussion of sexuality, safe sex was viewed by early AIDS activists, not merely as a practice to be imposed on the reluctant, but as a form of political resistance and community building that achieved both sexual liberation and sexual health.[44]

Ultimately, the effect of AIDS on the gay community and of the community's own efforts has been to render gay sexuality more like that favored by the wider society. That is, there has been an increased emphasis on monogamy and closer relationships and a decreased emphasis on mulitiple sexual partners and wide sexual experience. Concomitantly, those community institutions where sexuality was freely available have declined in importance. That is, a smaller proportion of the community now frequents them, and they have become less significant to gay identity and the process of "coming out" into the gay world. At the same time, the newer caregiving, social support, welfare, legal, and political action groups organized around AIDS have become far more significant to the community—not only because of their overt purposes but because they serve as places to socialize and meet other gay people—and have become central to the identity of a large proportion of gay men and lesbians.

Changes of this sort in gay institutions have had major effects on various subgroups within the community—particularly older gay persons, for whom the muting of the sexual aspects of gay life has meant an opportunity to reenter the mainstream of the community as providers of care, money, and labor.

AIDS has also played an important role in restructuring gender relationships within the community. Hostility between gay men and lesbians has become considerably less visible, giving way to a variety of cooperative efforts to meet the challenge of AIDS. Many lesbians threw themselves into the struggle against AIDS at its beginning and have continued to play a major role in all gay AIDS-related institutions, even though, from an epidemiological point of view at least, AIDS mainly affects them indirectly. Their response to the suffering and death of their male friends and to a potential political disaster for the wider gay community has been little short of heroic.[45]

The renewed ability of lesbians and gay men to work together fruitfully, if not always without significant tensions (largely, it appears, because of the persistence of sexism among many gay men), is attributable to the decline of sexuality as a major component of gay identity. Whether this working relationship will continue in the future, as AIDS ceases to be the predominant issue of importance to the community, is uncertain. In large measure the outcome depends on the success of efforts currently being made by AIDS organizations—particularly the newer and more radical ones (which we will deal with in the section headed "The Present and Future")—to eliminate sexism in their operations, to be more attentive to issues of concern to lesbians and other women, and to integrate women more fully into positions of leadership.

RELATIONSHIP TO THE OUTSIDE WORLD

AIDS has had a paradoxical effect on the relationship of the gay community to the wider society. On the one hand, because of the close identity of gay people and a deadly disease, it has distanced the community from the heterosexual majority. On the other hand, it has brought the two closer through the need of the wider society to deal directly and explicitly with AIDS and its etiology, which naturally involves more open discussion of homosexuality and an end to gay invisibility; through the need of the wider society to work directly with the gay community to combat the crisis; and through those changes, already noted, that have made the community more like the straight world than ever before.

Two aspects of the community's relationship to the wider society, one that illustrates the distancing effect of AIDS and one that illustrates the opposite effect, will make these points clearer.

AIDS has created a situation in which antipathy toward persons with AIDS as well as gay people in general has become a serious problem. The community has, through its political and legal structures (such as

the National Gay and Lesbian Task Force and Lambda Legal Defense
Fund), struggled against public hostility toward gay people—hostility
created or intensified by AIDS—as well as the many forms of discrimination and prejudice directed against people with AIDS and HIV-positive persons. These organizations have opposed particular instances of
discrimination (for example, in housing, employment, or insurance);
advocated the passage of protective legislation and the use of public
agencies to protect the civil rights and other interests of gay people and
persons with AIDS; and insisted that the gay community has the right
to determine whether specific public health and related measures proposed as weapons in the fight against AIDS (most notably the HIV antibody–testing controversy) will have adverse or positive effects on its
civil rights or liberties.[46]

The links between the gay community and the scientific and professional communities also define the relationship of gay people to the
outside world. As a group, scientists, physicians, and other professionals have tended to monopolize control over the definition of, and response to, illness and other problems of social welfare in our society.
This monopoly is precisely what the gay community has attempted to
rupture in its desire to empower itself and act as a fully active subject
in the case of AIDS. The problem for the community from the start of
the epidemic was how to use the power and resources of medical and
other professionals as well as government and private philanthropic
bodies—resources that the community could scarcely muster by itself—
without allowing those groups to attain, or regain, significant power
over the community, its sexuality, and its institutions. This problem
placed the community in a difficult position, one that Ronald Bayer, in
a felicitous phrase, has described as "between the specter and the promise of medicine," a description that could be expanded to all areas of
science, healing and caring, and social welfare.[47] The necessity to use
the promise and resources of the scientific and professional worlds forced
the community to eschew total distrust and distancing and attempt to
work closely with them without granting them total trust or authority
over AIDS.

This attempt was made in two closely interrelated manners. First, the
community has insisted, both explicitly and implicitly, that professionals must provide their expertise to persons with AIDS and to gay people
in general but that they must act in partnership with the persons they
serve. Second, the community has in general attempted to learn as much
as possible about medical care, epidemiology, and clinical research re-

garding AIDS. It has clearly believed—as did the women's movement before it—that only through knowledge can it deal with professionals on a basis of relative equality and prevent them from simply imposing their interests, aims, and methodologies on the community and on individuals with AIDS.[48] Such an approach probably has a better chance of working in the applied spheres of the provision of care and social welfare than in those of "purer" scientific research, but even in the latter areas (for example, in pharmaceutical research and trials) the community has made unusual and often successful efforts not to allow professionals to monopolize knowledge and its applications.[49]

These approaches to the scientific and professional communities were handled through a complex process of negotiations over the terms of research into the nature of AIDS. The community could, in fact, enforce it role in this process precisely because its members were needed by scientists as research subjects, just as the community itself required the expertise of scientists and medical researchers. One important illustration of this point involves negotiations over confidentiality of patient data within the research process, something that was naturally of great interest to a community concerned with the possibility of AIDS-related discrimination.

During the first years of the epidemic, the insensitivity of public health researchers forced the gay community into a defensive posture. For example, gay activists learned that the CDC maintained computerized files, with full identifiers, of all reported AIDS cases and had released names of such cases to local health departments and agencies not affiliated with the federal government—agencies such as the New York Blood Center.[50] Gay leaders demanded greater safeguards to protect the privacy of all AIDS patients and research subjects through strict confidentiality strictures. These included the reduction of identifiers, the control of AIDS data from the CDC and the health departments of origin to other agencies, and the creation of a consent form that clearly explained the degree to which the information provided could be protected against release.[51] To do less, according to gay leaders and their allies, would be to jeopardize the validity of epidemiological research, since many research subjects would, out of distrust or fear, provide inaccurate or incomplete information.

Because each needed the other, the gay community and the CDC negotiated. Having empowered itself by "owning" AIDS, the gay community was given de facto recognition as a partner by the U.S. government; the community's authority was therefore heightened. As a result, an almost unprecedented event occurred: the objects of scientific investigations helped define the conditions under which they would agree to participate in studies.

Given the realities of the actual social and historical environment in which it had to operate, the gay community was only partially successful in the efforts we have been discussing. In spite of the gay political movements of the 1970s, it had not yet achieved anything like full legitimacy in American society when AIDS struck. In addition, its search for legitimacy was hindered not only by AIDS itself but by the continued need to struggle on more than one front, most notably against the New Right.

The gay community had internal weaknesses as well. Not all cities or regions heavily affected by AIDS had equally visible or strong gay presences. Those in San Francisco, New York, and a few other large cities had the greatest success in creating caring institutions and in dealing with their local governments and societies. Others were often late in entering the struggle and sometimes failed to develop the full range of gay institutions needed to face the crisis. In this respect, the situation closely echoed the pattern of development of local gay communities and their strengths and weaknesses that had emerged in the 1960s and 1970s.

In addition, the community was never completely united. The community, is, as we have seen, a diffuse and diverse one without a single political voice, and much of its natural constituency is prevented from identifying with it publicly because of the persistence of homophobia and oppression. While the great majority of gays doubtless accepted the broad principles of dealing with AIDS that we have delineated here, many internal struggles arose over particular aspects of the crisis, the community's relationship to the non-gay world, and the community's own institutions. These differences were most notable, as we have seen, in the sphere of sexuality, where conflicts arose over the desirability of closing bathhouses and other sexual establishments. As a result, essential decisions were taken out of the hands of the community and were made instead by governmental and medical personnel.

Given these conditions and difficulties, the achievements of the gay community in the struggles surrounding AIDS have been substantial. Most notably, the community has provided services to persons with AIDS, has helped them to empower themselves, and has fought against discrimination. There have, in addition, been substantial successes even in the more difficult areas of scientific research and the procurement of funding from the federal and local governments. A gay voice has been established in most major aspects of the struggle against AIDS, and large numbers of the scientists, professionals, and government agencies most intimately involved in that struggle have learned to listen to it, at least to some degree. The community has successfully restructured many of its most important institutions and made them into relatively effective forces in the struggle against AIDS. Finally, although the community has not fully succeeded in changing the larger society's perception about AIDS (and about homosexuality itself), especially the perceptions among right-wing groups, it has done so to some degree; and it has certainly in large measure ensured that the crisis has not been ignored even among the most vociferous and powerful opponents of gay people and persons with AIDS.

The paradox seen here is that, just at the time when the wider society was distancing itself from AIDS and persons with AIDS and manifesting the greatest hostility toward gay people, gay people were able to exercise the greatest control over the crisis and to use what by any standard must count as a disaster to empower themselves within American society.

THE PRESENT AND FUTURE

If the anomalous features of the early period of the epidemic opened a window of opportunity for the gay community, that situation could not be expected to continue forever. By working to transform the crisis and render it more "normal," the community had helped draw other groups back into the AIDS epidemic. The window of opportunity that had opened in 1981 and 1982 thus began to close as early as 1983, with the beginning of large-scale interest in the syndrome on the part of researchers and clinicians. By 1985 and 1986 other groups—mainly professionals, the mainstream press, and certain government bodies—had discovered AIDS and were beginning to stake their individual claims to portions of it.

By themselves these factors might have had only minor effects on the situation. More recent developments have probably been of greater significance.

1. The epidemiology of AIDS and the public perception of its risk groups are changing substantially. While gay men continue to form the largest single number of AIDS cases, their numbers are declining as a percentage of total cases, steadily decreasing from over 90 percent dur-

ing the first years of the epidemic to a little more than 55 percent in recent years. [52] In contrast, there has been a dramatic and continuing demographic shift of the epidemic into the IV drug–using community. Although the public continues to associate AIDS and gays, the association is far weaker than in the early years of the epidemic. Indeed, among large parts of the population, an association with AIDS and minority communities appears to be replacing the earlier association with homosexuality.

Moreover, after a slow start, minority and drug-using organizations entered the AIDS struggle in a major way during the late 1980s.[53] These groups naturally sought a place for themselves and, to a certain degree, have come to believe that their place has been filled by gay AIDS organizations, which have garnered the money, talent, and attention, while gay persons with AIDS have been at the center of attention from scientists and researchers. This perception, by no means entirely unrealistic, has led to increasing tension between the two sets of groups. To date, serious conflict has largely been avoided, but whether that will remain the case is uncertain.

In large measure that may depend on the attitudes of the gay AIDS organizations themselves. Although jealous of the immense effort and money it took them to achieve their current position, they will inevitably have to share it with newer, non-gay groups. Many gay-founded groups are, indeed, beginning to do just that, and it is not an accident that gay AIDS organizations provide much of the care required by non-gay persons with AIDS. In addition, many AIDS organizations that are mainly gay are examining, and attempting to correct, their own internal racism. Even though a large proportion of persons with AIDS who are gay are also people of color, the leadership and membership of most gay AIDS organizations have remained largely, although by no means entirely, white. In part this disparity reflects the general tendency in American society to offer white men, and to a rather lesser degree white women, more opportunities to create and support organizations. In part it derives from what appears to be a traditionally lower gay consciousness among people of color. These factors are beginning to change, especially in the newer and more militant AIDS organizations, which have made a point of struggling against racism and sexism; but change is and will most likely continue to be slow in coming.

2. Professionals in general, along with government bodies, are rapidly reestablishing their control over the meaning and treatment of AIDS. Certainly, as we suggested above, by about 1985 both professionals and

the government had become more heavily involved in the epidemic than was earlier the case. Among them were many gay professionals, whose allegiance to their professions itself helped to create a bridge between the two groups. In addition, the institutions that the gay community was instrumental in creating were, in their methods of operation and ways of viewing the epidemic and the world, molded by the professional and scientific world in which they operated; not surprisingly, when one deals with and utilizes the power and resources of outside forces, one has to play by their rules, at least to some extent. It is significant that earlier attitudes of hostility toward professionals and scientists on the part of gay AIDS service organizations have generally given way to mutual cooperation and the rise of what some have begun to view as an "AIDS establishment" that cuts across the gay/straight division and has effectively "co-opted" much of the gay political struggle around AIDS.[54]

3.   Finally, some gay people themselves have begun to question what they consider a single-minded attention to AIDS on the part of the gay community to the detriment of other important issues. In 1989 an essay by Darrell Yates Rist, a gay activist, created a huge stir among gay people.[55] Rist suggested that it was time for the community to pay less attention to AIDS and more to other problems and, in addition, to share power over the crisis with minority and other non-gay groups. Many, although by no means all, of the respondents to the piece were hostile, but it would have been unthinkable for such a piece even to have been written in earlier years. A more measured 1990 essay, by Eric Rofes, has raised similar issues.[56] According to Rofes, professionalism and bureaucratization have tended to separate AIDS work from gay liberation, and AIDS has siphoned off gay funds and talent from other significant aspects of gay politics. Related suspicions about the responsiveness of AIDS organizations to the gay community have been voiced elsewhere.[57]

These voices, although they do not necessarily represent the majority of the gay community, indicate that at least elements of the gay community no longer want to own the disease outright and to focus on it in a single-minded manner. They also indicate that the ambivalence at the heart of the gay acceptance of the identification with AIDS has begun to have negative consequences. Many organizations that arose through the efforts of the gay community are indeed uncertain whether they are AIDS organizations, gay organizations, or both. This uncertainty has begun to affect some groups negatively. For example, AIDS caregiving groups risk losing their governmental and heterosexual connections if they appear to be "too gay"; at the same time, they risk losing their financial supporters and volunteers from the gay community if they appear to be professionally focused only on AIDS to the exclusion of other gay concerns. At least one organization, the San Francisco chapter of ACT UP, a radical AIDS activist group (which we discuss further below), has had to split into two groups—one focusing purely on AIDS; the other on wider social issues, especially those of concern to gay men but also those of concern to lesbians and people of color.[58]

While these indications themselves remain sketchy and the process is unfinished, the years from the beginning of the epidemic to roughly the present do seem to form a single period, one that has probably come to an end or is about to do so. Consequently, the role of the gay community in the epidemic will change significantly, and it will have to rethink its overall strategy if its aims and the principles upon which it based its response to AIDS in the first years of the epidemic are to continue to be even partially successful. In all probability, the entire community will no longer be involved in the struggle against AIDS; instead, there will be increasing bureacratization and professionalization, on both the gay and the non-gay sides, which will tend to exclude significant elements of the community.

That this change and other major changes are already under way is surely indicated by the rise, beginning in mid-1987, of a new style of gay AIDS organizing and struggle, epitomized by the ACT UP (AIDS Coalition to Unleash Power) groups that have arisen in New York and numerous other cities specifically to struggle against the tendencies just mentioned. This new style has less to do with the direct provision of care and lobbying for resources than with a far more confrontational demand for services, resources, and scientific intervention from government and professional bodies—including some established gay-founded and -run AIDS organizations—who are increasingly seen as in control of the epidemic.[59]

ACT UP represents a type of direct action that has rarely been seen so dramatically since the early post-Stonewall days. Indeed, many of its methods (careful attention to news media; use of highly effective, eye-catching graphics; direct participation; decision making by consensus; street demonstrations and confrontations; emphasis on the importance of women, minorities, and IV drug users in the AIDS movement) have much in common with the gay organizations of that period and with the New Left, black, and feminist groups that preceded them. As Douglas Crimp points out, "We [in ACT UP New York] see ourselves both as direct heirs to the early radical tradition of gay liberation and as a rejuvenation of the gay movement, which has in the intervening decades become an assimilationist civil rights lobby."[60]

Significantly, ACT UP has also shown its roots in the 1980s gay AIDS movement as well. It has, for example, managed to combine its radical methods with an extraordinarily impressive attention to the nitty-gritty, scientific aspects of the crisis. It is no exaggeration to claim that many of its members know as much about many aspects of AIDS as the professionals and scientists who have devoted their careers to it. Witness the skill with which ACT UP has managed—naturally, with a variety of allies in the professional worlds—to dramatically alter the manner in which new drugs are tested and introduced into the marketplace in the United States.[61]

ACT UP, with its roots in the gay past, has multiple aims, which, in a sense, recapitulate earlier gay experience:

1. To restructure the public and governmental conception of AIDS.

2. To intervene directly at specific junctures to ensure that AIDS is not ignored and that all persons with AIDS, whether gay or not, receive fair and adequate treatment.

3. To empower persons with AIDS, those with HIV-related illness, and gay persons and others, thereby raising their own consciousness and sense of power. In this respect ACT UP often functions as a kind of "town meeting" of (a part of) the gay community, a town meeting deciding its own identity and determining how to actualize that identity in practice.

The precise relationship between ACT UP, which has become increasingly important in the political and social life of the gay communities in which it operates, and the "first generation" of gay AIDS caregiving and lobbying organizations is only now being defined and remains difficult to describe. To date, there have been many instances of friction—intensified by the fact that the newer groups are led by "movement" activists while the older ones are led by professionals of various types[62]—but there have also been many cases of close cooperation. ACT UP has managed, to some degree, to push older groups into taking more radical, and often more clearly gay, stands on many issues, but the tendency toward absorption of those groups into the wider world of public health, medical, and governmental professionalism remains powerful. The potential for conflict remains large even though both sets of institutions have as their primary focus the AIDS crisis. In any case, the present conjuncture appears to be unique in gay history, in that the community for the first time, and largely as a result of the changing nature of the AIDS crisis, possesses at one and the same moment what we might term a "complete" set of political institutions, ranging from membership organizations practicing lobbying and pressure group activities to participatory groups engaging in direct action.

All this does not mean that the newer groups represent in any full sense a return to the politics of the early post-Stonewall period. The tactics and methods of the newer groups are indeed closely modeled on those of the earlier ones, and there is a certain tendency to share some of its concerns (such as the importance of combating sexism and racism). At the same time, the newer groups have by no means developed as universal a political approach as the earlier ones and still remain focused both on AIDS and the gay community as a legitimate minority rather than on any wider conception of human liberation.

These trends still possess great potential for further development, however, as can be seen in the most recent events within the gay community, events that again have begun to challenge the dominance of AIDS-related issues over other issues of importance to gay people. For the first time in some years, a major new group arose in New York in 1990 and has rapidly spawned chapters across the country. This group, which calls itself Queer Nation, was based not on AIDS organizing (even though most of its members' first political experience was in groups focused on AIDS) but on the success of ACT UP.[63] Using ACT UP's methods of operation and drawing on its gay membership, Queer Nation was created to focus purely on gay-related issues, leaving AIDS to ACT UP. Its membership does not believe that gays can now afford to ignore the AIDS crisis; most of its members remain in ACT UP as well. But it considers other gay issues (especially the fight against gay bashing, which has taken on epic proportions in the streets of many American cities)[64] of equal importance.

A renewed sense of gay militancy, emanating from the achievements of the AIDS struggles of the 1980s and the self-confidence and pride that went with them, infuses all of Queer Nation's activities. Without necessarily having a conscious social vision, Queer Nation is trying to steer the gay community back to a sense of its own uniqueness, to those needs that separate it from the majority community. Its name makes deliberate and proud use of what is, among straight people, a highly derogatory term, and its most favored slogan stresses gayness—and gayness in its most "offensive" form—rather than AIDS: "We're here, we're queer, we're fabulous, get used to it."

AIDS thus appears to be becoming less central to gay identity and gay struggle. Whether this trend will intensify and whether renewed gay activism of a broader sort will sit easily with more narrowly defined AIDS activism are questions that are impossible to answer at this time. The major changes in the political configuration and style of the gay community that will occur in the emerging period, in which gays no longer own AIDS, will only become fully apparent over time.

AIDS will, in any case, continue to affect the gay community and its members for the foreseeable future, and the community will continue to have to work out its relationship to the disease and the wider society while adapting its institutions to the struggle. And—if it is not to undo all the achievements of the gay struggle against AIDS—it will have to rethink that relationship without allowing outsiders simply to "de-gay" the epidemic on their own terms, as they have been inclined to do in the past.

Naturally, many broad and important questions that cannot at present be answered will have to be dealt with: What will the new style of gay politics look like, and will it be able to retain its relatively successful emphasis on self-empowerment? Will the community be able to retain its newfound visibility in the wider society, and will it move toward further integration within that wider society, in spite of continuing day-to-day prejudice and hostility? Will the noticeable "normalization" of the community—which has brought it closer to mainstream realities in terms of sexuality, politics, and social welfare needs—continue? How can the tension between such "normalization" and the self-definition of the gay community as "oppositional" be successfully resolved? Will the community be able to work out satisfactory relationships with minority, women's, and other new AIDS-oriented groups, with which it would seem to have many interests in common? The answers to these and other questions will, in part, depend on a new generation of gay men and lesbians and a new generation of gay leaders, a generation that scarcely remembers Stonewall or the "Dionysian" sexuality of the 1970s, except as the stuff of myths, and has not been devastated by AIDS nearly to the same extent as its predecessors.

This new generation will have to confront the fact that AIDS remains, in many ways, a tiger on whose back the gay community has been riding for years. If it was dangerous to mount the back of the tiger, it will be just as dangerous to get off it.

NOTES

1. Jean-Paul Sartre, *Saint Genet: Actor and Martyr*, trans. Bernard Frechtman (New York: Brazillier, 1963), p. 587. Originally published in French in 1952.

2. Jean-Paul Sartre, *Critique de la raison dialectique* (Paris: Gallimard, 1960), translated into English in two volumes: *Search for a Method*, trans. Hazel Barnes (New York: Knopf, 1963), and *Critique of Dialectical Reason*, trans. Aean Sheridah-Smith (London: New Left Books, 1976).

3. See Jonathan Katz, *Gay American History* (New York: Crowell, 1976), and *Gay/Lesbian Almanac* (New York: Harper and Row, 1983); Jeffrey Weeks, *Coming Out: Homosexual Politics in Britain from the Nineteenth Century to the Present* (New York: Horizon Press, 1977).

4. John D'Emilio, "Gay Politics and Gay Community: The San Francisco Experience," *Socialist Review* 11, no. 1 (January–February 1981): 77–104, *Sexual Politics, Sexual Communities: The Making of a Homosexual Minority in the United States, 1940–1970* (Chicago: University of Chicago Press, 1983).

5. On lesbian identity and sexuality, see Trudy Darty and Sandee Potter, eds., *Women-Identified Women* (Palo Alto, Calif: Mayfield, 1984); Elizabeth M. Ettore, *Lesbians, Women and Society* (Boston: Routledge and Kegan Paul, 1980); Sasha Gregory-Lewis, *Sunday's Women: A Report on Lesbian Life Today* (Boston: Beacon Press, 1979); and Ginna Vida, ed., *Our Right to Love: A Lesbian Resource Book* (Englewood Cliffs, N.J.: Prentice-Hall, 1978).

6. See Evelyn Hooker, "The Homosexual Community," in *Sexual Deviance*, ed. John H. Gangno and William Simon (New York: Harper and Row, 1967), pp. 176–94; Dennis Altman, "Sex: The Frontline for Gay Politics," *Socialist Review* 43 (September–October 1982): 3–17; Laud Humphreys, *Tearoom Trade: Impersonal Sex in Public Places*, expanded ed. (New York: Hawthorne, 1975); Edward Delph, *The Silent Community: Public Homosexual Encounters* (Beverly Hills, Calif.: Sage, 1978).

7. See Martin P. Levine, "Gay Ghetto," in *Gay Men: The Sociology of Male Homosexuality*, ed. Martin P. Levine (New York: Harper and Row, 1979), pp. 182–294; Edmund White, *States of Desire: Travels in Gay America* (New York: Dutton, 1980); and Neil Miller, *In Search of Gay America* (New York: Atlantic Monthly Press, 1989).

8. See J. V. Soares, "Black and Gay," in *Gay Men*, ed. Levine, pp. 263–74; and Michael J. Smith, ed., *Black Men/White Men: A Gay Anthology* (San Francisco: Gay Sunshine Press, 1983).

9. See Don Teal, *The Gay Militants* (New York: Stein and Day, 1971);

Toby Marotta, *The Politics of Homosexuality: How Lesbians and Gay Men Have Made Themselves a Political and Social Force in Modern America* (Boston: Houghton Mifflin, 1981); and Barry D. Adam, *The Rise of a Gay and Lesbian Movement* (Boston: G. K. Hall, 1987).

10. Teal, *The Gay Militants.*

11. See Ronald Bayer, *Homosexuality and American Psychiatry: The Politics of Diagnosis,* 2nd ed. (New York: Basic Books, 1988).

12. See Adam, *Rise of a Gay and Lesbian Movement,* chaps. 5–11.

13. Ibid., chap. 6.

14. See Anita Bryant, *The Anita Bryant Story: The Survival of Our Nation's Families and the Threat of Militant Homosexuality* (Old Tappan, N.J.: Revell, 1977).

15. Ronald Bayer, *Private Acts, Social Consequences: AIDS and the Politics of Public Health* (New York: Free Press, 1989).

16. Michael S. Gottlieb et al., "Gay-Related Immunodeficiency (GRID) Syndrome: Clinical and Autopsy Observations," *Clinical Research* 30 (1982): 349A.

17. Gerald M. Oppenheimer, "In the Eye of the Storm: The Epidemiological Construction of AIDS," in *AIDS: The Burdens of History,* ed. Elizabeth Fee and Daniel M. Fox (Berkeley: University of California Press, 1988), pp. 267–300.

18. *Morbidity and Mortality Weekly Report* 30 (1981): 250–52.

19. David T. Durack, "Opportunistic Infections and Kaposi's Sarcoma in Homosexual Men," *New England Journal of Medicine* 305 (1981): 1466.

20. *Morbidity and Mortality Weekly Report* 30 (1981): 409–10.

21. Oppenheimer, "In the Eye of the Storm," p. 282.

22. *Morbidity and Mortality Weekly Report* 32 (1983): 101.

23. Steven Seiddman, "Transfiguring Sexual Identity: AIDS and the Contemporary Construction of Homosexuality," *Social Text* 19–20 (Fall 1988): 187–206; cf. Dennis Altman, *AIDS in the Mind of America* (New York: Doubleday, 1986), and Cindy Patton, *Sex and Germs: The Politics of AIDS* (Boston: South End Press, 1985).

24. Cf. James Kinsella, *Covering the Plague: AIDS and the American Media* (New Brunswick, N.J.: Rutgers University Press, 1989).

25. Daniel Fox, "Aids and the American Health Polity: The History and Prospects of a Crisis of Authority," in *AIDS: The Burdens of History,* ed. Fee and Fox, pp. 316–43.

26. Randy Shilts, *And the Band Played On: Politics, People, and the AIDS Epidemic* (New York: St. Martin's Press, 1987); D. Guston, *Institutional Tensions in the Federal Government's Response to AIDS* (Cambridge, Mass: Department of Political Science, Program in Science, Technology, and Society, Massachusetts Institute of Technology, 1989); U.S. Congress, Office of Technology Assessment, *Review of the Public Health Service's Response to AIDS,* document no. OTA-TM-H-24 (Washington, D.C.: U.S. Government Printing Office, February 1985); General Accounting Office, *AIDS Education: Activities*

Aimed at the General Public Implemented Slowly, HRD-89-21 (Washington, D.C.: General Accounting Office, 1988).

27. Bayer, *Private Acts, Social Consequences.*

28. This is a phrase borrowed from Harlan Dalton, "AIDS in Blackface," *Daedalus* 118 (Summer 1989): 205–28, at p. 213.

29. Bayer, *Private Acts, Social Consequences,* pp. 20–29.

30. Shilts, *Band Played On.*

31. Larry Kramer, *Reports from the Holocaust* (New York: St. Martin's Press, 1989).

32. See Altman, *AIDS in the Mind of America,* chap. 8.

33. See Richard Goldstein, "AIDS and the Social Contract," in *Taking Liberties: AIDS and Cultural Politics,* ed. Erica Carter and Simon Watney (London: Serpent's Tail, 1989), pp. 81–94.

34. See Brian Wallis, "Aids and Democracy: A Case Study," in *Democracy: A Project by Group Material* (Seattle: Bay Press, 1990), pp. 241ff.

35. Bayer, *Private Acts, Social Consequences;* Shilts, *Band Played On.*

36. See Suzanne C. Ouellette Kobasa, "AIDS and Volunteer Associations: Perspectives on Social and Individual Change," *Milbank Quarterly* 68, Suppl. 2 (1990): 280–94, which provides further references.

37. On the absorption of "death" and the immense meanings AIDS has given it within the gay community, cf. Michael Bronski, "Death and the Erotic Imagination," in *Personal Dispatches: Writers Confront AIDS,* ed. John Preston (New York: St. Martin's Press, 1989), pp. 133–44.

38. Cindy Ruskin, *The Quilt: Stories from the NAMES Project* (New York: Pocket Books, 1988); Robert Dawidoff, "The NAMES Project," in *Personal Dispatches,* ed. Preston, pp. 145–51.

39. Dennis Altman, "Legitimation through Disaster: AIDS and the Gay Movement," in *AIDS: The Burdens of History,* ed. Fee and Fox, pp. 301–15, esp. 302.

40. See Peter S. Arno, "The Contributions and Limitations of Voluntarism," in United Hospital Fund, *AIDS: Public Policy Dimensions* (New York: United Hospital Fund, 1987), pp. 188–92; and Peter S. Arno and Karyn Feiden, "Ignoring the Epidemic: How the Reagan Administration Failed on AIDS," *Health-PAC Bulletin* 17, no. 2 (December 1986): 7–11.

41. See Shilts, *Band Played On;* Bayer, *Private Acts, Social Consequences,* pp. 21ff.; Michael Callen and Richard Berkowitz, "We Know Who We Are," *New York Native,* November 8–21, 1982, pp. 29ff.

42. See, e.g., J. Lynch, cited in Bayer, *Private Acts, Social Consequences,* p. 26.

43. Shilts, *Band Played On;* Bayer, *Private Acts, Social Consequences,* chap. 2.

44. Cindy Patton, "The AIDS Industry: Construction of 'Victims,' 'Volunteers,' and 'Expert,' " in *Taking Liberties,* ed. Carter and Watney, pp. 113–26, at p. 118.

45. Cf. Ines Rieder and Patricia Ruppelt, eds., *AIDS: The Women* (San Francisco and Pittsburgh: Cleis Press, 1988); and Kris Balloun, "Lesbians and the Epidemic," *San Francisco Sentinel,* August 24, 1990, p. 11.

46. Cf. Bayer, *Private Acts, Social Consequences,* pp. 101–36.

47. Ronald Bayer, "AIDS and the Gay Community: Between the Specter and the Promise of Medicine," *Social Research* 53 (Autumn 1985): 581–606.

48. Cf. Mark Harrington, "Let My People In: The Results of Direct Action Have Been Fruitful, Further Validating the Activist Approach to Medical Bureaucracy," *OutWeek,* August 8, 1990, pp. 34–37.

49. See Harold Edgar and David J. Rothman, "New Rules for New Drugs: The Challenge of AIDS to the Regulatory Process," *Milbank Quarterly* 68, Suppl. 1 (1990): 111–42.

50. Personal communication to G. Oppenheimer from Carole Levine, Executive Director, Citizens Commission on AIDS for New York City and Northern New Jersey, June 1989.

51. Ibid.

52. Centers for Disease Control, *HIV/AIDS Surveillance* (Washington, D.C.: CDC, September 1990).

53. See John Anner, "People of Color Define New AIDS Strategies," *Guardian,* September 26, 1990, p. 9; reprinted from *The Minority Trendsetter,* Fall 1990. See also Dalton, "AIDS in Blackface."

54. See, for example, Patton, "The AIDS Industry."

55. Darell Yates Rist, "AIDS as Apocalypse: The Deadly Cost of an Obsession," *Nation,* February 13, 1989, pp. 181ff., with letters to the editor in the March 20, May 1, May 8, June 19, 1989, issues of the *Nation.*

56. Eric Rofes, "Gay Groups vs. AIDS Groups: Averting Civil War in the 1990s," *OutWeek: National Lesbian and Gay Quarterly* 8 (Spring 1990): 8–17.

57. See, for example, Mark Harrington, "Life among the Ruins," *OutWeek,* October 3, 1990, pp. 32–33, calling for greater accountability from AIDS organizations.

58. See Rachel Pepper, "Schism Slices ACT UP in Two: San Francisco Chapter Splits in Debate over Focus," *OutWeek,* October 10, 1990, pp. 12–14; Tim Vollmer et al., "ACT UP/SF Splits in Two over Consensus, Focus," *San Francisco Sentinel,* September 20, 1990, pp. 1, 4–5. Cf. Donna Minkowitz, "ACT UP at a Crossroads," *Village Voice,* June 5, 1990, pp. 19–20: "As the group grows in size and power, a debate is raging: Should ACT UP be an AIDS lobby, a Gay Liberation front, a New Left collective, or all of the above?"

59. The remarks that follow on ACT UP derive, for the most part, from personal observation and participation in the New York City group's meetings and activities. An important published source of information about the group is Douglas Crimp, with Adam Rolston, *AIDS Demo-Graphics* (Seattle: Bay Press, 1990). See also David Handelman, "ACT UP in Anger," *Rolling Stone,* March 8, 1990, pp. 80ff.

60. Crimp and Rolston, *AIDS Demo-Graphics,* p. 98.

61. See Harrington, "Let My People In"; Edgar and Rothman, "New Rules."

62. Cf. Altman, "Legitimation through Disaster," p. 309.

63. See Guy Trebay, "In Your Face! Beyond AIDS, Beyond ACT UP: The Next Wave of Lesbian and Gay Activism Breaks Every Rule," *Village Voice,*

August 14, 1990, pp. 34–39; Robin Podolsky, "Birth of a Queer Nation," *The Advocate,* October 9, 1990, pp. 17ff.; and the various articles on Queer Nation in *OutLook* 11 (Winter 1991).

64. See, for example, the weekly reports on attacks on gays in New York and other cities in the pages of *OutWeek*. See, especially, Nina Reyes, "Reign of Terror," *OutWeek,* October 17, 1990, pp. 34–39.

The First City: HIV among Intravenous Drug Users in New York City

*Don C. Des Jarlais,
Samuel R. Friedman,
and Jo L. Sotheran*

The epidemic of human immunodeficiency virus (HIV) among intravenous (IV) drug users in New York is of particular public health importance because of both the size of the problem and the length of time that the virus has been present among IV drug users in the city. HIV has spread rapidly among drug injectors, not only in New York but also in many other cities, including Edinburgh, Scotland;[1] Bari, Italy;[2] and Bangkok, Thailand.[3] As in New York, many public health and drug abuse treatment systems are coping with the problems of preventing further HIV transmission among drug injectors and providing medical and substance abuse treatment for drug injectors who have developed HIV-related diseases.[4] New York is still, however, the most commonly used negative example of an HIV epidemic among drug injectors. No one wants the rapid transmission of HIV or the problems of coping with HIV seropositives that occurred in New York to be duplicated elsewhere.

Preventing problems of this scale from occurring in other cities requires an understanding of just what did happen in New York. In this essay we review the history of the spread of HIV among IV drug users and the responses of the drug abuse treatment system in New York. We focus on history rather than epidemiology or program administration. In a methods section we describe the personal actions and institutional contexts that shaped both the research on HIV transmission in New York and the translation of the research findings into information that the drug abuse treatment system could use to cope with the epidemic.

HISTORY OF HIV TRANSMISSION

Three cases of pediatric AIDS in children born in 1977 provided the first evidence for HIV infection among IV drug users in New York. These cases were retrospectively diagnosed by the New York City Department of Health AIDS Surveillance Unit. Their only known risk factor was that they were born to IV drug–using mothers.

The earliest-known case of AIDS in an adult IV drug user occurred in 1979 in a man who also had homosexual activity as a risk behavior. The first 5 known cases among heterosexual IV drug users occurred in 1980, when there were an additional 3 cases with IV drug use and male homosexual activity as risk behaviors. Known cases among IV drug users increased rapidly: 8 in 1980; 31 in 1981; 160 in 1982; and 340 in 1983. The 3 cases in 1977 of apparent perinatal transmission from IV drug–using women strongly suggest that HIV was introduced into the IV drug user group around 1975 or 1976, or perhaps even earlier. It was probably introduced into this group from homosexual/bisexual men, with homosexual/bisexual IV drug users serving as a bridge group. The earliest-known adult cases of AIDS all occurred among homosexual/bisexual men not known to have injected drugs, and a very high percentage of homosexual/bisexual men were among the first-known cases among IV drug users. If male homosexual/bisexual IV drug users did serve as a bridge from homosexual/bisexual men who did not inject drugs to heterosexual IV drug users, it is likely that there were multiple points of introduction of HIV into the heterosexual IV drug–using group in New York.

During 1975 to 1978, the initial phase of the epidemic among IV drug users in New York, HIV undoubtedly was being transmitted, but most risk behavior—the sharing of drug injection equipment and unsafe sexual activity—was probably among persons who had not been exposed to the virus. Without extensive serum samples from this time period, we cannot be certain about the spread of HIV among IV drug users, but later samples suggest that the seroprevalence rate remained below 20 percent prior to 1978 among IV drug users in the city.

Seroprevalence data from samples collected in Manhattan from 1978 through 1983 and the rapid rise in cases from 1980 through 1983 indicate that a second phase occurred from approximately 1978 through 1982.[5] During this phase the seroprevalence rate rose rapidly, from less than 20 percent prior to this phase to about 50 percent at the end of the period. In New York City several factors may have contributed to this rapid spread beyond the simple increase in the probability that a partner with whom one shared injection equipment had been exposed to the virus. During the late 1970s and early 1980s, there was a substantial increase in the supply of both heroin and cocaine in the New York area. This increase in supply led to increases in the injection of both drugs, primarily among persons who already had histories of injecting heroin. Frequency of injection of these drugs has been linked to seropositivity among IV drug users in New York City.[6] New York City also has numerous "shooting galleries," places where one may rent drug injection equipment, use it, and then return it to the gallery owner for rental to the next customer. The use of shooting galleries provides a mechanism for the spread of HIV to large numbers of other IV drug users and also has been linked to HIV exposure.[7]

Since 1983 the seroprevalence rate among IV drug users entering treatment in Manhattan appears to have stabilized. No increase has been observed in the seroprevalence rates from 1984 through 1987.[8] (Preliminary analysis of more recent data indicates that this stabilization has persisted through 1990.) In spite of this relative stabilization, new HIV exposures are occurring. Our own cohort study shows an annual rate of new infections of approximately 2 percent among subjects who were initially seronegative,[9] and a cohort study in the Bronx has found a similar seroconversion rate.[10] The current seroprevalence rate among IV drug users in Manhattan may best be understood as a balance among the rate of new infections, presumed "saturation" in IV drug users engaged in very high levels of risk behavior for long time periods, and three additional factors.

One additional factor is the loss of HIV-seropositive drug users from the pool of active IV drug users. Loss of seropositives both reduces the spread of the virus to uninfected IV drug users and, of course, reduces the absolute number of seropositives likely to be found in any sample of recent or current IV drug users. Seropositive drug users may stop injecting, either through their own effort or through a variety of other mechanisms, including successful drug abuse treatment, development of disease, and death from any of a variety of causes. From our ongoing cohort study, we would estimate that approximately 3 percent of seropositives per year are lost from active IV drug use through the development of AIDS and other fatal illnesses.[11]

Conscious AIDS risk reduction would be a second factor reducing the rate of new HIV infections. AIDS-related behavior change is believed to be the primary cause of stabilization of HIV seroprevalence rates among homosexual/bisexual men in San Francisco,[12] and risk reduction is likely to be playing a part in the observed stability of HIV seroprevalence among IV drug users in Manhattan. Several studies have shown AIDS risk reduction among IV drug users in New York City.[13] There is also evidence of increasing behavior change among IV drug users in Manhattan over the period in which the seroprevalence rates have remained at their current level. In 1984, 59 percent of the methadone patients in one sample stated that they had made some form of behavior change in order to reduce the risk of AIDS.[14] When the same question was asked in 1986 of persons who had recently entered methadone treatment, 75 percent stated that they had changed their behavior; and when the question was asked in 1987 of patients entering an experimental methadone program, 85 percent replied that they had changed their behavior.[15]

The final factor that is probably contributing to the observed stability of seroprevalence rates among IV drug users in Manhattan is the entry of new IV drug users into the group. Persons who begin injecting drugs are very unlikely to be HIV seropositive before they begin; continued entry of new users into the IV drug use group would therefore help stabilize the seroprevalence rate below 100 percent saturation.[16]

RESPONSE OF TREATMENT SYSTEM

In New York City the drug treatment system is not integrated with medical treatment. The staff of drug programs had little experience in providing treatment for infectious diseases, and most of the actual spread occurred prior to an AIDS problem. The awareness that did exist was based on cases of AIDS among IV drug users, since antibody testing to monitor spread of the virus itself did not become available until 1984. The first cases among IV drug users that were recognized as AIDS occurred in the second half of 1981, shortly after the syndrome was recognized in homosexual men. The number of cases of AIDS among IV drug users then increased rapidly, doubling approximately every six months over the next three years. When antibody testing did become available in the summer and fall of 1984, the early results indicated that half or more of the IV drug users in the city were already exposed to the virus.[17] These results were communicated to the staff of New York City drug treatment programs through an extended series of training seminars, informal consultations, and an extensive rumor network. The training sessions also presented the "best" scientific data then available on HIV infection and AIDS: that there was no evidence for casual-contact transmission, that all persons carrying the virus must be assumed to be able to transmit it, that AIDS itself was essentially untreatable and fatal, and that only a minority of persons exposed to the virus were expected to develop full AIDS.

The rapid increases in the number of cases, as well as the early antibody test results, caused strong emotional reactions within the drug abuse treatment system. These reactions tended to follow a staged pattern, somewhat similar to the stages outlined by Elisabeth Kübler-Ross in her study of reactions to death and dying.[18]

STAGE ONE: DENIAL

The first stage, occurring from 1982 through 1984–85, can best be termed denial. In this stage programs tried to carry on business as usual in the treatment of drug abuse. AIDS was seen as a special medical problem that did not need to be integrated into the everyday functioning of drug abuse treatment programs. Intake and provision of treatment occurred as before, and no special effort was made to inform staff or clients about AIDS.

AIDS did not easily fit into the normal operation of drug abuse treatment programs. Organizationally, treatment of infectious diseases had not been integrated with therapy and counseling for drug abuse or dispensing medication for methadone maintenance. The number of AIDS cases among IV drug users was relatively small, and most program staff (and clients) associated the disease with male homosexuality. The IV drug use subculture tends to denigrate homosexuality, and the association between AIDS and homosexuality impeded frank discussions of the syndrome. There were concerns that dealing with AIDS would detract from or even contradict the primary business of getting drug abusers to stop using drugs.

Two aspects of this denial stage are particularly worth noting. First, the treatment staff believed that any emphasis on AIDS, because of its association with death, would undermine the hope an individual needs to overcome drug abuse problems. In their view, the hope for a new and better life is a vital part of giving up the short-term pleasures of illicit drug abuse and working through the difficult aspects of drug abuse treatment; if this hope was undermined, drug abusers might discontinue treatment. Second, the treatment staff believed that discussions about AIDS would highlight the difficulties in completely eliminating drug abuse

in any given episode of treatment, thereby reducing the clients' belief
that they might be able to eliminate their IV drug use. A large percentage of persons in ambulatory drug abuse treatment continue to use
illicit drugs while in treatment, and a large percentage of persons in
residential treatment do leave and return to illicit drug abuse. Acknowledgment of a need to prevent AIDS among persons with a history of IV
drug use would require confronting explicitly the discouraging evidence
that a single episode of treatment does not result in complete abstinence
from IV drug use in the majority of persons who enter treatment with
a history of illicit drug injection. Treatment does serve to reduce IV
drug use greatly, both during and after treatment, but complete elimination of IV drug use is a very difficult treatment goal, which often
requires multiple episodes of treatment.[19] This is not just a problem of
working with embarrassing evidence of the difficulties in treating IV
drug use (as well as other forms of addiction). To discuss AIDS with a
person in treatment raises the possibility of treatment failure. Indeed, a
full education about AIDS, including information that the sharing of
drug injection equipment spreads the virus, was often seen as planning
for the failure of treatment to eliminate IV drug use.

    During the "denial" stage the treatment system largely tried to carry
on as usual; that is, by providing drug abuse treatment without any
special education of staff or clients about AIDS. The cognitive beliefs
supporting this behavior were that the staff was not properly equipped
for working with fatal infectious diseases and that making AIDS an
issue in drug abuse treatment would likely undermine the success of
treatment. Providing good drug abuse treatment, however, would reduce IV drug use and thus help to alleviate the AIDS problem. Under-
neath this behavior pattern and belief system, however, there was considerable anxiety about AIDS. This anxiety would become evident in
the "panic" stage.

STAGE TWO: PANIC

    As the AIDS epidemic continued in New York, particularly during
1985 and 1986, it became very difficult for a treatment program to
continue "normal" operations after a person in the program developed
AIDS or AIDS-related complex. Development of HIV disease raised both
realistic and unrealistic fears about AIDS. For clients and staff with
histories of IV drug use, the appearance of AIDS or ARC served as a
warning that they too might develop the disease. Since the person who

developed AIDS typically had been asymptomatic for a considerable time prior to the development of the disease, present health could not be taken as an indication of freedom from AIDS. The presence of AIDS or ARC in a client or staff member also set off fears of casual-contact transmission of AIDS. At the time, the official U.S. Public Health Service description was that AIDS was transmitted through "exchange of bodily fluids." The lack of clarity in this phrase accentuated fears that AIDS could be transmitted through urine, saliva, and sneezing or through such activities as preparing food or sharing the same bathroom facilities.

The occurrence of AIDS in a person associated with a client, such as a relative or sexual partner, was also likely to provoke panic in the program. For example, one client was asked to leave a residential treatment program because the client's husband, who was not in treatment at the time, had developed AIDS.

The panic phase was characterized by a search for information on AIDS. Information about routes of transmission was primary. Other information included the likely outcomes of full AIDS, ARC, and asymptomatic infection; the specific symptoms of ARC and pre-AIDS conditions; and the resources for meeting the practical needs of persons with AIDS, such as arranging medical care and social support from AIDS service organizations in the city.

From the beginning of the epidemic, there has been no evidence for any casual-contact transmission of the virus. This lack of evidence has not prevented widespread fears of casual-contact transmission. Drug abuse treatment staff are particularly susceptible to such fears because they are frequently involved in the handling of "body fluids" when collecting urine specimens for drug testing, and in communal living within residential programs. The lack of clarity in the phrase "exchange of bodily fluids" and the difficulties of proving that casual-contact transmission could not occur exacerbated the fears among drug abuse treatment personnel. As a result, they would sometimes try to get rid of the offending person with AIDS or ARC or the person associated with AIDS. A client who had clinical illness would be sent to a hospital and then would not be permitted to reenter the program even when his or her health would have permitted it. A clinically ill client who was receiving methadone would not be permitted to attend the clinic during normal hours but would be required to attend after normal hours, or not attend at all and be given the medication at home. Refusal to collect urines from persons with AIDS or ARC also occurred.

During the panic phase the treatment staff were forced to confront their fears—the specific fear of possibly contracting AIDS and a generalized fear of death that the epidemic was provoking even in persons who did not believe themselves to be at any risk for contracting the disease. To get through the panic phase, they had to do more than simply acquire new information. They also had to express fears and feelings, receive support for the legitimacy of the fears, develop "guidelines" for the handling of AIDS cases, invoke the authority structure of the program to reestablish professional behavior, and learn how to work with people who were dying. Working through the panic stage involved not only written communications and formal training but also staff meetings, the rumor network within programs, and interpersonal confrontations. Successful working through the panic phase led to the coping phase.

STAGE THREE: COPING

The coping stage has been occurring since 1986, and involves incorporating AIDS issues into the day-to-day operation of drug abuse treatment programs. In programs that are fully in the coping stage, all levels of the staff and clients receive AIDS education and training; and all clients with HIV disease receive drug abuse treatment. Typically, an AIDS coordinator or an AIDS task force is appointed for each program or clinic, and this person or group has ongoing responsibility for formulating policies regarding AIDS issues and for continuing education of the staff and clients regarding AIDS.

The education and counseling of clients are aimed at both reducing AIDS risk behavior and reducing unrealistic fears of casual-contact transmission. Information is provided about heterosexual and *in utero* transmission as well as transmission through sharing drug injection equipment. There is also active encouragement of "safe-sex" behavior through the distribution of condoms to clients. At this stage the treatment staff realize that preventing HIV transmission and AIDS is an integral part of working with persons with a history of IV drug use and with persons who are at risk for future IV drug use. The goal of preventing further HIV transmission (that is, preventing needle-sharing transmission by stopping drug injection) overrides any potential conflict between providing AIDS education and eliminating illicit drug injection.

Coping with the epidemic also involves expanding drug abuse treatment capacity. The AIDS epidemic has increased the demand for treatment among IV drug users, and it is clearly a human and public health tragedy not to provide for the increased demand for treatment. New formats for treatment might need to be developed, to permit larger numbers of IV drug users to be taken into treatment for a given amount of resources. Treatment program staff have been generally supportive of expanding treatment capacity but often express concern that the present programs are already underfunded and that more resources are needed to enrich the quality of the existing programs. Consequently, they also support other efforts at preventing HIV infection among IV drug users. For example, they support a variety of prevention efforts, aimed primarily at IV drug users not in treatment, that do not involve elimination of drug injection. These include public education campaigns (in which IV drug users are informed about the risk of sharing drug injection equipment; or are given bleach, along with instructions on how to decontaminate used injection equipment; or are actually provided with sterile equipment) and programs to prevent persons at risk from starting to inject drugs. A syringe exchange program was started by the New York City Department of Health in 1988 and received mixed support from the drug treatment programs (prior to its termination in 1990 after a new mayor was elected). Some programs quietly supported the exchange, while others publicly opposed it as "condoning" illicit drug use or possibly taking resources away from the drug treatment system.

Treatment programs in the coping stage are also providing drug abuse treatment to persons with AIDS and with ARC, and to asymptomatic HIV seropositives. Fears of casual-contact transmission are well under control and are not permitted to interfere with humane treatment of persons with HIV disease. Staff have developed expertise in counseling regarding death and dying and in meeting the many practical needs of persons with AIDS when such persons are neither sufficiently ill to require hospitalization nor well enough to handle all tasks of daily living. Providing drug abuse treatment to persons with AIDS and/or ARC requires developing close liaison with hospitals that provide inpatient treatment for AIDS, as well as making some changes in the normal operations of the drug abuse treatment program. Clients with AIDS or ARC do have special medical and psychological needs, and providing for those needs requires alteration of program functioning.

In addition to providing treatment for IV drug users with AIDS and ARC, staff of programs in the coping stage frequently serve as consultants to infectious disease specialists who provide inpatient treatment for IV drug users with AIDS. Infectious disease staff are not likely to have much experience with extended treatment for IV drug users. They will often need expert advice on how to recognize the behavior patterns associated with drug abuse and how to avoid discriminating against persons with a history of IV drug use. Closer cooperation between infectious disease personnel and drug treatment personnel has also occurred with the recent increase in HIV counseling and testing in drug abuse treatment programs. Clients who test positive need to be referred for medical treatment of their HIV infection, including antiviral treatment. As of mid-1990, however, only a comparatively small number of such clients were receiving antiviral treatment, so that this is clearly an area of needed improvement.

This coping stage sounds quite idealistic, and certainly not all programs that we have observed are managing to cope with all aspects of the AIDS epidemic all of the time. The AIDS epidemic has, however, led to increased dedication and skill levels among many drug abuse treatment staff. At the same time, there is a possibility that the staff may progress to a potential fourth stage.

A POTENTIAL STAGE FOUR: BURNOUT

Coping with the AIDS epidemic has high costs, both in financial and in human terms. The episodes of burnout that we have observed have been in individuals rather than in programs as a whole, and in those individuals the burnout has not been permanent. The burnout has involved a sense of being overwhelmed, depression, hopelessness, inability to set priorities and organize work, and a confusion of purpose. Staff suffering from burnout typically have been in programs with numerous cases of AIDS or ARC among clients. These clients require considerable extra counseling as they face death; and they have many practical needs, such as housing, that can be difficult to meet. If the client has young children, there are the additional problems of potential HIV infection and AIDS in the children and/or providing for the children after the death of the parent.

Part of the strain involved in potential burnout comes about because the staff feel obligated to be optimistic and hopeful about the outcomes of clients' HIV disease and about preventing infection among the unexposed; but they do not have any clear indicators of success in either of these areas. A second part of the strain comes from their sense that the needs created by the epidemic have completely taken over their professional lives. It seems as though they went from working in a drug abuse treatment program into working in an AIDS program without a conscious choice in the matter.

From our observations, protection against burnout is possible. Recognition of burnout as a potential problem is critical; in particular, those experiencing burnout must be given legitimacy for expression of their feelings within an appropriate setting. Peer counseling/self-help groups, both within and across programs, appear to be particularly useful in working with symptoms of burnout. Reducing burnout also requires realistic limitations on what program staff can be expected to do regarding the epidemic. Unfortunately, realism will often mean that many things that need to be done regarding the AIDS epidemic among IV drug users will be beyond the resources of drug abuse treatment programs.

DISCUSSION

One of the pleasures of writing history is drawing analogies between what happened in one location and time and what may happen in other locations in the future. We will refer readers to recent reviews of HIV transmission among intravenous drug users, and restrain ourselves in this respect, leaving much of this task to persons in those other locations.[20]

We do, however, wish to make a few brief comments about possible analogies. First, the current relative stabilization of HIV seroprevalence among IV drug users in New York indicates that there has been a substantial slowing of HIV transmission among IV drug users in the city. Similar stabilization has also been observed in San Francisco, Amsterdam, Stockholm, and Innsbruck.[21] The relative importance of the factors leading to this slowing has not been determined. This development does, however, indicate that AIDS risk reduction among IV drug users may be effective, and efforts to prevent the spread of HIV among IV drug users should be undertaken or strengthened in many different areas.

Second, given the availability of antibody testing, the reaction of drug abuse treatment systems to an AIDS epidemic is less likely to be closely tied to the development of cases of AIDS. From our observation of drug abuse treatment systems in other areas, however, we do believe that many of the stages we saw in the New York drug abuse treatment system are being repeated elsewhere. Denial is more likely to be based on a low seroprevalence rate rather than a small number of cases, and the exclusionary procedures we observed in a panic stage are more likely to be occurring in a denial stage, with antibody testing used as a method for exclusion.

The increased use of HIV antibody testing and the development of medical treatments that retard HIV immunosuppression and reduce the chances of opportunistic infections also mean that "coping" with a local HIV epidemic will require providing drug users with access to at least the currently approved medical treatments for persons with HIV infection. A better understanding of the reactions of drug abuse treatment systems to a local AIDS epidemic will require data from many more cities. We hope that this staging system will at least provide an adaptable framework for collecting such data.

METHODS

The source for almost all the work described here—the research on the spread of HIV among drug injectors in New York City, the research on behavioral change by drug injectors in response to the AIDS epidemic, and the information that served as a basis for the training sessions for the staff of the drug treatment programs—was a single research grant (R01 DA03574) from the National Institute on Drug Abuse (NIDA). It is appropriate for us to include a brief history of this grant as a "methods" section for the above data.

Work on writing this grant began in 1982, and the first funding was obtained in 1983. With continued funding through competing renewals, the grant is currently funded through 1994, making it undoubtedly the longest continuous study of AIDS among intravenous drug users. It was also the first NIDA-funded study of AIDS among intravenous drug users. Institutions cooperating in the grant included the New York State Division of Substance Abuse Service (DSAS) and its affiliated nonprofit research corporation, Narcotic and Drug Research, Incorporated (NDRI). Because the DSAS is responsible for the funding and oversight of the drug abuse treatment programs in New York, and because the NDRI, under a contract from the Division of Substance Abuse Services, is responsible for providing in-service training for drug abuse treatment staff, these two organizations were well situated for incorporating results from AIDS research into the operations of drug abuse treatment programs. Another participating institution was Beth Israel Medical Center, where blood samples from intravenous drug users had been collected in 1978 through 1983 and stored for later research. The testing of these stored blood samples for HIV was critical in developing an understanding of the early history of the spread of HIV among drug injectors in New York.[22]

Work on developing the grant was initiated by Charles Sharp, a project officer at NIDA. During 1982 Dr. Sharp made several trips to New York City to meet with researchers and encourage them to develop and submit a proposal to study AIDS in intravenous drug users. Researchers from the New York State Division of Substance Abuse Services, New York University Medical Center, Beth Israel Medical Center, and Rockefeller University began meeting irregularly to develop the grant proposal. These researchers became the investigators for grant R01 DA03574. The group included Don C. Des Jarlais and Douglas S. Lipton, New York State Division of Substance Abuse Services; Michael Marmor, New York University Medical Center; Usha Mathur, Donna Mildvan, and Stanley R. Yancovitz, Beth Israel Medical Center; Mary Jeanne Kreek, Rockefeller University; Thomas Spira, Centers for Disease Control; Waffa M. El-Sadr, Veterans Administration Medical Center of New York; and Robert S. Holzman, New York University School of Medicine. The group represented a wide variety of disciplines, including drug abuse, epidemiology, immunology, and infectious diseases. Don Des Jarlais assumed overall responsibility for preparation of the grant proposal, because of his personal intellectual interest in AIDS and his ability to reduce other work demands, and because no one else volunteered for the task.

The study was originally designed as a case-control study in which intravenous drug users with diagnosed AIDS were compared with intravenous drug users without diagnosed AIDS. The proposal was submitted in the spring of 1983 and was reviewed by a special review group at NIDA that summer. Of the forty-four proposals submitted for review at that time, it was the only proposal funded to study AIDS in intravenous drug users. At that time, the NIDA policy toward AIDS research was that, while drug users were at greatly increased risk for AIDS, they were also at greatly increased risk for other diseases, such as hepatitis B and endocarditis. Even though it was the lead agency for research on drug abuse in the United States, NIDA research rarely focused on medical complications of drug abuse. Research on these diseases was generally left to the National Institutes of Health.[23] Grant R01 DA03574 was the only NIDA-funded study of AIDS in intravenous drug users for approximately two years.

Samuel Friedman joined the study early in 1984 as a data analyst. He was quickly promoted to project director and then became a coprincipal investigator. Jo Sotheran joined the grant as a research associate in the fall of 1984 and was later promoted to project director. One of the original components of the study was to compare lymphocyte subsets of the cases to the controls. This comparison required a cell sorter, which was to be purchased at one of the participating institutions. Difficulties in finding a suitable location for the cell sorter led to an indefinite delay in purchasing the machine. Dr. David Sencer, commissioner of the New York City Department of Health, then offered the services of the New York City Health Laboratory for cell sorting at no charge to the grant. The Health Department became an official collaborating institution for the grant.

Through an affiliation with Dr. Thomas Spira of the Centers for Disease Control, developmental HIV antibody testing was provided for the grant in the spring and summer of 1984. The antibody tests revealed that more than half of the "control" group had already been exposed to the AIDS virus; the research design was then changed to a seroprevalence study followed by a cohort study of seronegative and seropositive intravenous drug users. It was these data on seroprevalence that provided the first information about the extent of HIV infection among drug injectors in New York. These data were very useful in assisting treatment programs to begin coping with the magnitude of the AIDS epidemic among drug users in New York City.

CONCLUSION

Writing about the history of the AIDS epidemic among drug injectors in New York from the perspective of researchers leads us to reflect on how little has been written about the epidemic from the perspective of the drug injectors themselves. The mass media, a number of scholarly works, and a number of artistic works have presented the epidemic from the perspectives of gay men. In contrast, the mass media, in their coverage of the AIDS epidemic, have paid relatively little attention to drug injectors, and much of that attention has been on drug injectors as sources of infection for women, heterosexual men, and children.[24] A small number of ethnographic studies of drug injectors have incorporated drug injectors' perspectives on the epidemic,[25] but even these are clearly filtered through the research methods employed in studies of other people with AIDS and are usually focused on finding ways of reducing HIV transmission rather than capturing the experiences of the drug injectors. Oral histories[26] or autobiographies[27] may provide the best methods for presenting the perspectives of drug injectors during the epidemic, but it will be necessary for such projects to be undertaken immediately to avoid permanent loss of much historical information.

NOTES

An earlier version of this paper was presented at the Colloque International SIDA et Toxicomanie: Repondre, Paris, December 9, 1988. The section on transmission of the virus is adapted from Don C. Des Jarlais et al., "HIV-1 Infection among Intravenous Drug Users in Manhattan," *Journal of the American Medical Association* 261, no. 7 (1989): 1008–12. The section on the response of the treatment system is adapted from Don C. Des Jarlais, "Stages in the Response of the Drug Abuse Treatment System to the AIDS Epidemic in New York City," *Journal of Drug Issues* 20, no. 2 (1990): 335–47.

1. J. R. Robertson et al., "Epidemic of AIDS Related Virus (HTLV-III/LAV) Infection among Intravenous Drug Users," *British Medical Journal* 292 (1986): 527–29.

2. G. Angarano et al., "Rapid Spread of HTLV-III Infection among Drug Addicts in Italy," *Lancet* 2, no. 8467 (1985): 1302.

3. S. Vanichseni et al., "Second Seroprevalence Survey among Bangkok's Intravenous Drug Addicts (IVDA)," paper presented at the Fifth International Conference on AIDS, Montreal, June 4–9, 1989.

4. For reviews of current epidemiology and treatment efforts, see C. F. Turner, H. G. Miller, and L. E. Moses, eds., *AIDS: Sexual Behavior and Intravenous Drug Use* (Washington, D.C.: National Academy Press, 1989); and Gerry V. Stimson, "The Prevention of HIV Infection in Injecting Drug Users: Recent Advances and Remaining Obstacles," paper presented at the Sixth International Conference on AIDS, San Francisco, June 23, 1990.

5. Des Jarlais et al., "HIV-1 Infection among Intravenous Drug Users in Manhattan"; David M. Novick et al., "Cocaine Injection and Ethnicity in Parenteral Drug Users during the Early Years of the Human Immunodeficiency Virus (HIV) Epidemic in New York City," *Journal of Medical Virology* 29 (1989): 181–85.

6. Michael Marmor et al., "Risk Factors for Infection with Human Immunodeficiency Virus among Intravenous Drug Abusers in New York City," *AIDS* 1 (1987): 39–44.

7. Ibid.

8. Des Jarlais et al., "HIV-1 Infection among Intravenous Drug Users in Manhattan."

9. See the following papers by Don C. Des Jarlais et al.: "Development of AIDS, HIV Seroconversion, and Co-factors for T4 Cell Loss in a Cohort of Intravenous Drug Users," *AIDS* 1 (1987): 105–11; "HIV-1 Infection among

Intravenous Drug Users in Manhattan"; and "HIV-1 Is Associated with Fatal Infectious Diseases Other Than AIDS among Intravenous Drug Users," paper presented at the Fourth International Conference on AIDS, Stockholm, June 1988.

10. Gerald Friedland, personal communication, April 1991.

11. Marmor et al., "Risk Factors for Infection"; Des Jarlais et al., "HIV-1 Is Associated with Fatal Infectious Diseases Other Than AIDS."

12. W. Winkelstein et al., "The San Francisco Men's Health Study, III: Reduction in Human Immunodeficiency Virus Transmission among Homosexual/Bisexual Men, 1982–1986," *American Journal of Public Health* 77 (1987): 685–89.

13. Don C. Des Jarlais, S. R. Friedman, and W. Hopkins, "Risk Reduction for the Acquired Immunodeficiency Syndrome among Intravenous Drug Users," *Annals of Internal Medicine* 103 (1985): 755–59; Don C. Des Jarlais and William Hopkins, "Free Needles for Intravenous Drug Users at Risk for AIDS: Current Developments in New York City," *New England Journal of Medicine* 103 (1985): 313–23; S. R. Friedman et al., "AIDS and Self-Organization among Intravenous Drug Users," *International Journal of the Addictions* 22 (1987): 201–20; P. A. Selwyn et al., "Knowledge about AIDS and High-Risk Behavior among Intravenous Drug Abusers in New York City," *AIDS* 1 (1987): 247–54.

14. Friedman et al., "AIDS and Self-Organization among Intravenous Drug Users."

15. Des Jarlais et al., "HIV-1 Infection among Intravenous Drug Users in Manhattan."

16. Samuel R. Friedman et al., "AIDS and the New Drug Injector," *Nature* 339 (1989): 333–34.

17. T. J. Spira et al., "Prevalence of Antibody to Lymphadenopathy-Associated Virus among Drug-Detoxification Patients in New York," *New England Journal of Medicine* 311 (1984): 467–68.

18. Elizabeth Kübler-Ross, *On Death and Dying* (New York: Macmillan, 1980).

19. D. R. Gerstein and H. J. Harwood, eds., *Treating Drug Problems* (Washington, D.C.: National Academy Press, 1990); R. L. Hubbard et al., *Drug Abuse Treatment: A National Study of Effectiveness* (Chapel Hill and London: University of North Carolina Press, 1989); U.S. Congress, Office of Technology Assessment, *The Effectiveness of Drug Abuse Treatment: Implications of Controlling AIDS/HIV Infection* (Washington, D.C.: OTA, 1990).

20. Turner, Miller, and Moses, *AIDS: Sexual Behavior and Intravenous Drug Use;* Stimson, "Prevention of HIV Infection in Injecting Drug Users."

21. Turner, Miller, and Moses, *AIDS: Sexual Behavior and Intravenous Drug Use.*

22. Any discussion of the early history of research on AIDS among intravenous drug users in New York City must also acknowledge the critical work done at the Montefiore Medical Center under the leadership of Gerald Friedland. The Monefiore research included important studies of the different modes of transmission for AIDS. Of particular importance to understanding the spread

of the virus and to modifying the response of drug abuse treatment program staff were the studies showing that AIDS is not transmitted through ordinary household contact. The consistency of the research results from the DSAS-NDRI–Beth Israel–New York University research and the Montefiore research enabled us to incorporate research results into training for drug abuse treatment staff. Had there been substantial disagreements in the research results, none of the studies would have been credible to nonresearchers.

23. This policy dramatically changed with the growing importance of AIDS; by the late 1980s AIDS research accounted for approximately half of all NIDA research.

24. James Kinsella, *Covering the Plague: AIDS and the American Media* (New Brunswick, N.J.: Rutgers University Press, 1989); Don C. Des Jarlais, "Pride and Prejudice" (Review of *Covering the Plague: AIDS and the American Media; AIDS: A Moral Issue;* and *AIDS and the Courts*), *Nature* 346 (1990): 521–22.

25. For example, Sheigla Murphy and Dan Waldorf, "Kickin" Down to the Street Doc: Shooting Galleries in the San Francisco Bay Area," manuscript submitted for publication, 1989.

26. For example, David Courtwright, H. Joseph, and Don C. Des Jarlais, *Addicts Who Survived: An Oral History of Narcotic Use in America, 1923–1965* (Knoxville: University of Tennessee Press, 1989).

27. For example, William Burroughs, Jr., *Kentucky Ham* (New York: Berkley Publishing Corp., 1973); and Art Pepper and Laurie Pepper, *Straight Life: The Story of Art Pepper* (New York: Schirmer Books, 1979).

PART IV

International Perspectives

AIDS Policies in the United Kingdom: A Preliminary Analysis

Virginia Berridge and Philip Strong

In a paper on the intellectual agenda surrounding the AIDS epidemic, Jeffrey Weeks comments that "AIDS has . . . provided important insights into the complexities of policy formation in pluralist societies."[1] But, with some notable exceptions,[2] most of the burgeoning social science research on AIDS has necessarily focused not on policy formation but on studies of sexual behavior or disease transmission.[3] Historians, as social scientists, have been prominent in bringing the historical record into debates on AIDS. But, as Daniel M. Fox and Elizabeth Fee observe, they have played relatively little part in writing and analyzing the "contemporary history" of AIDS.[4]

In this essay we focus both on AIDS policy development and on "contemporary history." We chronicle the development of AIDS policies in the United Kingdom in the 1980s and focus on three distinct stages of policy development. In particular we show how an initial policy vacuum in the AIDS area gave rise to a new "policy community" and how that community has changed over time. We outline some themes for future policy research and examine the potential role that historians could play in the study of AIDS policies. "Contemporary history," in the United Kingdom at least, has so far focused almost exclusively on "high politics."[5] Indeed, some practitioners have argued that the term *contemporary history* applies only to conventional political history. We will argue that the study of AIDS policies can provide a model, too, for the way in which the "contemporary history" of health and science policy could develop.[6]

This essay is a preliminary analysis based on a survey of the historical material already available: in part published sources, in part a round of initial interviews with participants in the AIDS arena—among them a senior civil servant; gay community activists; those involved in voluntary organizations, both gay and non-gay; clinicians; an actuary; and representatives of a pharmaceutical company. Its purpose is not to convey direct policy advice or to lay down a policy message—much of the social science research on AIDS has necessarily been funded with such an aim—but to identify the nature and determinants of issues, to raise questions about policy rather than to suggest solutions. Nor is its purpose to praise or to assign blame. As Roy Porter commented in a review of Randy Shilts's *And the Band Played On*, " 'Heroes and villains' history only gets you so far. . . . We need a much more reflective grasp of the dialectics of making decisions. . . . Shilts typically reduces complex issues to personalities, and neglects the social and structural. By all means let's blame Reagan and media homophobia. But let us also see that the appalling slowness and ineptitude of the U.S. response to AIDS arose out of the mixed blessings of the decentralised state and of City Hall caucus politics."[7] The focus of this study is, by contrast, British AIDS policies, but the emphasis on the necessity for structural rather than personal levels of analysis is the same.

First, the basic epidemiological story of AIDS in the United Kingdom needs to be quickly outlined. The disease was first diagnosed there in 1981, and the first AIDS death in the United Kingdom was reported in 1982. By the end of 1983, there had been 29 cases; there were 106 by 1984, 271 by 1985, and 610 by 1986. By the end of April 1989, there had been 2,228 cases in total, of which 1,190 had resulted in death. London remained the primary center for AIDS cases; the majority of cases came from the Thames regions of the National Health Service. These comprised 70 percent of the total number of cases in the first quarter of 1989. As for the types of people with AIDS, 95 percent were men, and the great majority of these were homosexual or bisexual; 6 percent of these cases were hemophiliacs, and 6 percent were drug users or had acquired the disease through heterosexual intercourse. For HIV-positive persons the percentages were different. Here 14 percent were drug users, nearly half of them women. Drug users are a growing category of the seropositive. Consequently, because of the high proportion of seropositive IV drug users in Scotland, Edinburgh and Dundee in particular, its geographical importance is increasing.[8]

CHRONOLOGY OF AIDS IN THE UNITED KINGDOM

The periodization assigned to the epidemic varies. Jeffrey Weeks, for example, sees 1981–1982 as "the dawning crisis." Then followed (in 1982–1985) a period of "moral panic," when AIDS "became the bearer of a number of political, social and moral anxieties, whose origins lay elsewhere, but which were condensed into a crisis over AIDS." This period was followed by a period of "crisis management," beginning in 1985 and lasting until the present.[9] Weeks uses evidence both from the United States and the United Kingdom to support his case; the death of Rock Hudson in 1985 marked a turning point in public perceptions of AIDS in both countries. Other policy studies have focused on the "crisis management" period—the period when AIDS became a direct and immediate concern for politicians. The emphasis in these studies is on policy as a top-down process; on AIDS as exemplifying the role of the state in sending signals to the public, as well as receiving them; on the consensual nature of policymaking and the handling of AIDS within traditional British policy structures.[10]

We emphasize different aspects to the AIDS story and specify three distinct policy phases. In the first phase (1981–1986), AIDS slowly became a national policy issue. Policy was essentially, particularly at the beginning, formed in a bottom-up rather than a top-down way. It was initially formed at the local level, both through gay groups and through the construction of clinical and scientific expertise. These groups coalesced to form an initial "policy community" around public health interests in the Department of Health. In the second and briefer phase (1986–1987), a period of "wartime emergency," AIDS came to be viewed as a clear political priority rather than simply a departmental matter, and sections of society were put on almost a wartime footing to meet what was regarded as a national emergency. This phase has been followed (1987–1988 to the present) by a phase of "normalization," where AIDS and the reaction to it are becoming part of the normal policy and institutional processes. The threat of immediate epidemic spread has receded; and the threat of widespread heterosexual infection no longer appears imminent. Changes in therapy and the time scale of disease progression have helped to bring about a model of chronic, rather than acute, disease, which has aided, but not determined, the process of normalization.

1981–1986: CONSTRUCTION OF A POLICY COMMUNITY

In the early 1980s there was little by way of a reaction from central government. In 1981 the *Annual Report of the Chief Medical Officer* noted that for the first time there had been more than half a million new cases of venereal disease, concentrated particularly in the more recently recognized sexually transmitted diseases.[11] However, at that time this increase was not regarded as so significant that it required political action. Ironically, too, the same report contained the conclusions of an advisory group on the management of patients with spongiform encephalopathy—namely, that "Creutzfeldt-Jakob disease was the only disorder caused by a transmissible slow virus agent which is likely to be encountered in the UK."[12]

Initial knowledge of and reactions to AIDS had instead a volunteer ethos; knowledge of the disease was transmitted through existing gay networks and served also to consolidate them. New organizations also began to be founded. How did this gay response develop? Some gay men were in the United States in the early 1980s and began to hear about people dying of strange cancers. A member of a student gay group at Cambridge recalled that the groups's gay helpline began to get calls after a BBC *Horizon* program, "Killer in the Village," in 1983. The students began to look around for information and to hold weekly meetings on AIDS and health issues. "We were groping in the dark. There was no sense of there being anyone other than us to turn to."[13] That television program, like others later in the epidemic, appears to have had a key impact on the gay response. Volunteers at the Gay and Lesbian Switchboard in London arranged to open up a special line after the program, and volunteers were specifically briefed. "For a number of days after, a lot of very worried people were ringing. . . . The 'Killer in the Village' program was absolutely crucial."[14]

The Gay and Lesbian Switchboard was of central importance in the initial response. In May 1983 more than two hundred attended the country's first public conference on AIDS organized by the Switchboard. Mel Rosen, director of the New York–based Gay Men's Health Crisis, spoke. Some present at the conference remembered his words: "There's a train coming down the track and it's heading at you." A member of the audience recalled: "I was struck by the potential gravity of what was happening and the absolute silence on what was happening. There was very little in the mainstream press."[15] The *Horizon* program also led to the refounding (in 1983) of the Terrence Higgins Trust, originally established in 1982 by friends of Terrence Higgins, who had died of AIDS in abject circumstances in a London hospital. When the trust was refounded, many of the Switchboard volunteers—including Tony Whitehead, later chairman of the Steering Committee of the trust—moved over to it. By the end of 1983, the trust was producing its first leaflets on AIDS, and it opened its own AIDS helpline early in 1984. Articles in the gay press—for example, by Julian Meldrum, the trust's press officer and also a *Capital Gay* correspondent—forced discussion of issues such as safe sex and the role of promiscuity within the gay community. One gay man recalled, "Safe sex really hit London at the end of 1984."[16]

Also involved in the initial gay response was the Gay Medical Association, which produced a leaflet early on directed at doctors dealing with AIDS. Its response was to stress the potential and actual heterosexual nature of the disease. In April 1983 a letter in the *British Medical Journal* put this point strongly. In an AIDS review article, A. P. Waterson, a virologist, had compared the syndrome to diseases of overcrowded poultry, relating it, as was common at that time, to the use of nitrites and the high number of sexual contacts among some gay men.[17] Gay Medical Association representatives commented: "Of course, promiscuity is an important factor in the spread of communicable diseases, but promiscuity is not the prerogative of homosexuals. . . . The homosexual community has demonstrated its awareness of its own health problems. We are confident that it will respond to health education programmes which are not underwritten by any prejudice or moralising." The correspondents pointed out that this condition could potentially affect the whole of society; already around 25 percent of cases to date had not been in homosexual males.[18]

Many dimensions of the initial gay response remain to be documented. But its voluntaristic, self-helping ethos is clear—with meetings in gay men's houses and flats and in gay pubs. "We formed an ad hoc committee . . . and I called a public meeting in the upstairs bar of the London Apprentice at Hoxton, a gay pub. It wasn't an education meeting, it was a recruitment meeting."[19] The "gay freemasonry," the already existing networks of gay men, operated to spread advice and information and to develop reactions to the disease. By 1983 organized sections of the activist gay community had developed specifically around the AIDS issue. (Such phrases are, of course, shorthand. We are wary of monolithic interpretations such as "gay community" or "medical profession," being aware of debates and tensions within these groups.)

The policy aims were threefold: to convey the message of the dangers of AIDS to gay men; to develop a more public role (but without thereby sacrificing credibility among gays) by raising public and political awareness of the dangers of an AIDS epidemic; and to prevent the danger of an anti-gay backlash by stressing—as the Gay Medical Association had done—the idea of AIDS as potentially and actually a heterosexual disease.

Another policy lobby was also forming at around the same time. Clinical and scientific expertise on AIDS was also in the process of being established. The human immunodeficiency virus was first identified in 1983. Up to and for some time after that date, there was an absence of the kind of scientific knowledge and scientific certainty that had come to be an expected concomitant of any normal fight against disease. Professor Waterson's 1983 summary demonstrated the uncertainty: "The most sinister feature of this acquired immune deficiency is that it appears to be communicable, perhaps principally by intimate physical contact." This scientific vacuum led to explanations couched in terms of morality rather than of science: "The traffic in human material in certain quarters by abnormal routes has reached such a level that, combined with the effects of drug abuse of various kinds, the sheer weight of chemical and microbial insult to the body in general, and to T-lymphocytes in particular, goes beyond the tolerable limit."[20] The *Annual Report of the Chief Medical Officer for 1983* did not moralize but was no less tentative: "Expert opinion suggests that there is no risk of contracting AIDS as a result of casual or social contact with AIDS patients eg. on public transport, in restaurants, or in private dwellings. The spread of AIDS appears to require intimate contact."[21] The explanations being advanced in the scientific and medical press—links with African swine fever; the virus emerging from Africa or Haiti—show that scientific knowledge of the sort normally taken for granted was in the process of being constructed.[22]

Expertise also requires experts; and the AIDS experts initially came from a range of areas, such as immunology and virology, and from cancer research, where work on retroviruses had been undertaken for the previous twenty years and where the change from studying chicken viruses to studying human retroviruses had already been made because of new directions in leukemia research. Significantly, too, AIDS brought the area of sexually transmitted diseases and genitourinary medicine in from the cold. One participant commented: "It was a 'Cinderella specialty' with poor facilities and second-rate people working in it. . . . You could go into genitourinary medicine without a higher medical qualification. . . . It was a pretty poor service in terms of the quality of physicians and facilities. . . . AIDS has helped—it's made genitourinary medicine a primary career option." [23]

AIDS meant, too, that a specialty not normally close to the center of policy formation in the health arena was drawn directly into a policy advisory role. The early researchers in the AIDS area in Britain came from this mixed type of background. Jonathan Weber and Robin Weiss at the Institute of Cancer Research were viologists; Anthony Pinching at St. Mary's and Richard Tedder at the Middlesex were immunologists; Michael Adler at the Middlesex and Charles Farthing at St. Stephen's were specialists in genitourinary medicine. The Social Services Committee report noted in 1987 the "haphazard recruitment" of expertise to AIDS.[24] There were undoubted tensions and differences, as there are in any scientific community; but these new-fledged scientific and medical experts also developed a consistent policy line and a means of airing it. Particularly noticeable was the high media profile they adopted in order to press the case for urgent action on the part of government. Certain of them adopted an overt public lobbying style, which was initially characteristic of the AIDS area. In the absence of the type of established policy consultative machinery that would exist in a well-established area of health policy, the experts resorted to the press and to television. In doing so, they were consolidating existing patterns of health reporting, which rely heavily on the small circle of medical "experts."[25] But they were also joined by gay AIDS activists. The Terrence Higgins Trust in particular was aware of the value of using the media. It became "pretty clued up about news management," as one activist put it.[26] Gay activists and the medical and scientific experts were prepared to be openly critical of lack of action on the part of government or the research councils. Anthony Pinching, for example, in his evidence to the Social Services committee, attacked the Medical Research Council's funding of AIDS research—peer review was in fact "peer refusal."[27] Jonathan Weber criticized its roles as "leading from behind."[28]

The type of public reaction that would normally lead to exclusion from the "corridors of power" in this case brought admission to them. For the external policy lobbies were complemented by the "public health" reaction to AIDS within the Department of Health. AIDS was initially dealt with through classic public health routines of monitoring and surveillance. From 1982 onward AIDS cases were monitored on a voluntary basis by the Communicable Disease Surveillance Center at Colindale (part of the Public Health Laboratory Service, whose uncertain future was saved by its role in monitoring AIDS).[29] CDSC doctors early on developed links with gay activists in the Terrence Higgins Trust. Sir Donald Acheson, the chief medical officer, as a public health epidemiologist himself, was also well aware of the disease's potential for spread. His annual reports made conscious references to the role of the great nineteenth-century public health pioneers, such as Sir John Simon, medical officer to the Privy Council Office. AIDS was, in his view, a disease that belonged in this great tradition of the public health fight against disease: "While the scourge of smallpox has gone and diphtheria and poliomyelitis are at present under control, other conditions such as legionellosis and AIDS have emerged. The control of the virus infection (HTLV III) which is the causative agent underlying AIDS is undoubtedly the greatest challenge in the field of communicable disease for many decades."[30]

Acheson also spoke of "the need for the control of the spread of infection" as "an issue of prime importance to the future of the nation." Universally hailed for his role in AIDS by members of the policy lobbies ("If any honours are deserved for AIDS, he deserves one"), Acheson had held a meeting in late 1983 with gay activists to register support for the nascent Terrence Higgins Trust and its activities in the gay community. His department also issued a number of warning and advisory circulars: a circular issued by the Advisory Committee on Dangerous Pathogens to laboratory workers in 1984; a leaflet issued by the Health Education Council, *Facts about AIDS;* and advice for doctors in 1985.[31] Also in 1985 the Public Health (Infectious Disease) regulations, made under the Public Health (Control of Diseases) Act of the previous year, were extended to cover AIDS.[32] AIDS was, significantly, not made a notifiable disease. Acheson was strongly opposed to notification; and the strength of the historical record in the area of sexually transmitted diseases seemed to indicate that a voluntary approach would, for the moment, lead to the best results. But the regulations did allow some draconian precautions, such as the removal and detention in hospital of a person with AIDS (used only once) and restrictions on the removal of bodies from hospitals (for example, a requirement that body bags be used).

The department's public health stance was given added impetus by the question of potential and actual heterosexual spread of the disease. This was part of the gay lobby's position; it also arose through the blood tissue, which first developed in 1983. There had previously been criticism of the government because it had failed to develop self-sufficiency in Factor VIII and other blood products after an outbreak of hepatitis B among children at a special school in Hampshire in 1981. The development of self-sufficiency, critics argued, was being hindered by failure adequately to invest in the expansion of the Blood Products Laboratory at Elstree and by health service cuts that were preventing the regional health authorities from supplying the laboratory with the extra blood it would need.[33] Heat-treated Factor VIII, introduced originally because of hepatitis, was available by 1984, but there were technical problems in getting it into mass production. In the spring of 1983, reports of the possibility of the transmission of AIDS through blood first began to appear in the medical press and thereafter in the press in general. In May 1983 a report in the *Mail on Sunday* on hospitals that were using "killer blood" noted that two men in hospitals in London and Cardiff appeared to be suffering from AIDS after routine transfusions for hemophilia.[34] Exact knowledge of the virus and its transmissibility was limited at this stage; and both the Health Department and the Haemophilia Society, the voluntary organization concerned, gave priority to encouraging hemophiliacs to continue with treatment.[35] A DHSS spokesman was quoted in May 1983 as saying that "the advantage of using imported blood products far outweighs the 'slight possibility' that AIDS could be transmitted to patients through Factor VIII."[36] The department's initial reaction was to issue a leaflet, in August 1983, asking high-risk donors not to give blood. Heat-treated Factor VIII was not available from the United States until the end of 1984. Dr. Charles Rizza, an Oxford hematologist, was reported as saying that, until it was available, "I'm afraid our haemophiliacs are in the lap of the gods."[37] The domestic supply came on stream in the following year. By October 1985, too, a British HIV antibody test had been developed, and all blood donations began to be screened.

By late 1984 the policy lobbies were beginning to coalesce into more established policy advisory mechanisms. The Department of Health began to set up administrative and policy advisory machinery focused on the new disease. The Expert Advisory Group on AIDS (EAGA) first met in January 1985 to advise the chief medical officer. Its members came from the clinical and scientific areas of new expertise on AIDS. A "social" group dealing with prevention and health education issues had a mixture of medical and gay activists. There was overlap between the groups. The expert group met seven times in 1985 and set up a number of associated groups: groups on counseling, screening, and resources; a working group on health education in relation to AIDS; a group on AIDS and drug abuse; a subgroup composed of surgeons, anesthetists, and dentists; and groups on employment, renal units, artificial insemination, and immunoglobulin.[38] In addition to external links, the department developed its own internal policy machinery on AIDS. In 1985 a direct phone line for professional inquiries was linked to a special AIDS unit in the department. By 1985 AIDS had clearly become a departmental policy issue, with its emergent gay/medical/scientific policy community linked to the department. The policy lines that most clearly united the community were a stress on the need for urgent action and for public education to highlight the heterosexual nature of the disease rather than the "gay plague" angle of the popular press.

1986–1987: PERIOD OF WARTIME EMERGENCY

The governmental reaction until 1986 was primarily at a departmental level. But in 1986 AIDS was recognized as a clear political (in the sense of being a concern for party politicians) priority as well. No longer regarded as a problem for civil servants, volunteers, and medical and scientific experts, AIDS became a political issue—indeed, a national emergency. This reaction was marked in a number of ways, most notably by the formation in October 1986 of an interdepartmental Ministerial Cabinet Committee on AIDS, chaired by William Whitelaw, who was then deputy prime minister. The state of urgency was such that Whitelaw was on the steps of Number 10 Downing Street briefing the press on the (normally secret) meeting before the Cabinet Secretariat had finished typing the minutes.[39] The first full-scale debate on AIDS in the Commons was held in November.

The health education campaign on AIDS was also enormously upgraded. Until 1985 the Terrence Higgins Trust had been the main source of information and advice on AIDS, but the Department of Health now began to expand its earlier series of leaflets and professional guidance into a public education campaign. In March 1986 a series of full-page advertisements appeared in the national press. These were widely criticized for poor presentation and lack of public impact, but in October, following the creation of the Whitelaw Committee, a public campaign costing twenty million pounds was announced, involving television as well as newspapers and wide distribution of a leaflet to all households in the country. The theme of the campaign—"Don't die of ignorance"—was the potential heterosexual spread of AIDS. This campaign culminated in an AIDS week in the spring of 1987. There was cooperation, perhaps unparalleled since wartime, between two broadcasting companies, the BBC and ITV. One participant recalled, "If what was known about AIDS was true, then we had to educate the public fast. If it was left, it might be too late." The commitment of the broadcasting companies was wholly exceptional. After the sense of urgency had lessened, however, other considerations became uppermost: "People were beginning to ask, what next? Broadcasters by then had more or less given up editorial rights, were more or less acting as the government's mouthpiece. It made broadcasters reflect on the dangers of giving up editorial freedom and control—not because of AIDS but because of the dangers of being on the slippery slope to government control."[40]

In late 1986 the Health Education Council was replaced by a new Health Education Authority, a special health authority under much more direct political control and with specific responsibility for the public education campaign on AIDS. And early in 1987 the Commons Social Services Committee began an extensive series of meetings dealing with problems associated with AIDS. The potential for heterosexual spread of the disease was further underlined by the discovery of the virus among injecting drug users in Edinburgh. In the autumn of 1986 the report of the McClelland Committee on HIV in Scotland declared the prevention of HIV among drug users to be of the highest priority.[41]

Everywhere, indeed, there was an air of emergency. Norman Fowler, then social services secretary, paid a visit to San Francisco with the chief medical officer early in 1987. Princess Diana's opening of the first purpose-built AIDS ward in the country at the Middlesex received widespread press publicity. The professional guidelines became a flood, and extra funding began to flow. AIDS became a target for increased resources rather than, as previously, a potential drain on existing finance. The £680,000 for AIDS services that had gone to the North East, North West, and South East Thames Regional Health Authorities in 1985–86 rose to £2.5 million in 1986–87.[42] The Medical Research Control received a million pounds from the Whitelaw Committee at the end of 1986 for research on AIDS. Early in 1987 a further £17.5 million was approved for AIDS research, £14.5 million of which was to go to a special Directed Programme on AIDS, aimed primarily at developing an AIDS vaccine. In wartime the pharmaceutical industries had collaborated. "It's a war-type coalition where everyone gets their jackets off and mucks in," commented a participant.[43] Funding also went to the newly established Global Programme on AIDS, set up by the World

Health Organization. In 1987 over £200 million also went from the
Overseas Developmental Administration to the European Community's
developing program on AIDS.

AIDS was already defined as a problem at the policy community/
departmental level before 1986. But how did it become defined as a
problem at the political level? How did it become feasible for Conservative politicians to become closely involved in an issue which, in many
of its aspects, would appear to have little appeal to the ethos of the
Thatcher government? There are a number of possible explanations,
none of them mutually exclusive and all warranting further investigation. There is an explanation based on personalities—either the concern
of influential public and political figures or the particular involvement
of politicians such as Norman Fowler at the DHSS. Fowler was regarded as an astute politician who could use an emergency such as AIDS
to attract extra resources to his department. He has also been closely
involved in the department's previous continuing activity on drugs, which
in some respects—for example, the creation of an interdepartmental
Ministerial Cabinet Committee and the development of a mass media
campaign—prefigured many of the political responses to AIDS. Lessons
from abroad—in particular the danger of heterosexual spread of the
disease—also weighed heavily. Dispatches from the British ambassador
in Kinshasa had drawn attention to the rapid heterosexual spread in
Zaire and the possibility that Britain might share the same fate. The
drugs issue in Scotland fueled those concerns. In 1986 the CMO's report pointedly noted that the current sex ratio of the disease in England
and Wales was 33:1 (male to female), but in Africa it was 1:1 and in
Scotland the ratio was different because of the higher proportion of
intravenous drug abusers.[44]

The role of the media was also clearly important. As John Street has
remarked, AIDS is perhaps the first "media disease."[45] Particular media
stories punctuate the early history of the disease—the death of the chap-
lain in Chelmsford prison in 1985, for example, and the death of Rock
Hudson in the same year. Television programs that followed the pattern
of the 1983 Horizon broadcast also appear to have made a particular
impact—for example, the Panorama news analysis series devoted an
entire program to AIDS in 1985. These programs were reacting on a
particularly media-conscious government, with a general preference for
mass advertising and market research and a reliance on particular media entrepreneurs. Just before the second mass media campaign was
announced, there had been a spate of programs dealing with the AIDS

issue, *Weekend World* among them; and there is evidence that these programs fueled the concern of government ministers.

But the pressure for emergency action also came in traditional bureaucratic ways, from the internal workings of the Department of Health and through the role of both medical and generalistic civil servants. For them, too, as one commented, AIDS just "gradually bubbled up."[46] The role of Sir Donald Acheson has already been mentioned. AIDS was, in that context, essentially part of a revival of infectious disease since the 1970s, with outbreaks of salmonella and of hepatitis B as well as the arrival of AIDS. It also was part of the apparent revival of public health medicine, which had been severely downgraded in the postwar period. Acheson was chairing a committee on the public health function within the department at the same time that he was chairing the Expert Advisory Group on AIDS. This committee, which reported in January 1988, placed great emphasis on the role of AIDS in legitimating the revival and extension of public health powers. The legacy of Sir John Simon and the nineteenth-century "heroic phase" of public health was again to the fore; this committee's report, too, was remarkable for its historical consciousness. Acheson also appears to have had the support of the policy and generalist side of the Department of Health and of the civil servants in the Cabinet Office. An interdepartmental committee of officials preceded the Cabinet's interdepartmental political committee. In this sense, the period of national emergency conformed to a fairly classic model of bureaucratic policymaking.

But the public context of the political reaction should also be recognized. Governmental activity took place against a background of increasing public fear, which should be distinguished from the "moral panic" and anti-gay feeling to which other writers have drawn attention. This kind of panic undoubtedly existed—in particular in the pages of the popular press, with its talk of "gay plague." But there was also a public fear of contagion. A senior London probation officer recalled, "If we had an HIV-positive person in those days, we'd clear the court."[47] In the letter pages of the *Guardian* and the *British Medical Journal* in the early months of 1987, the safety of kissing was debated by Dr. John Seale, a Harley Street consultant; Sir Donald Acheson; and Dr. Joe Smith, director of the Public Health Laboratory Service. Although the virus had been discovered and scientific knowledge about transmission was proceeding apace, knowledge was not finally constructed and the boundaries with popular knowledge were undefined. A psychologist recalled: "X, consultant at Y hospital, came to see us at the beginning of the epidemic. I asked about transmission through sexual intercourse with women. That was seen as no risk then; now it's high risk. There were the arguments about deep kissing and how you'd need a liter of saliva. . . . Some doctors in Italy think you can and if it is the case, it's very serious. How do you know? There's sloppy talk—and no acknowledgment of doubts. They're full of certainties, and these change."[48] Scientific and popular perceptions of the disease appeared to have equal credibility; science itself, early on, was only folklore in relation to AIDS. There was in a sense a popular decline in confidence in the authority of science and of official pronouncements about the disease. How far this decline impinged on the emergency policy reaction remains to be investigated. But certainly the vastly expanded health education campaign appears to have achieved an important, if partial, transformation in public knowledge about the virus and its means of transmission.[49]

1988 ONWARD: NORMALIZATION OF THE DISEASE

In one sense, the wartime reaction was relatively short-lived. Some of the leading politicians moved on. Norman Fowler left the DHSS in 1988; William Whitelaw relinquished the chairmanship of the Cabinet Committee on his retirement in the same year; Tony Newton, who as minister of health had taken a particular interest in the AIDS issue, also moved on. Some witnesses to the Social Services Committee demanded an expansion of the wartime model of response. A memorandum from the Terrence Higgins Trust urged a national body to control and integrate all services, both voluntary and statutory.[50] But Britain did not appoint a minister for AIDS or an AIDS supremo. The first report of the government's Advisory Council on the Misuse of Drugs—which argued for an extension of the harm-minimization approach to drugs and in particular for the establishment and extension of needle exchange projects—almost missed the emergency boat when it was presented to ministers in the autumn of 1987. It took ministers until March 1988 to decide on the publication of the report because of doubts within the government about the measures proposed.[51] The emergency reaction had become less appropriate.

In the new phase, which began around 1988, AIDS gradually came to be perceived more as a "normal" nonepidemic chronic disease, and reactions to it became professionalized and institutionalized. Clearly, however, the high-level reaction has not disappeared. In January 1988, for example, the British government and the World Health Organization jointly presided over a World Summit of Ministers of Health on programs for AIDS prevention. Delegates from 148 countries, three-quarters of them ministers, attended; 1988 was declared the year of communication and cooperation on AIDS.[52] But in other ways the period of wartime emergency was over. After the departure of Whitelaw, Fowler, and Newton at the Department of Health, no government minister was quite so publicly associated with the issue. The meetings of the Cabinet Committee were no longer publicized, and the committee itself was disbanded in 1989. Some of the earlier key committees were reconstructed, and some of the early actors became less central in policy development. "EAGA was a force in developing policies very quickly. . . . Now most are developed in the Department of Health and rubber-stamped," recalled an ex-member.[53]

The policy community around AIDS was visibly changing to accommodate new experts; it, too, was part of the process of normalization. "The new people represented institutions—but then they all became experts."[54] The volunteer ethos remained important, but it was a rather different type of voluntary sector that became involved in AIDS. The Terrence Higgins Trust continued to expand after some internal changes. But it lost its place in the policy sun and became more marginal to policy development. It was to a degree displaced by a voluntary sector that was partly government funded—as exemplified in the establishment of the National AIDS Trust in 1987. (An earlier U.K. AIDS Foundation had failed to get off the ground in 1986 and had fallen apart amid recriminations.) "It's all become much more mainstream," commented one participant.[55]

The normalization process was at work in the research arena, too. The Medical Research Council's AIDS Committee was re-formed—"The old-boy network of British science" moved in.[56] The Economic and Social Research Council developed an AIDS program that did something similar for British sociology: established non-AIDS/non-gay networks began to develop research. One early actor took these developments phlegmatically: "We have to learn that AIDS is everybody's business. . . . No one can be Mr. AIDS. No one can hang on to AIDS as their own. A lot of us find that difficult if we were involved from the very beginning. It's very hard to let other people get in on the turf."[57]

Normalization and institutionalization were also demonstrated in the way that AIDS became seen as a long-term issue for services and treatment, rather than an emergency issue. In 1988 the Cox report on the short-term prediction of HIV infection revised figures downward:

"Continued exponential growth would lead to about 10,000 new cases diagnosed in 1992. While this cannot be totally excluded, there are a number of reasons for expecting slower growth and predictions in the range of 2,500–5,000 are more likely."[58] Once the threat of epidemic heterosexual spread had passed, AIDS became a normal part of the public health administrative machinery established after the Acheson report. In each health district a standing action group accountable to the Health Authority through a nominated community physician was now responsible for coordinating the relevant services.[59] AIDS care quickly moved from the specialist to the community care model, with a conference in 1987 on community care followed by the setting up of a Departmental Working Party on the subject. When the British Medical Association AIDS Foundation began to produce videos on the subject aimed at general practitioners, AIDS moved into the primary care arena. The stress on "early treatment"—the use of Zidovudine in asymptomatic disease—made clear that AIDS was regarded as a chronic disease, encompassed within a conventional spectrum of medical reaction. "AIDS will become a chronic disease requiring maintenance doses throughout life, but consequently less debilitating than multiple sclerosis," predicted one observer.[60] The discourse on AIDS began to emphasize AIDS in the spectrum of chronic rather than infectious or sexually transmitted disease; "a disease like diabetes" was one comment, with AZT as a latter-day insulin. By 1989 AIDS still raised some burning issues—notably the debates, in particular in the gay community, about the ethics of clinical trials and the ethical and practical issues surrounding testing. But other issues—for example, housing and care in the community— were common to many other conditions.[61]

SOME THEMES IN BRITISH AIDS POLICY

In this section we outline some themes arising from the preliminary research and then propose an agenda for future policy research on AIDS.

POLICYMAKING FROM BELOW: THE RISE—AND PARTIAL FALL—OF A NEW POLICY COMMUNITY

Fox, Day, and Klein, in their study of AIDS policymaking, emphasize the essential consensual nature of the policy reaction to AIDS and, by implication, the formation of policy in a top-down manner. "Governments," they argue, "have employed their standard procedures for hearing, acknowledging, and, to a very limited extent, accommodating the dissenters." Like Fox, Day, and Klein, John Street, in his analysis of AIDS policies, emphasizes the medical and clinical input into policy-making and tends to downplay the impact of the gay lobby.[62] Both sets of authors focus in particular on the period characterized here as the wartime emergency. In another paper Day and Klein comment on the "normality" of the policy process in relation to AIDS: "Health policies in Britain have generally been developed in a closed arena, where action tends to be limited to professional groups and technical experts . . . so that in this respect also AIDS falls into a familiar and predictable pattern."[63] But if the initial period of policymaking in 1981–1985 is brought into the picture, then the relative—if temporary—openness of policy-making is more striking. The concept of policy communities, the way in which subsystems in particular government departments develop relationships with outside pressure groups with shared priorities, is of relevance.[64]

The AIDS story clearly demonstrates how a new policy constituency was formed. There was an initial policy vacuum and a genuine initial openness about what forms of policy might be developed. Groups outside the normal policy arena—the gay lobby and the specialists in sexually transmitted diseases—were admitted to positions of power and policy advice. A three-way alliance, albeit a temporary one, was formed between public health interests in the Health Department and the new scientific and medical experts and the gay lobby. AIDS policy at this early stage perhaps exemplified a genuine pluralistic model, where all groups had potential power in the policy marketplace. But in 1986–1987, with the politicization of policy, power was taken away from that particular policy constituency and given back to more traditional actors and institutions. Thus, the nominal "depoliticization" of AIDS since 1988 has seen a change toward a more conventional model, where established scientific and medical interests play a more central role, as do established voluntary organizations.

CONTINUITY AND CHANGE IN POLICY

Much of this essay has emphasized the essential newness of some aspects of AIDS policymaking. There is no denying the essential novelty that AIDS presented to many in policymaking circles, even at the senior civil servant level. But the element of continuity as well as the newness of policymaking also needs emphasis. How much was new in policy development and how much was not? Here one can use the analogy of the historical debates on the impact of war on social policy. Historians have, in recent years, tended to downplay the impact of war and the supposed construction of a wartime consensus for social and political reform; instead, they have traced, for example, the roots of the National Health Service in prewar debates and blueprints for health care. The effect of war was to enable change to occur more quickly than might otherwise have been the case.[65] This analogy can be applied to AIDS. How far has AIDS changed existing policies—and how far has it been a means whereby developments in existing policies have been achieved perhaps more quickly than before? AIDS and drug policy offers one example. Fox, Day, and Klein, in their analysis of AIDS policies, see drugs as the single exception to the general theme of consensus, the one example where existing policy was overthrown. "The only instance of AIDS overriding established policy objectives has been in the field of drugs. . . . The Government had abandoned its previous stance of augmenting its restrictive and punitive policies on drugs now that AIDS had come to be seen as the greater danger."[66] But AIDS has not overthrown government penal policy; Britain remains part of an international system of legal control; at the European level in particular, the commitment to control is stronger as 1992 approaches. Nor is the harm-minimization (or secondary prevention) approach anything new in British drug policy. It had already been enunciated as an official objective of policy—for example, in the 1984 report of the Advisory Council on the Misuse of Drugs.[67] Because of AIDS, what was previously an objective of researchers, service workers, and some civil servants has now become politically feasible.[68]

AIDS AND THE RENAISSANCE OF "PUBLIC HEALTH"

The language of public health has become a commonplace in relation to AIDS. Day and Klein emphasize the definition of AIDS as a public health issue; Gerry Stimson, in a recent commentary on British drug policy, says that AIDS has brought about a redefinition of drugs as a public health matter.[69] AIDS can indeed be seen as part of the pattern whereby the dominance of chronic, noninfectious disease in postwar health planning has been challenged by the rise of communicable disease over the last two decades. AIDS needs to be set in the context of legionnaires' disease and hepatitis B as well as the rise in sexually transmitted diseases. As we have already noted, the Acheson report on public health was produced in tandem with the developing AIDS issue in the Department of Health.[70] But "public health" is not an unchanging absolute. Its definition has narrowed in the twentieth century, as the nature of state intervention in social issues has itself shifted.[71] In the early twentieth century, concerns for personal hygiene and health education replaced more wide-ranging nineteenth-century concerns for social and environmental reform. The "new public health" of the 1970s and 1980s, with its focus on the individual and on prevention, has revived these earlier social hygienist concerns. AIDS policies—with their emphasis on the voluntary sector, prevention, and epidemiology—have epitomized some key elements of this redefined "public health" and have served to legitimate them.

AN AGENDA FOR POLICY RESEARCH

The "social history" of AIDS raises a number of issues that have long been of interest both to social historians of medicine and to medical sociologists. For example, the relationship between doctor and patient has entered a new phase, with debates over clinical trials and the use of alternative remedies publicized through alternative information networks. The "revolt of the patient" has reached a climax through AIDS. The early public reaction to AIDS—the debates on transmission of the new disease, the belief in contagion—is relevant to the way in which scientific knowledge is constructed and the relationship, often symbiotic, between popular and official perceptions of science. But in this section on agenda we will concentrate in particular on some policy issues that merit further research.

AIDS AND THE CHARACTER OF PUBLIC POLICY

Preliminary studies of policymaking and theories of AIDS policy formation need more detailed empirical examination. The rise of a policy community and its change over time have already been discussed. More specifically, we need to look at, for example, the role of expert groups in policy formation. AIDS policymaking has been marked by the use of such groups: the Expert Advisory Group on AIDS, CAPE, the health education advisory committee, the Advisory Committee on Dangerous Pathogens, the Advisory Council on the Misuse of Drugs. The recruitment, membership, activities, and impact of such groups need analysis. But there are other, equally important, elements in the structure of power:

the role of civil servants; relationships within, and between, government departments; and the role of politicians. According to Day and
Klein, AIDS has been defined as a technical problem evoking classic
public health responses, such as public education campaigns. But how
far did these responses also derive from the political agenda of the
Thatcher government, which had already laid stress on mass media
campaigns in health and other policy areas? The impact of the media
and of public opinion on policy also enters into the equation. What has
AIDS meant for the new policy lobbies that have developed around it?
Dennis Altman, for example, has perceptively commented that the United
States gay community, although decimated by AIDS, has achieved greater
legitimacy and political acceptability through the disease.[72] What function has AIDS performed for the British gay community and for the
medical and scientific experts involved in policymaking?

THE OWNERSHIP OF AIDS

AIDS, as a new disease, has engendered professional tensions over
who should have control over treatment and services. The range of differing specialties involved has already been discussed. Within drug clinics AIDS has led to a new emphasis on physical examination and general health, with consequent awakening of medical interest not just among
drug specialists but among other areas of clinical expertise as well. There
has been a debate on whether there should be separate "AIDS consultants." New occupations have appeared or have been enhanced. Counseling is a prime example—with divisions between the contact tracers
re-formed as sexually transmitted disease health advisers and the new
professional groups of counselors.[73] Gerald Oppenheimer has noted that
the balance of power in U.S. AIDS policies shifted from epidemiology
to virology with the discovery of the nature of the disease and the development of testing for it.[74] The processes at work in the British medical and scientific community likewise need examination.

AIDS POLICY DEBATE AND RESOURCE ALLOCATION

Part of the necessary analysis must concern the allocation of resources to different areas of activity. Some interesting differentials have
already emerged—for example, in the much lower allocation of funding
for drug services to Scotland despite the overwhelming preponderance

of seropositive drug users in Scottish cities. How far has resource allocation actually reflected the nature of the AIDS debate?

THE ROLE AND PROFESSIONALIZATION OF THE VOLUNTARY SECTOR

AIDS policies, as this essay has demonstrated, have stressed the role of the voluntary sector. But the role and nature of that sector have changed as AIDS policy has developed. Ben Pimlott has commented, provocatively, that the Conservative government, with its emphasis on voluntarism, has in fact presided over the decline of any real voluntary sector and the rise of a government-funded and -controlled new "voluntary movement."[75] How far is this perspective applicable to AIDS?

PREVENTION POLICY AND THE ROLE OF HEALTH EDUCATION

As already noted, AIDS has increased the focus on prevention in health policy and on health education as a means of achieving it. But the "politics of health education" in relation to AIDS needs examination—for example, the replacement of the Health Education Council by the Health Education Authority and the relationships between these bodies and the Departments of Education and of Health; the controversies over the health education "packages," *Teaching about AIDS* and *Learning about AIDS;* the debates about the utility and effectiveness of mass media campaigns; and the impact of market research and the relationship between commercial and academic forms of research and evaluation. AIDS provides, in microcosm, a demonstration of some more general prevention policy issues in the 1980s.

RESEARCH POLICY AND AIDS

AIDS has had a clear impact on science policy. The Medical Research Council's Directed Programme on AIDS offers an example of an integrated program, from basic science to the clinical level, which scientists had long wanted in other areas. But it also raised other issues, many of which were already inherent in research policy—for example, the relationship of commerce and industry to academic research and a focus on policy-relevant research.

THE LOCAL DIMENSION OF NATIONAL POLICIES

This interpretation of AIDS policy has emphasized the initial bottom-up rather than top-down nature of policy formulation. The local dimension must also enter into this approach. In the early years local policies stimulated national attention; for example, the Oxford City Council appointed the country's first AIDS liaison officer. The geographical dimension has also been important in the different nature of the epidemic, and the policy response, in Scotland and in England. Policy is also a question of implementation and impact as well as of formation; here, too, the local dimension is important. How have national policies had an impact at the local level?

THE INTERNATIONAL DIMENSION OF NATIONAL POLICIES

British AIDS policies have also interacted with policy formation at the international level. Among the major issues are the role of the World Health Organization; British participation in European Community AIDS initiatives; and the impact of AIDS in Africa on British policy. It is easy enough to assess British policy in isolation; but cross-national comparisons, as one study has already demonstrated, are fruitful means of exploring different (and similar) time scales of response.[76]

CONCLUSION: WHAT ROLE FOR HISTORY?

As we initially noted, historians have been prominent in their initial contribution to AIDS issues. The historical record of epidemics such as cholera, plague, and the Black Death; the area of sexually transmitted disease; and the public health issues of quarantine, screening, and notification entered centrally into the debates.[77] In Britain history was a matter not just for historians but for key policy actors as well. The chief medical officer's reports stressed the voluntaristic tradition in management of sexually transmitted disease; in evidence presented to the Commons Social Services Committee in 1987, the 1916 Royal Commission on Venereal Disease was cited with similar intent.[78] Public health doctors are in general historically conscious; but the readiness to quote, and to pay attention to, the historical argument also underlines the relative openness of policy at that stage.[79]

But history can, as this essay has indicated, make two further contri-

butions: in outlining the "prehistory" of AIDS and in writing and analyzing the "social history" of AIDS and AIDS policies. We cannot assess
the elements of continuity or of change in AIDS policies without some
assessment of what has gone before. For example, we need prehistories
of virology, of immunology, and of developments in science research
policy and drug policy.[80] AIDS has, in fact, highlighted a striking lack
of research on the postwar history of medical and clinical specialties
and of health and science policy. A "contemporary history" of AIDS
itself also needs to be written. The dangers of such approaches are clear—
a potential return to the "bad old days" of Whig internal histories of
medicine, or a focus on institutional history. But the "combat history"
both of AIDS and of postwar and contemporary health policy is a potentially valuable new historical direction.[81]

NOTES

Another version of this essay, which is reprinted with permission, has been
published in *Twentieth-Century British History* (2 [1991]). The authors are
grateful to the Nuffield Provincial Hospitals Trust for financial support for the
research on which this essay is based and to Ingrid James for secretarial assistance. Thanks are also due to audiences at the conference on AIDS and the
Historian, National Institutes of Health, Bethesda, and at the Wellcome Institute for the History of Medicine in London, where versions of this essay were
presented.

    1. Jeffrey Weeks, "AIDS: The Intellectual Agenda," in *AIDS: Social Rep-
resentations, Social Practices,* ed. P. Aggleton, G. Hart, and P. Davies (Brighton:
Falmer Press, 1988), pp. 1–20.
    2. Among recent studies are Daniel M. Fox, Patricia Day, and Rudolf Klein,
"The Power of Professionalism: AIDS in Britain, Sweden, and the United States,"
Daedalus 118 (1989): 93–112; John Street, "British Government Policy on
AIDS," *Parliamentary Affairs* 41 (1988): 490–508; Ewan Ferlie and Andrew
Pettigrew, "Coping with Change in the NHS: A Frontline District's Response
to AIDS," *Journal of Social Policy* 19 (1990): 191–220; and Patricia Day and
Rudolf Klein, "Interpreting the Unexpected: The Case of AIDS Policy Making
in Britain," *Journal of Public Policy* 9 (1990): 337–53.
    3. For the range of British research, see *Register of Behavioural Research
on AIDS, MRC AIDS Behavioural Research Forum,* ed. Mary Boulton (London: Health Education Authority, 1989).
    4. Elizabeth Fee and Daniel M. Fox, "The Contemporary Historiography
of AIDS," *Journal of Social History* 23, no. 2 (1989): 303–14.
    5. See, for example, Anthony Seldon, ed., *Contemporary History: Practice
and Method* (Oxford: Blackwell, 1988).
    6. Our focus here is primarily historical. Another paper deals with issues

from the sociological perspective. See Philip Strong and Virginia Berridge, "No one Knew Anything: Some Issues in British AIDS Policy," in *AIDS: Individual, Cultural and Policy Dimensions*, ed. P. Aggleton, P. Davies, and G. Hart (Brighton: Falmer Press, 1989).

7. Roy Porter, "Epidemic of Fear," *New Society*, March 4, 1988, pp. 24–25.

8. For details of the epidemiological picture, see Department of Health, Press release 89/201, May 8, 1989.

9. Weeks, "AIDS: The Intellectual Agenda."

10. For examples of these interpretations, see Fox, Day, and Klein, "The Power of Professionalism"; Day and Klein, "Interpreting the Unexpected"; and Street, "British Government Policy on AIDS."

11. *Annual Report of the Chief Medical Officer of the Department of Health and Social Security for 1981* (London: Her Majesty's Stationery Office [HMSO], 1982), p. 40.

12. Ibid.

13. Interview, gay community worker, February 1989.

14. Interview, gay community worker, March 1989.

15. Interview, gay activist, July 1989.

16. Interview, gay journalist, November 1988.

17. A. P. Waterson, "Acquired Immune Deficiency Syndrome," *British Medical Journal* 286 (1983): 743–46.

18. M. R. Farrell et al. (members of Gay Medical Association), "Acquired Immune Deficiency Syndrome," *British Medical Journal* 286 (1983): 1143.

19. Interview, gay activist, July 1989.

20. Waterson, "Acquired Immune Deficiency Syndrome," pp. 743–46.

21. *Annual Report of the Chief Medical Officer of the Department of Health and Social Security for 1983* (London: HMSO, 1984), p. 45.

22. See, for example, the range of articles in the *Lancet* or *British Medical Journal* in 1983 dealing with the origins of AIDS in Haiti and in swine fever.

23. Interview, genitourinary medicine consultant, February 1989.

24. Social Services Committee, *Third Report: Problems Associated with AIDS*, vol. 1 (London: HMSO, 1987), p. viii.

25. See, for example, Anne Karpf, *Doctoring the Media: The Reporting of Health and Medicine* (London: Routledge, 1988), for the role of medical experts in structuring the reporting of health matters. A particular example vis-à-vis hepatitis B is given by William Muraskin, "The Silent Epidemic: The Social, Ethical and Medical Problems Surrounding the Fight against Hepatitis B," *Journal of Social History* 22 (1988): 277–98.

26. Interview, gay activist, July 1989.

27. Social Services Committee, *Problems Associated with AIDS: Minutes of Evidence*, vol. 2 (London: HMSO, 1987), p. 153.

28. Ibid., p. 53.

29. B. H. O'Connor, M. B. McEvoy, and N. S. Galbraith, "Kaposi's Sarcoma/AIDS Surveillance in the UK," *Lancet* 1, no. 2 (1983): 872.

30. *Annual Report of the Chief Medical Officer of the Department of Health and Social Security for 1984* (London: HMSO, 1986), pp. 35–37.

31. See *Annual Report of the Chief Medical Officer of the Department of Health and Social Security for 1985* (London: HMSO, 1986), p. 46.

32. Public Health (Control of Disease) Act, 1984, chap. 22; Public Health (Infectious Diseases) Regulations, 1985, No. 1546.

33. Andrew Veitch, "Extra £30 Million Could Have Kept Out AIDS," *Guardian*, May 3, 1983.

34. Susan Douglas, " 'Virus' Imported from U.S. Hospitals Using Killer Blood," *Mail on Sunday*, May 1, 1983.

35. Interview, Haemophilia Society worker, June 1989.

36. Quoted in John Hamshire, "Probe on Imports of 'Killer Blood,' " *Daily Mail*, May 2, 1983.

37. Stephen Cantle, "Haemophilia Alert over AIDS Factor," *Doctor*, May 12, 1983.

38. *Annual Report of Chief Medical Officer for 1985*, p. 46; John Street, "AIDS Policy Advice in the UK" (forthcoming).

39. Peter Hennessy, *Whitehall* (London: Secker and Warburg, 1989).

40. Interview, media worker, January 1989.

41. *HIV infection in Scotland: Report of the Scottish Committee on HIV Infection and Intravenous Drug Misuse* (Edinburgh: Scottish Home and Health Department, 1986).

42. *Annual Report of Chief Medical Officer for 1985*, p. 46.

43. Interview, MRC research worker, November 1988.

44. *Annual Report of the Chief Medical Officer of the Department of Health and Social Security for 1986* (London: HMSO, 1987), pp. 53–61.

45. Street, "British Government Policy on AIDS." Obviously, other diseases—such as tuberculosis and influenza—have had considerable media salience. In AIDS, however, the political response was unusually (for Britain) determined by the media representations of the nature of the disease. Politicians derived their definitions of the problem directly from television in particular. See V. Berridge, "AIDS and Media Policy in Britain," *Social History of Medicine*, 3 no. 1 (1990): 144.

46. Interview, senior civil servant, 1988.

47. Interview, senior probation officer, 1988.

48. Interview, hospital psychologist, February 1989.

49. Department of Health and Social Security, *AIDS: Monitoring Responses to the Public Education Campaign* (London: HMSO, 1987).

50. Social Services Committee, *Problems Associated with AIDS* (Memorandum Submitted by Terrence Higgins Trust), 2:101. The original memorandum, submitted by Michael Adler of the Middlesex Hospital, also argued along these lines, but Adler withdrew this suggestion when he gave evidence to the committee.

51. Department of Health and Social Security, *AIDS and Drug Misuse, Part 1* (London: HMSO, 1988).

52. *Annual Report of the Chief Medical Officer of the Department of Health and Social Security for 1987* (London: HMSO, 1988), p. 8.

53. Interview, consultant, February 1989.

54. Interview, scientific research worker, February 1989.

55. Interview, voluntary-sector worker, January 1989.

56. Interview, scientific research worker, February 1989.

57. Interview, consultant, February 1989.

58. Department of Health/Welsh Office, *Short-Term Prediction of HIV Infection and AIDS in England and Wales: Report of a Working Group* (London: HMSO, 1988), p. 41.

59. *Annual Report of Chief Medical Officer for 1987*, p. 125.

60. Interview, gay journalist, November 1988.

61. On housing see Raynsford and Morris, *Housing Is an AIDS Issue* (London: National AIDS Trust, 1989).

62. Fox, Day, and Klein, "The Power of Professionalism," pp. 93–112; Street, "British Government Policy on AIDS." Fox, Day, and Klein do comment, however, that the gay lobby may have lacked visibility in Britain because it had fairly easy access to the department.

63. Day and Klein, "Interpreting the Unexpected."

64. A. G. Jordan and J. J. Richardson, *British Politics and the Policy Process* (London: Allen and Unwin, 1987); see also Christopher Ham, *Health Policy in Britain: The Politics and Organisation of the NHS*, 2nd ed. (London: Macmillan, 1985).

65. See Charles Webster, *Problems of Health Care: The National Health Service before 1957*, vol. 1 of *The Health Services since the War* (London: HMSO, 1988); also Daniel M. Fox, "The National Health Service and the Second World War: the Elaboration of Consensus," in *War and Social Change: British Society in the Second World War*, ed. H. L. Smith (Manchester: Manchester University Press, 1986), pp. 32–57.

66. Fox, Day, and Klein, "The Power of Professionalism."

67. Home Office, *Prevention: Report of the Advisory Council on the Misuse of Drugs* (London: HMSO, 1984).

68. For a fuller discussion of these points, see Virginia Berridge, "AIDS and British Drug Policy: History Repeats Itself . . . ," in *Policing and Prescribing*, ed. David Whynes and Philip Bean (forthcoming).

69. Gerry Stimson, "AIDS and HIV: The Challenge for British Drug Services" (forthcoming in *British Journal of Addiction*).

70. Department of Health and Social Security, *Public Health in England: The Report of the Committee of Inquiry into the Future Development of the Public Health Function* (London: HMSO, 1988).

71. Jane Lewis, *What Price Community Medicine? The Philosophy, Practice and Politics of Public Health since 1919* (Brighton: Wheatsheaf, 1986).

72. Dennis Altman, "Legitimation through Disaster: AIDS and the Gay Movement," in *AIDS: The Burdens of History*, ed. Elizabeth Fee and Daniel M. Fox (Berkeley: University of California Press, 1988), pp. 301–15.

73. David Silverman, "The AIDS Crisis and Its Impact on Counselling: The Social Organisation of Understanding," paper presented at the third conference on the Social Aspects of AIDS, London, 1989.

74. Gerald M. Oppenheimer, "In the Eye of the Storm: The Epidemiological Construction of AIDS," in *AIDS: The Burdens of History*, ed. Fee and Fox, pp. 267–300.

75. Ben Pimlott, paper presented at the Institute of Contemporary British History seminar on Ten Years of Thatcherism, London School of Economics, 1989.

76. Fox, Day, and Klein, "The Power of Professionalism."

77. One paper may stand for many. See Roy Porter, "History Says No to the Policeman's Response to AIDS," *British Medical Journal* 20, no. 7 (December 1986): 1589–90.

78. Social Services Committee, *Third Report,* p. viii.

79. A point made by David Musto at the conference on AIDS and the Historian, NIH, Bethesda, March 1989. The "openness" of AIDS policy was contrasted with the currently closed nature of drug policy and consequent lack of input from historians.

80. For one example of a "prehistory," see Muraskin, "Silent Epidemic."

81. The term *combat historians* was used by Daniel M. Fox at the conference on AIDS and the Historian.

Foreign Blood and Domestic Politics: The Issue of AIDS in Japan

James W. Dearing

Japan is, by any measure, a country with a low incidence of acquired immune deficiency syndrome. As of September 1, 1990, the Japanese Ministry of Health and Welfare reported a total of 285 cases out of a population of over 120 million. Estimates by the World Health Organization in Geneva place the number of actual cases in Japan at about 500. Despite the low number of AIDS cases in Japan relative to some other countries, the issue of AIDS took Japan by storm for fourteen months beginning in January 1987. The short-lived yet remarkable salience of the issue of AIDS, juxtaposed with few actual AIDS cases in Japan, offers several insights concerning the Japanese society's reaction to an epidemic and to minority demands.

The issue of AIDS has gone through three distinct phases in Japan. The first phase was dominated by the international problem of AIDS and the policies of the Japanese Ministry of Health and Welfare; the second, by aggressive mass media coverage and public-interest groups that reacted to the threat of AIDS in Japan. In the third and current phase, the issue of AIDS has become routinized in Japan. After telling this three-phase story of AIDS in Japan, I then compare the history of the issue of AIDS in Japan and the United States.

AIDS IN JAPAN

AIDS was first detected in Japan in 1982.[1] Through August 1988 1,048 AIDS carriers were identified by the Ministry of Health and Welfare. Current unofficial estimates by the World Health Organization are higher, but questionable epidemiological extrapolations by the Ministry of Health and Welfare make the number of people in Japan carrying the HIV virus very difficult to determine. Of the 1988 official total, 1,029, or 98 percent, were male. There were 90 identified persons who had developed AIDS, 46 of whom had died. Virus infection in Japan began later than in Africa, the United States, and Europe; although the rate of infection was similar through mid-1987, there is reason to believe that it has grown more slowly in Japan than in other countries since then.[2]

In Japan the disease has overwhelmingly been contracted through the use of imported blood-clotting coagulant by hemophiliacs. Hemophilia is a genetic disorder, inherited from the mother, of immoderate bleeding even from slight injuries. The disorder is inherited almost exclusively by males. In 1988 over 92 percent of all AIDS carriers in Japan were thought to be hemophiliacs.[3] Therefore, the vast majority of AIDS carriers in Japan are male. It is the regulation, prescription, importation, and use of blood coagulant which came to define the issue of AIDS in Japan.

Throughout the 1980s Japan imported one-third of the world's blood products, 90 percent of which came from the United States. Japan itself has a high rate of blood donation, but until recently donations to the Japanese Red Cross have been used only for whole-blood transfusions, not for making blood products for commercial sale.[4] Commercial blood products for sale in Japan are manufactured by several large companies in Japan as well as a few firms in the United States and West Germany. Patient prescriptions for blood products are controlled by physicians and hospitals, many of whom maintain their own blood dispensaries; so in Japan the profit in blood products is shared by manufacturers, hospitals, and doctors. The cost of blood coagulant to Japanese hemophiliacs is about four times higher than for hemophiliacs in the United States. Because of the dependence on U.S. manufacturers of blood coagulant, whose blood supply was contaminated with the AIDS virus, the Ministry of Health and Welfare estimates that up to 40 percent of Japan's 5,000 hemophiliacs are carriers of AIDS. Nongovernmental estimates suggest that as many as 60 percent of hemophiliacs are infected.[5] In 1988 about 44 percent of hemophiliacs identified by the Ministry as carrying the AIDS virus were twenty years of age or younger;[6] 30 percent of them were under fifteen years of age.[7]

THE MASS MEDIA AGENDA

In modern societies the mass media often determine what issues policymakers and citizens think about, as well as the relative importance they ascribe to those issues.[8] The influential newspapers and television networks serve as the forum in which the issues of the day are shaped and debated, much as town squares, country markets, and coffee shops served this public function in preindustrial societies. Thus, an understanding of the "life" of a public issue requires an analysis of mass media coverage. How important has the issue of AIDS been in the mass media's news agenda in Japan? And how have the mass media covered this issue?

Our analysis suggests that for several years AIDS was considered strictly a foreign problem. When it was made public in 1983 that the disease had been identified in Japan one year earlier, responsibility for bringing the disease to Japan was attributed to non-Japanese, even though tens of thousands of Japanese businessmen travel abroad every year on organized group "sex tours."[9] The first newspaper articles on AIDS tended to frame the disease as an international curiosity. Most articles were from international wire services.

With the first case of AIDS in Japan, domestic coverage began. NHK, the dominant national (and public) television network, broadcast a fifty-minute informational program in 1983. By 1985 about 30 percent of AIDS stories in the general-interest *Asahi Shimbun* and about 55 percent of AIDS stories in the four financial Nikkei newspapers (including the *Nihon Keizai Shimbun*, often referred to as "Japan's *Wall Street Journal*") were about AIDS in Japan. As the number of Japanese AIDS patients increased, the percentage of domestic-based articles increased, to over 50 percent for the *Asahi Shimbun* and over 60 percent for the Nikkei newspapers in the second quarter of 1988. Meanwhile, the percentage of articles about AIDS cases outside of Japan clearly declined. Many of the articles in the Nikkei group of newspapers centered on new product developments and the public stock values of domestic and foreign pharmaceutical companies.

The over-time distribution of the number of articles in these same newspapers is shown in figure 4. As this figure makes clear, early coverage of AIDS tended toward the foreign problem of AIDS, but the issue was of little importance in the print media. The first AIDS story to capture the public's attention occurred in November 1986: A Filipino nightclub prostitute working in the Nagano Prefecture city of Matsu-

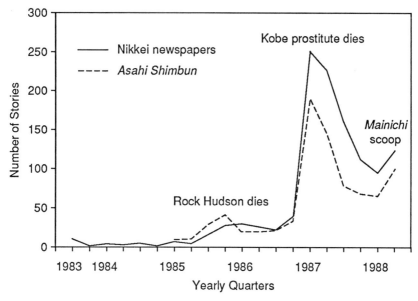

4. Japanese Newspaper Coverage of AIDS

SOURCE: Adapted from data from Nikkei NEEDS data base (an electronic source owned by the Nikkei Corporation for accessing mass media stories).

moto was found to have AIDS, and it was suspected that she may have transmitted the disease to men in the area. The prefectural government quickly deported the woman back to the Philippines, declaring her visa expired.[10]

With the death of a single woman in January 1987, AIDS became a dominant issue in Japan. The January 1987 story had all the right news angles to propel the issue of AIDS to the top of the news agenda: it was domestic, it was about sex and death, and it implied that approximately one hundred anonymous Japanese men might be transmitting a deadly disease to their wives and other partners (extramarital sex is quite common in Japan).

The January story also involved a Kobe prostitute, but she was Japanese. She, her illness, and the public issue they would give rise to could not just be deported. Nevertheless, the AIDS Surveillance Committee of the Ministry of Health and Welfare did not release news of her illness until two days prior to her death on January 20, 1987, though she had been too sick to work for six months. She was the eighteenth Japanese to die from AIDS, and the first woman. In describing the woman as a "habitual" prostitute, the Ministry said that she might have had sex with about one hundred men.[11] This announcement and its aftermath were widely covered by all the mass media in Japan. The most sensational news treatment was in the weekly tabloids, which have a circulation of more than one million. One of these tabloids had been tipped off about the family's funeral arrangements, and it subsequently published a photograph on its front page showing the woman in her coffin. Thus, she did for AIDS in Japan what Rock Hudson and the ostracized schoolboy Ryan White did for AIDS in America. Whereas the five newspapers of study printed a total of 2 stories about AIDS in January of 1985, in March of 1987 the same newspapers ran 189 articles about AIDS (the *Asahi Shimbun* alone printed 76 of these). The peak in mass media coverage in the first quarter of 1987 (fig. 4) represents this story and its aftershock, which included a sensational story about a pregnant Japanese woman with AIDS who refused to abort her child. These three heavily covered stories domesticized the issue of AIDS in early 1987 and represented the beginning of the second phase of the issue in Japan.

How did the Japanese mass media cover the issue of AIDS? The major mass media, with the exception of the *Nihon Keizai Shimbun* and perhaps NHK, have a reputation for liberalism and sensationalism. According to the present research, early AIDS coverage was dominated by international wire service stories, which stressed homosexual and intravenous drug transmission. When cases first were diagnosed in Japan, staff-written stories and special reports appeared. Yet very few received print space or broadcast time prior to the Ministry of Health and Welfare's announcement that the Kobe prostitute was dying of AIDS. Overnight a maelstrom of AIDS stories dominated the news. For example, on January 19, 1987—one day after the Ministry announcement—NHK began a week of nightly seven-minute informational segments on AIDS on its *Today* show. Television ratings indicated that 20 percent of the Japanese population saw all or a part of the segments.[12] Certainly a part of the mass media fascination with the Kobe prostitute story centered on the means of transmission, which was heterosexual and thus strikingly different from what reporters and editors had been previously conditioned to think about AIDS transmission. They were forced to interpret AIDS in a new way, framing the issue with a new meaning. The Ministry of Health and Welfare, which served as the primary news source for AIDS information, had steadfastly framed the epidemiology of AIDS transmission in Japan as paralleling the spread of AIDS in the United States.

An analysis of the *Asahi Shimbun* articles on AIDS, in which the articles were coded into twenty-two "subissue" categories, indicates that stories were most often about (1) government spending and policy responses, (2) the epidemic spread of the disease, (3) explanation of the disease and new information reported by medical scientists, (4) tests for AIDS antibodies and the effects of such tests on civil rights and privacy, and (5) means of transmission of the virus, including blood coagulant infection. Table 1 shows that the *Asahi Shimbun*'s coverage is quite similar to that of four major mass media in the United States.[13] The Pearson's rank-order correlation between the Japanese and American coverage is .86, which is significantly different from zero at the .001 level.

Figure 5 compares the distribution of stories by Japanese mass media (the *Asahi Shimbun* and the four Nikkei newspapers) with the distribution of stories by U.S. mass media (the *New York Times*, the *Washing Post*, ABC, and NBC) from January 1985 through June 1987. The distributions are somewhat similar ($r = .69$, significantly different from zero at the .001 level), although they clearly peak at different times.

Through 1987 Japanese news reporters generally did not question what their sources told them about AIDS. As in the United States, there was little if any investigative reporting about AIDS. But as the disease spread, mass media coverage became more aggressive. Reporters began writing stories about AIDS patients. And Japanese AIDS patients were angry.

On February 5, 1988, the general-circulation *Mainichi Shimbun* published the first article in a comprehensive series of front-page investigative reports. And these reports changed the direction of influence in the relationship between the Ministry of Health and Welfare and, on the other side, the mass media and public-interest groups. The *Mainichi* ran a banner-headline interview with a university vice-president, Takeshi Abe, who was also a medical doctor and who had chaired the Ministry's AIDS Surveillance Committee. In the interview Abe stated that clinical testing in Japan of heat-treated blood coagulant (which had been on the market in the United States and in West Germany since late 1983) for use by hemophiliacs had been delayed twenty-eight months (clinical trials had been completed in one month in the United States). Abe, who had been completely in charge of the testing, defended the delay:

> When one company is ahead of the others in the research and development of a new drug, the duty of a research council is to coordinate things among

TABLE ONE   COMPARISON OF JAPANESE AND
AMERICAN MASS MEDIA STORY THEMES ABOUT AIDS

Categories	Number and (Rank) of Story Themes	
	U.S.	Japan
Government spending and policy responses	624 (1)	185 (1)
Transmissibility of AIDS	507 (2)	66 (6)
Testing, civil rights, privacy	347 (3)	77 (5)
Discrimination	275 (4)	52 (7)
Knowledge about AIDS	250 (5)	106 (4)
Cures, medical breakthroughs	236 (6)	32 (9)
Epidemic spread to the general population	204 (7)	123 (3)
Children with AIDS in school, threat to children	166 (8)	7 (17)
Other	147 (9)	128 (2)
Medical care	143 (10)	32 (9)
Sex education, teaching about AIDS	134 (11)	8 (16)
Importance of AIDS, how worried	129 (12)	41 (8)
Public figures with AIDS	90 (13)	22 (13)
Condom usage and advertisements	87 (14)	4 (19)
Compassion for people with AIDS	73 (15)	27 (11)
Nongovernment spending on AIDS	57 (16)	18 (14)
Life-style changes, precautions	51 (17)	21 (12)
God's punishment, religion and gays	47 (18)	1 (20)
Responsibility of virus carriers, noncarriers	43 (19)	14 (15)
Scientific dispute over discovery of AIDS virus	24 (20)	5 (18)
Media coverage	17 (21)	1 (20)
Personally know anyone with AIDS	16 (22)	1 (20)
Totals	3667	981

NOTE: The U.S. analysis includes the *New York Times,* the *Washington Post,* ABC, and NBC; the Japan analysis is of the *Asahi Shimbun.*

the companies to make them even, for the drug inspection by the Ministry of Health and Welfare. At least two or three companies should be bound together. . . . We needed to give patients the impression that all pharmaceutical companies are reliable to the same degree. . . . All companies must compete fairly. . . . It was for the sake of the patients. Those who complain don't understand things.[14]

Apart from what these comments imply about the Japanese coordination of industrial policy, epidemiologists estimate that Abe's delay may have infected over one thousand Japanese hemophiliacs with the AIDs virus. Ministry of Health and Welfare sources anonymously suggested that, although the policy may have led to an increased number

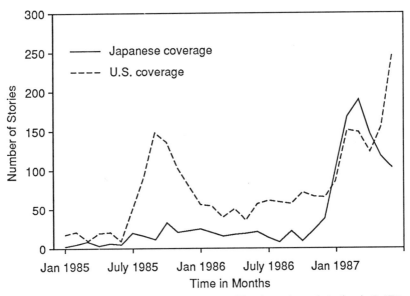

5. Mass Media Coverage of AIDS in Japan and the United States, January 1985–June 1989

of hemophiliacs' contracting the AIDS virus, their experts worried that heat-treated blood coagulant might cause a degeneration of protein. Moreover, they said, AIDS had never been a priority within the Ministry.[15]

The *Mainichi* did not stop with Abe's explanation—damning as it was. The newspaper also revealed that the leading Japanese blood company, which had not yet developed the heat-treatment process, had paid Abe $850,000 to set up a nonprofit corporation (the headquarters of which was a two-bedroom apartment that was usually empty) and that Abe had induced two of the foreign firms to pay money to the corporation. The implication was clear: Abe had delayed the clinical testing process to allow a Japanese firm, which had paid him a large amount of money, to develop heat-treatment technology so that the firm would not lose market share to foreign rivals. Meanwhile, the foreign firms were pressured into paying Abe money in order to stay in the race for access to the lucrative Japanese market.[16]

The trail of deceit, scandal, and profiteering was lengthened in March 1988, when the *Mainichi* broke the closely related story that imports of untreated blood coagulant actually increased during the two years of Abe's delay, while other nations were phasing out untreated blood co-agulant for fear of AIDS infection.[17] American blood suppliers, seeing that their markets for untreated blood had evaporated in the United States, discounted their prices to rid themselves of untreated coagulant inventories. Japanese hospitals bought the discounted coagulant and resold it to hemophiliac patients for large profits.[18]

The *Mainichi Shimbun* stories fundamentally changed the public is-sue of AIDS in Japan. Prior to the newspaper's breakthrough, the im-portance of the issue and the way that it was interpreted were con-trolled by the Ministry of Health and Welfare. After the *Mainichi* series the previously vocal but ineffective hemophiliac association became more successful in having its own goals adopted by both the Ministry and the national Diet. Other, more traditionally efficacious, interest groups joined hemophiliacs in denouncing Ministry policy. Legal suits were filed by hemophiliacs. And news coverage of AIDS policy became more critical. A news editor at another Japanese daily newspaper said, "The *Mainichi* did the best job of any of the media. It was a big scoop and they really pursued it."[19] The three reporters who worked on the stories received the *Mainichi Shimbun* Editor-in-Chief's Award for outstanding report-ing. By and large, however, while acknowledging the *Mainichi* scoop, other mass media did not accord the scandal a high position on their news agendas. The *Asahi Shimbun*, for example, reported on the scan-dal on page 26, three days after the *Mainichi Shimbun* broke the story.[20] A news director at NHK was unaware of any particularly outstanding mass media coverage of AIDS, except for NHK's own reports.[21] Though hemophiliacs and their supporters have sued corporations and the gov-ernment, the traditionally slow pace of litigation in Japan has helped to drop the issue of AIDS to what most media observers describe as a "nonissue." Nevertheless, control over the definition and shared inter-pretation of the issue had been wrested away from the government by the newspaper.[22]

The distribution over time of the number of articles about AIDS (fig. 4) in the Japanese mass media shows a positive correlation with the distribution over time of the number of articles about AIDS in the U.S. mass media.[23] This similarity is perhaps accounted for by the juxtapo-sition of two variables. First, the United States has approximately 500 times more AIDS carriers and AIDS patients than Japan. Whereas the U.S. mass media underreacted to the issue of AIDS in relation to the large number of patients,[24] it appears that the Japanese mass media overreacted. In January 1987, when media coverage in Japan began to peak, there were fewer than twenty deaths nationwide attributed to AIDS. Theoretically, we would have expected less of a media response (or at least a more moderate one) to the threat of AIDS. But the scarce real-world evidence of AIDS was perhaps little heeded because the Japanese mass media were "primed" for the disease; that is, reporters and editors were aware of what was happening in the United States and in Africa, where the number of AIDS cases was multiplying rapidly. If either of these two conditions (few actual cases but awareness of the U.S. experience with the disease) had occurred separately, such a similarity between the distribution over time of the number of mass media stories about AIDS in each nation would not be expected.

PUBLIC OPINION AND PUBLIC-INTEREST GROUPS

Whereas in the United States mass media organizations and public opinion pollsters had asked representative samples of the American adult population over 400 questions about AIDS midway through 1987,[25] relatively few surveys of Japanese public opinion about AIDS have been collected. In the present research, therefore, survey results have been supplemented with other indicators of public opinion, such as the public activities of affected interest groups.

In August 1983 the National Hemophiliac Society petitioned the Ministry of Health and Welfare to stop the importation of untreated blood coagulant. One month later the society requested the drafting of special legislation to facilitate the quick changeover to heat-treated blood coagulant. Both initiatives ended in vain. Instead, the Ministry required all untreated blood products to be certified not to contain blood from groups of people at high risk of contracting the AIDS virus. In October 1983 about fifty mothers of hemophiliac children banded together and entered a Tokyo factory of Nihon Pharmaceutical, where only domestic blood was used for making coagulant. The mothers pleaded and then screamed for the firm to increase its production of domestic coagulant. Again they were rebuffed.[26]

In October 1984, when the U.S. National Hemophilia Foundation recommended that only heat-treated coagulant be used, the new product had already been on the U.S. market for one year. Almost all Japanese doctors assured their hemophiliac patients and their families that imported untreated blood from the United States was safe. Most Japanese doctors would continue to give such assurances until 1986.[27] Even so, one Tokyo hospital alone tested 1,400 walk-up volunteers for the presence of AIDS antibodies between October 1985 and September 1986.[28]

The death of the Kobe prostitute and its ensuing media storm brought AIDS to the forefront of public concern. Within six days of the Kobe woman's death, more than 10,000 local citizens there approached public health officials to inquire whether they too might have the AIDS virus.[29] This panic was repeated throughout Japan.[30] AIDS discussions drew overflow crowds.[31] One week after the death of the Kobe woman, a Tokyo metropolitan AIDS hotline had received 170,000 calls.[32] After their business had declined by more than half, seventy owners of massage parlors in Gifu Prefecture held a lecture on the prevention of AIDS and the testing of employees.[33] Ministry of Health and Welfare officials soon realized that calming the public would be one of their main tasks.

Public apprehension led to suspicion of foreigners as AIDS carriers. Public baths and massage parlors posted signs saying "No Westerners admitted." Hostess clubs advertised "Japanese girls only" and "No foreign items work here." In Tokyo's Kabuki-cho red-light district, two previously popular sex nightclubs which featured foreign women closed for lack of business. Newspaper articles mentioned that non-Japanese had lost their jobs because they were suspected of having AIDS. A survey of 390 Japanese high school students in early 1987 found that when asked which ideas they associated with AIDS, the students most often mentioned (1) homosexuality, (2) death, and (3) foreigners.[34] Government attempts to educate the public about AIDS prevention stressed the danger of sexual intercourse with foreigners, and may have perpetuated the ready association of foreigner with AIDS carrier. According to Feldman, the Kobe city government distributed a comic book to 70,000 high school students which showed "a map of the world with a large finger pointed at Africa, and a boatload of devilish-looking creatures sailing toward Mount Fuji."[35]

Public opinion surveys show that awareness of, and personal concern about, contracting AIDS stabilized by at least May 1987.[36] As in the United States, the distribution over time of data about the means of transmitting the AIDS virus indicates a certain degree of confusion on the part of the public. For example, in a sample of 1,400 blood donors in February 1988 at twenty-one Red Cross donation centers across Japan, 13 percent of the respondents who said they would not donate blood in the future cited the possibility of getting AIDS as their reason.[37] The number of blood donors fell by nearly 5 percent in 1987, the second consecutive yearly decline.[38] One media analyst suggests that public response to sensational mass media coverage of AIDS has counterbalanced other effects from the mass media; specifically, the fear of contracting AIDS may have reversed a trend toward increased extramarital sex by Japanese women, a trend influenced by exposure to popular television soap operas featuring married women involved in extramarital sex.[39]

Respondents to a May 1987 survey about AIDS said that they had learned about AIDS from (1) television, (2) daily newspapers, (3) weekly newsmagazines and tabloids, and (4) other people. The weeklies, which carried the most sensationalistic and perhaps inaccurate coverage of AIDS, were cited as an information source about AIDS by 53 percent of respondents aged twenty to twenty-nine, who are most sexually active.[40]

NATIONAL AIDS POLICY

After January 1987 Japanese government officials were aware that the government had to play a role in AIDS education and prevention. Official collection of AIDS data was entrusted to the Ministry of Health and Welfare's AIDS Surveillance Committee. This committee served as a coordinating body for linking the efforts of other groups, such as the Ministry's Blood Products Division, its AIDS Patients and Virus Carriers Future Estimate Research Group, the private AIDS Prevention Foundation, the Japan Public Health Association, the Japan Society for AIDS Education, the Tokyo Metropolitan Research Group on AIDS, and prefectural public health departments.

Despite this intra-Ministry coordination, traditional animosity between the Ministry of Health and Welfare and the Ministry of Education has prevented any cooperation regarding AIDS prevention and education. The Ministry of Health and Welfare has jurisdiction over epidemiological research and patient treatment for the disease, and has received supplementary funding from the Ministry of Finance for both tasks. Although the Ministry of Education has supported some educational programs on AIDS awareness and prevention, it has not received supplementary funding for AIDS education from the Ministry of Finance. There is, then, a lack of funding for AIDS education in Japan; there is also virtually no money for educational campaigns about discrimination against individuals perceived by Japanese to be at high risk. Because of the low incidence of sexually transmitted AIDS in Japan, this task of defusing discrimination among Japanese has been identified as by far the most important aspect of AIDS in Japan by the Japan AIDS Prevention Association.[41] Between 1987 and 1988 the amount of money allocated by the national government for AIDS doubled, from $7.2 million to $15.7 million, but subsequent annual funding has not increased at such a high rate.

By late January 1987 the Ministry of Health and Welfare had published 1.5 million copies of two AIDS pamphlets. One was distributed to the general public through local governments, medical institutions, and public health centers; the other pamphlet was for public health center counselors. In early February another pamphlet was produced for the general public.[42] By late February the Ministry proposed AIDS legislation that included (1) fines and prison sentences for AIDS carriers who continued to have sex or to donate blood, (2) fines for doctors who failed to report AIDS cases, and (3) the right to refuse entry into Japan to foreigners previously identified as AIDS carriers.[43] A watered-down version was soon passed by the Social Affairs Subcommittee of the ruling Liberal Democratic Party. The bill eventually stalled in the Diet.

The Ministry of Health and Welfare soon directed local governments to assist in the dissemination of AIDS educational materials, set up AIDS consultation centers for concerned people, and provide special counseling services for AIDS carriers.[44] Acupuncturists were ordered to use only disposable needles.[45]

A nationwide public health campaign included the distribution of 340,000 AIDS prevention posters, a toll-free telephone counseling service, and AIDS reference books for physicians.[46] The Japan AIDS Prevention Association distributed videos and sponsored seminars on AIDS.[47] The national government also distributed public service announcements, which were aired on television stations.[48] Schools were instructed to distribute teaching manuals and videos about AIDS prevention to teachers in March 1988. Apparently, little use was made of these materials. Many teachers refused to talk about a topic that they were unfamiliar with and regarded as offensive. The Ministry reported that the anti-AIDS video was shown at only 3 percent of big-city schools and at less than 1 percent of rural schools. The opposition of school teachers was understandable, since sex education had not previously been a topic discussed in junior or senior high school.

After the *Mainichi Shimbun* exposé in February 1988, hemophiliacs found it easier to influence national health policy. Hemophiliacs successfully defeated national legislation that they considered discriminatory. They also demanded monetary compensation from the national government and from pharmaceutical companies, as well as a formal apology from the Ministry of Health and Welfare.[49] Though the national government has steadfastly refused to accept blame or to apologize, Japanese pharmaceutical companies finally decided to "donate" 200,000 yen per month (about 1,500 U.S. dollars at an exchange rate of 130 yen to the dollar) to each hemophiliac eighteen years of age or over, and 80,000 yen per month to those under eighteen, who have been infected with the AIDS virus through blood coagulant.[50] Persons in the general public not personally affected by the disease may have sensed that the issue of AIDS in Japan had reached a stage of resolution.

Noboru Takeshita, then prime minister, promised that the government would financially assist hemophiliacs by covering the costs of treating asymptomatic patients as well as some inpatient hospital costs.[51] By September 1988 this promise was specified as paying up to 180,000 yen (about 1,500 U.S. dollars) per month to hemophiliacs with AIDS, payments of about $45,000 to families of hemophiliacs who have died of AIDS, about $1,000 for funeral expenses, and about $80 per month to hemophiliacs who test positive for antibodies to the HIV virus.[52]

So the national government, mostly through the Ministry of Health and Welfare, did take action on AIDS. Yet its public response was not only slow but also, for several years, directed toward the wrong risk groups. Many Ministry statements about AIDS referred to the threat of disease spread by homosexuals and drug users; in effect, the Ministry was echoing the epidemiology of AIDS in the United States and seemingly refusing to acknowledge that the disease was following a completely different epidemiology in Japan. This mistargeting of risk groups led some critics, particularly hemophiliacs and their representatives, to charge that Ministry AIDS policy was deliberately deceitful. Perhaps a more likely explanation is that the Ministry had not conducted epidemiological research about AIDS in Japan prior to 1987, and there were few reported cases of AIDS.

The Ministry of Health and Welfare refused to criticize the activities of its former AIDS Surveillance Committee chairman, Dr. Abe. Somewhat remarkably, Abe has not been the target of official sanction by either the Ministry, the Japanese medical association, or his university.

THE NONISSUE OF AIDS IN JAPAN

The previous three sections suggest that the issue of AIDS has reached a certain "maturity" on the mass media news agenda, in the public consciousness, and in the minds of policymakers in Japan. If the salience of public issues can appropriately be thought of as cyclically rising and falling,[53] then the issue of AIDS is clearly ebbing at present in Japan. Because of a unique epidemiology (in that most AIDS cases were transmitted nonsexually), the disease is not as much of a public health threat in Japan as it is in some other countries.

The real threat as a result of AIDS in Japan is the generalized perception, demonstrated through public opinion surveys, that anyone other than a "normal" Japanese—meaning foreigners, Japanese hemophiliacs, Japanese homosexuals, and Japanese IV drug users—is likely to have AIDS and should be avoided. In interviews during 1988 Japanese respondents said that they avoided grasping subway handles or using toilets, public telephones, and water fountains after non-Japanese had done so.

Even though it has fallen from importance on the agendas of the mass media, the general public, and policymakers, the issue of AIDS, like the disease itself, has not gone away. The issue has been routinized and institutionalized. Consider the following points:

1. *In mass media organizations* AIDS is now one of the health problems about which health and science reporters must consider writing. For journalists the issue stands as another example of why reporters must critically appraise the information they receive from authoritative news sources.

2. *For the Japanese hemophiliacs* who will live through the epidemic, the issue may bring legitimacy to their public identity. The unified response to the disease and to the government has led to far greater efficacy for the National Hemophiliac Society. Though the persons infected by coagulant have yet to receive the full apologies and money that they have demanded, the government and the blood companies have acknowledged some degree of fault. These acknowledgments, which have been reported by the mass media, may suffice as indications to the general viewer and reader that the problem has been handled (and thus that the issue is cognitively routinized).

3. *The national government* now has a network of offices, counseling centers, and hospitals which deal explicitly with AIDS. Routes for diffusing information about the disease are now established. The Ministry of Health and Welfare has a coordinating AIDS Office. The government has financially contributed (although modestly) to the efforts of the World Health Organization in attempting to curb the worldwide spread of AIDS.

This evidence that the issue of AIDS has been routinized in Japan represents a somewhat typical response to social problems. By this process of institutionalization, issues are legitimized. Legitimization is a goal of issue proponents. In the present case hemophiliacs sought to legitimize the idea that they had been victimized by the government, blood companies, and their doctors. The legitimization process, made visible through institutionalization, transforms an issue into a nonissue. The perception results that "something is being done" and finally that "the problem has been resolved." As early as February 1988, the *Japan Times* editorialized that "the AIDS problem is being marginalized" and that there is a "growing complacency" about the disease.[54]

A COMPARATIVE CONCLUSION ABOUT SOCIETY AND AN EPIDEMIC

The present essay has told the story of AIDS in Japan by focusing on how the mass media, public-interest groups, and government policymakers influence one another in defining and controlling a public issue. When this history is compared with the history of the issue of AIDS in the United States,[55] several comparative conclusions can be drawn about how societies deal with an epidemic.

1.   Both national governments responded very slowly to the threat of AIDS. In both countries groups assumed to be at high risk for AIDS had been ostracized from society prior to the threat of AIDS; when they were identified as at high risk for AIDS, they were stigmatized even further. A main reason for slow government action was that the disease primarily affected groups outside of mainstream society. In Japan, a relatively homogeneous society, little accommodation by the national government was offered to minority or ostracized societal groups whose members are most affected by AIDS. In the United States, a relatively heterogeneous society, the national government has been far more accommodating of the demands of affected societal groups. The egregious government AIDS scandal in Japan faded from the public consciousness after media coverage subsided, the villain never punished. Competition from other public issues (such as the Recruit Cosmos scandal in which public officials were given large amounts of corporate stock), combined with a lack of new sensational information about AIDS, drove this issue down the agendas of producers, news editors, and reporters. Such a scandal most certainly would have been rectified more in line with the demands of the affected societal groups if it had occurred in the United States.

2.   Certain of the mass media in each country provide examples of outstanding investigative journalism centered on government inaction. In each country such media coverage led to changes in national government policy regarding AIDS. In Japan heroic journalism was largely ignored by the other, competing mass media. In the early 1990s AIDS is a nonissue in Japan. In the United States heroic journalism by a few sources eventually put AIDS on the news agenda of virtually all the mass media. The disease has remained on the U.S. news agenda, no doubt influenced by editors' perceptions of issue salience. In comparison with Japan, the United States has a far greater number of people with AIDS, persons carrying the virus, and especially people who know someone with AIDS.

3.   In each country the amount of mass media coverage skyrocketed when perceptions spread that AIDS was a threat to the general heterosexual population. In Japan people perceived that the disease was relevant to them when it became known that Japanese prostitutes had AIDS. Extramarital sex is common in Japan. In the United States the illness of Rock Hudson, a movie star who was a stereotype of masculinity, and especially the illness of a teenage schoolboy, Ryan White, gave people the impression that anyone could get AIDS.

4.   Policy solutions to AIDS have not satisfied claimants in either country, particularly in Japan. Policy actions in response to mass media coverage of an issue provoke an image of issue resolution to the general public, regardless of whether the issue has really been resolved. In Japan hemophiliacs are still very angry at the government, but the lack of current attention in the mass media means that the government need not respond. In the United States the sheer number of AIDS patients, as well as extrapolations of future patient loads, demands a more proactive government set of policies toward AIDS. Yet, aside from the much greater real-world problem of AIDS in the United States, the present results suggest that in the United States well-organized public-interest groups, such as gay political activists, have been able to affect policy (in contrast, IV drug users are paid little heed by the U.S. government because their interests and needs are not represented by a well-organized political action group), whereas in Japan such groups (even the well-organized National Hemophiliac Society) apparently play a much lesser role in the formation of national policy.

NOTES

The present essay is based on research carried out in Japan with the support of a grant from the University of California University-Wide Task Force on AIDS, University of California, Berkeley, and was first presented to the 1988 Symposium on Science Communication: Environmental and Health Research, December 15–17, Los Angeles. The author acknowledges the assistance of the following persons: Reimei Okamura, head, International Affairs, Asahi Broadcasting Corporation; Dr. Bin Takeda, Department of Education, Chiba University; Rika Mazaki, news director, Japan Broadcasting Corporation (NHK); Yasushi Saeki, Information Service Department, Databank (NEEDS) Bureau, *Nihon Keizai Shimbun;* Yoshiaki Takeda and Osamu Murayama, staff writers, *Mainichi Shimbun;* and Yasuo Nakagawa, news editor, and Tai Kawabata, staff writer, *Japan Times.* Helpful criticisms on an earlier draft were offered by Dr. Everett M. Rogers, Annenberg School for Communication, University of Southern California; Dr. Youichi Ito, Institute for Communications Research, Keio University; Kiyoshi Nomura, Dentsu Institute for Human Studies; and Dr. Shigehiko Shiramizu, Takachiho Commercial University. The present essay benefited from advice from editors Dr. Elizabeth Fee and Dr. Daniel M. Fox, as well as anonymous reviewers.

1. John Roberts, "AIDS in Japan," *Japan Journal,* November 1987.

2. *Medical Immunology* 14, no. 3 (September 1987). In most countries AIDS has spread primarily through sexual relations. In Japan the majority of people infected with AIDS and carrying the HIV virus contracted the disease through contaminated blood products. Ensuring a safe blood supply is relatively simple compared to the difficult task of convincing people to change their sexual behavior; so the rate of new AIDS cases, especially among hemophiliacs, should be very low in Japan compared to the rate of new cases in other countries.

3. Ministry of Health and Welfare, AIDS Surveillance Data Sheet (1988).

4. "U.S. Blood Blamed for AIDS Spread," *Japan Times,* June 25, 1988.

5. Eric Feldman, "AIDS in Japan," *PHP Intersect,* November 1987.

6. "Total of AIDS Carriers Exceeds 1,000 for First Time," *Japan Times,* February 21, 1988.

7. "Four Become Japan's First Child AIDS Fatalities in 1987," *Japan Times,* February 14, 1988.

8. Everett M. Rogers and James W. Dearing, "Agenda-Setting Research: Where Has It Been, Where Is It Going?" in *Communication Yearbook 11,* ed. James A. Anderson (Newbury Park, Calif.: Sage, 1988), pp. 555–94). The mass media can also determine how people think about issues and how they evaluate presidential performance. See Shanto Iyengar and Donald R. Kinder, *News That Matters* (Chicago: University of Chicago Press, 1987). For a study of mass media influence on national policymaking, see Martin Linsky, *Impact: How the Press Affects Federal Policymaking* (New York: Norton, 1986).

9. Personal interview with Yasuo Nakagawa, news editor, and Tai Kawabata, staff writer, *Japan times,* July 19, 1988, Tokyo.

10. "News of AIDS-Infected Hostess Provokes Fear," *Japan Times*, November 15, 1986.

11. "Ministry Reports 1st Diagnosis of Female AIDS Patient Here," *Japan Times*, January 18, 1987; "First Woman AIDS Victim Dies," *Japan Times*, January 21, 1987.

12. Personal interview with Rika Mazaki, news director, Japan Broadcasting Corporation, July 26, 1988, Tokyo.

13. This coding scheme of twenty-two categories was initially developed for comparing the mass media news coverage of AIDS in the United States with public opinion survey questions about AIDS in the United States. As might be expected, a larger percentage of stories about AIDS from the Japanese mass media fell into the "other" category. Many of these articles dealt with announcements of international AIDS conferences or of joint Japan–foreign country research initiatives. In some of the articles in this category, translations from Japanese to English were insufficient to permit precise codification.

14. "Coordination for Clinical Testing Normal: Q & A with Dr. Abe, Vice-President of Teikyo University," *Mainichi Shimbun*, February 5, 1988.

15. "Measures against Hepatitis Contamination Developed in West Germany 7 Years Ago," *Mainichi Shimbun*, February 5, 1988.

16. David Swinbanks, "Japanese AIDS Scandal over Trials and Marketing of Coagulants," *Nature* 331 (February 18, 1988): 552.

17. "Actual Conditions over Suddenly Increased Import of Untreated Blood Products Made Clear," *Mainichi Shimbun*, March 12, 1988.

18. David Swinbanks, "Pharmaceutical Companies Profit from Japan's Blood Boom," *Nature* 332 (March 17, 1988): 193.

19. Interview with Nakagawa and Kawabata.

20. "Government and Company Compensation Demanded for AIDS Coagulant Disaster," *Asahi Shimbun*, February 8, 1988.

21. Interview with Mazaki.

22. See Stephen Hilgartner and Charles L. Bosk, "The Rise and Fall of Social Problems: A Public Arenas Model," *American Journal of Sociology* 94, no. 1 (1988): 53–78.

23. For a detailed qualitative and quantitative analysis of American mass media coverage of AIDS, see Everett M. Rogers, James W. Dearing, and Soonbum Chang, "AIDS in the 1980s: The Agenda-Setting Process for a Public Issue," *Journalism Monographs* 12B (April 1991): 1–47.

24. Ibid.

25. James W. Dearing, "The Polling Agenda for the Issue of AIDS," *Public Opinion Quarterly* 53 (1989): 309–29.

26. "Forced to Choose AIDS or Death: Cruel Choice for Patients," *Mainichi Shimbun*, February 5, 1988.

27. Roberts, "AIDS in Japan."

28. "Hospital Finds 21 People with AIDS Virus," *Japan Times*, April 3, 1987.

29. "Over 10,000 People Come to AIDS Counseling Center in Hyogo Prefecture," *Asahi Shimbun*, January 26, 1987.

30. Interview with Nakagawa and Kawabata.

31. "Yokosuka AIDS Talk Draws Crowd," *Japan Times*, January 21, 1987.

32. "170,000 Call Tokyo AIDS Information Number," *Asahi Shimbun*, January 28, 1987.

33. "Gifu 'Soapland' Group Sponsors AIDS Talk," *Japan Times*, February 7, 1987.

34. "Teachers, Students Want to Keep Out Foreigners with AIDS," *Japan Times*, April 30, 1987.

35. Feldman, "AIDS in Japan," p. 15.

36. Prime Minister's Office, "Public Opinion about AIDS," May 1987; Gallup Organization, "AIDS: A Multi-Country Assessment," *Public Opinion*, May–June 1987.

37. Japanese Red Cross Society, Questionnaire on Blood Donation, February 1987.

38. Jennifer J. Lin, "Attitudes and Awareness on AIDS in Japan," Master's Thesis, School of Medicine, Case Western Reserve University, Cleveland, 1987.

39. Shigehiko Shiramizu, personal correspondence, November 11, 1988.

40. Prime Minister's Office, "Public Opinion about AIDS."

41. Personal interview with Bin Takeda, October 27, 1988; *AIDS Education I*, March 1988, entire issue.

42. "Health Ministry Issues AIDS Booklet," *Japan Times*, February 3, 1987.

43. "Proposed AIDS Legislation to Be Presented to Diet," *Japan Times*, February 27, 1987; "Law Would Bar Aliens with AIDS," March 27, 1987.

44. "Directive on AIDS Sent to Local Governments," *Japan Times*, March 19, 1987.

45. "Use Needles Once: AIDS Notice to Acupuncturists," *Japan Times*, March 25, 1987.

46. "Gov't Outlines AIDS Information Campaign," *Japan Times*, March 28, 1987.

47. "Know-Your-Enemy AIDS Campaign," *Japan Times*, April 19, 1987.

48. Interview with Mazaki.

49. "Hemophiliac Association Demands Compensation for Wrongdoing," *Mainichi Shimbun*, February 9, 1988.

50. NHK Television Evening News, "Pharmaceutical Companies Make Offer," October 20, 1988.

51. David Swinbanks, "Relief in Sight for HIV-Carrying Japanese Haemophiliacs," *Nature* 333 (May 5, 1988): 5.

52. "Gov't to Compensate Hemophiliacs with AIDS," *Mainichi Daily News*, September 15, 1988.

53. Anthony Downs, "Up and Down with Ecology: The Issue-Attention Cycle," *Public Interest* 28 (1972): 38–50.

54. "AIDS and Complacency," *Japan Times*, February 29, 1988.

55. See Rogers, Dearing, and Chang, "AIDS in the 1980's."

Medical Research on AIDS in Africa: A Historical Perspective

Randall M. Packard and Paul Epstein

The history of Western medical research on AIDS in Africa closely resembles earlier attempts by Western-trained medical researchers to understand the epidemiology of infectious diseases, such as tuberculosis and syphilis, that were known in the West but that appeared to exhibit different epidemiological patterns in Africa. Like research into TB and syphilis, early inquiries into AIDS in Africa attempted to understand why African experience with the disease differed from Western experience. All of these efforts were handicapped by the limited state of Western knowledge about these diseases, an absence of adequate epidemiological data for Africa, and a lack of knowledge about the African societies and cultures within which these diseases occurred. Despite these shortcomings, early medical researchers quickly constructed theories to explain the peculiarities of the African disease experience. These theories were strongly influenced by cultural assumptions about Africa and Africans and tended to focus on the peculiarities of African behavior.[1] Once these theories were constructed, they shaped the course of subsequent research, privileging certain lines of inquiry while largely excluding or marginalizing other potentially important areas of research.

In this essay we compare the development of AIDS research in Africa with the history of earlier efforts by Western medical professionals to understand the epidemiology of TB and syphilis. By drawing these parallels, we hope to contribute to a clearer understanding of how Western medical ideas about AIDS in Africa developed and how these ideas have shaped the direction and boundaries of African AIDS research and, ultimately, our understanding of the epidemiology of AIDS in Africa.

TUBERCULOSIS AND THE "DRESSED NATIVE"

Early discussions about the causes of black susceptibility to TB centered on the problem of explaining why Africans had higher rates of morbidity and mortality than Europeans. At the time little was known about the nature of host resistance to the disease or about the role of cofactors in the transmission of infection and in the progression of infection to active disease. Research on TB was in fact in transition from the hereditary arguments of the late nineteenth century to Koch's germ theory. In addition, knowledge of African social and economic life was limited and was infused with racial and cultural stereotypes. Predictably, the explanations of European medical authorities came to reflect the perceptions about Africans that were current in European colonial society.

Central to these perceptions was the image of the "primitive native" making a difficult adjustment to conditions of a "civilized" industrial world. This image, embedded in European discussions of African morality, political participation, and labor skills, came to influence early explanations of TB in Africa. Africans were viewed as more susceptible to TB because they had not adjusted to the conditions of a civilized industrial society; their incomplete adoption of Western clothing and their failure to observe "proper" dietary and sanitary laws symbolized this lack of adjustment.

At the same time, it was argued that Africans who remained in their customary rural environment, working in the open air and wearing traditional attire, were generally healthy. These explanations for African sickness and health, focusing attention on the Africans' maladjustment to civilization, placed responsibility for the adverse living conditions of Africans squarely on the shoulders of Africans themselves and deflected attention from the low wages and inadequate housing policies of employers and government officials. More importantly, these explanations shaped the development of TB control measures, which came to focus naturally on education rather than on social and economic reform. Blacks had to be taught about the dangers of living in overcrowded housing and eating nutritionally inadequate diets, as if they chose to do so out of perversity rather than out of economic necessity.

Later on, discussions about African susceptibility to TB became infused with biological arguments that focused on the Africans' lack of experience with the disease and their consequent lack of physiological resistance to it. Like earlier behavioral arguments, physiological models defined the African as essentially different from the European, as the "other," and at the same time placed responsibility for the disease on the victim.[2] Not until the middle of this century did health officials come to see that the adverse environmental conditions under which Africans lived were not of their own making. Even then, environmental reform efforts continued to be hampered by behavioral explanations that emphasized the Africans' difficult adjustment to the conditions of Western industrial civilization. Typical of this discourse is the following statement by the director of Kenyan medical services in 1963:

> The African in his rural setting is strictly bound by tribal patterns of behavior, beliefs and customs. He is an integral part of his community and his thinking tends to be communal. . . . With the transposition to the town he forsakes the communal life for an individualistic life, unsupported by tribal rules and regulations. While forsaking these supports, he is not yet ready to adopt the codes and rules which have brought social stability to western civilizations. Furthermore, he is abandoning ingrained centuries of agricultural and pastoral tradition and learning the technical skills of an industrial world quite strange to him.[3]

Even today TB control programs in Africa continue to view TB as a behavioral problem, attributing treatment failures to "patient default" rather than to the government's failure or inability to cope with environmental factors that continue to generate new cases of this disease.

SYPHILIS AND AFRICAN SEXUALITY

The recent work of the historian Marc Dawson on the history of syphilis in East Africa provides another example of how earlier Western medical researchers came to construct a behavioral paradigm to explain the peculiarities of African disease experience and how these models shaped medical responses to this experience.[4] The epidemiology of syphilis, like that of tuberculosis, was not well understood by Western medical researchers during the first decades of this century. Specifically, the epidemiological and pathological differences between yaws, venereal syphilis, and endemic or nonvenereal syphilis had yet to be sorted out. As a result, there was considerable confusion among early medical personnel working in Africa. This confusion led early European observers to regard the African experience with the disease as different from the European and to look for the reasons for this difference. As with TB, early theories about syphilis in Africa focused on behavioral theories that were infused with racial stereotypes.

Early medical researchers in East Africa concluded that between 50 and 90 percent of the African population in parts of Kenya and Uganda were infected with venereal syphilis. Col. F. J. Lambkin, a leading British expert on syphilis, who was seconded to Uganda to study the problem, concluded in 1906: "As things are at present, the entire population is in danger of being exterminated by syphilis in a very few years, or of being left a degenerate race fit for nothing."[5] In explaining this extraordinary situation, Lambkin concluded that the major cause of the epidemic was a breakdown of various Ganda social institutions. In this respect he echoed early medical opinions about the spread of TB, as well as later theories about AIDS. Specifically, Lambkin argued that Christianity had broken down customs that restricted the social movement of women. At the same time, sanctions against adultery had been eliminated at the behest of the British colonial government. These changes, he argued, had permitted Ganda women to engage in *"promiscuous sexual intercourse and immorality,"* resulting from *"their natural immoral proclivities"* (emphasis added). Lambkin further indicted the Bahima of Ankole as primary disseminators of the disease because of their practice of allowing a man's age-mates and visitors to have sex with his wife.[6]

Similar claims were made by observers in western Kenya. G. L. Gilks, discovering what he believed to be a major epidemic of venereal syphilis in Kavirondo, concluded: "The whole attitude of the native toward sexual matters renders it certain that venereal disease, once introduced, is bound to spread among old and young."[7]

On the basis of subsequent studies and a careful reexamination of the medical evidence, Dawson suggests that what Lambkin and Gilks were observing was not an epidemic of venereal syphilis but nonvenereal or endemic syphilis, which is caused by the same *Treponema pallidum* spirochete that causes venereal syphilis. Endemic syphilis, however, spreads through bodily contact in warm climates and in the absence of adequate sanitation. According to Dawson, syphilis was clearly being spread sexually into various parts of East Africa as a result of the development of migrant labor, commercial centers, military movements, and a growing population of African prostitutes; however, its subsequent spread among large numbers of men, women, and children in rural and urban areas was via bodily contact.

The point of this episode is not simply that the disease was misdiagnosed. After all, the differences between yaws, venereal syphilis, and endemic syphilis were difficult to sort out and in fact were not clearly understood until the 1930s. The importance of this episode lies instead in the way these early medical observers constructed the medical evidence they were observing to fit preexisting assumptions about African sexuality and disease. Seeing a disease, which they assumed to be venereal syphilis, Lambkin, Gilks, and others readily constructed a theory to explain its extraordinary rate of spread. That theory was based on assumptions about the extreme sexuality of Africans—assumptions for which they had virtually no empirical evidence. This is not surprising. As Sander Gilman notes, the association of Africans with sexuality and the tendency to link African sexuality with disease have a long history in Western thought.[8] By the end of the nineteenth century, when European powers began carving out African colonies, the association could be found in many works of literature and art in continental Europe and held a central position in the constellation of ideas that made up European perceptions about Africans. As a result, early medical authorities, missionaries, and colonial administrators came to Africa with certain strong assumptions about African sexuality. There can be little doubt that these presumptions colored both their epidemiological findings and their control efforts. Following this behavioral explanation, these authorities advocated public health policies that centered largely on the development of measures, often draconian in nature, to control the behavior of prostitutes. At the same time, problems associated with living conditions and sanitation, which were in fact centrally important to the spread of endemic syphilis, were ignored.

AIDS AND THE "SEXUAL LIFE OF THE NATIVES"

Early discussions of AIDS in Africa developed in an intellectual environment similar to that in which early inquiries into TB and syphilis were conducted. When medical researchers first began studying AIDS in Africa, they quickly realized that the epidemiology of the disease was different from that in the West. The ratio of male to female cases was 13:1 in the West, whereas the ratio in Africa was nearly 1:1. This fact, combined with an apparent absence of known risk groups in the form

of either IV drug users or homosexuals, led early researchers to con-
clude that AIDS transmission in Africa was different from that in the
West. They therefore tried to determine what it was about Africa and
Africans that accounted for its peculiar pattern of transmission.

In trying to explain transmission patterns in Africa, AIDS researchers
were handicapped by limited knowledge about the etiology of the disease. Thus, when African AIDS cases (or what seemed to be AIDS cases)
first began appearing in Belgium in 1983, the infectious agent causing
AIDS had not yet been identified. In addition, early discussions of AIDS
in Africa occurred, and in fact continue to occur, in the absence of any
clear understanding about the role of various cofactors in either the
transmission or the progression of HIV infection. Finally, early AIDS
researchers had only limited experience or knowledge of the societies
and cultures within which AIDS was occurring in Africa.

This lack of social and medical knowledge, combined with the suspicion that the key to understanding AIDS in the West might lie in
Africa, contributed to a great deal of speculation about the epidemiology of AIDS in Africa and encouraged researchers to construct hypotheses that often were based on extremely limited data. It is therefore
not surprising that stereotypic images of Africa and Africans entered
into the discourse on the epidemiology of AIDS in Africa.

Early reports on AIDS in Africa took a somewhat eclectic approach
to the question of why African populations exhibited an epidemiological pattern different from that of populations in the West.[9] However, a
number of influential Western AIDS researchers concluded early on that
the apparently equal sex ratio of AIDS cases in Africa was most easily
explained by a pattern of heterosexual transmission, a phenomenon relatively rare in the West at that time. This conclusion was supported by
early prevalence studies, which seemed to indicate that both cases and
HIV seropositivity were most frequent among sexually active adults.
But why, then, was HIV occurring through heterosexual transmission
in Africa and not to any great degree in Europe or America?

This question quickly led to two theories. The first argued that AIDS
had existed in Africa for a longer period of time than in the West and
therefore had reached a different stage in its epidemiological history.
This theory—combined with the virological research of Essex, Gallo,
and others on Simian T-Lymphocyte Retrovirus III in African green
monkeys—led to arguments that AIDS originated in Africa.[10] This hypothesis was hotly debated on scientific grounds. More important, it
ignited a political firestorm among African political leaders, who re-

garded the theory as imperialist scapegoating.[11] This produced a political environment in which the cooperation of African governments in further AIDS research appeared to be in jeopardy. As a result, the Western medical research community appears to have put aside the question of African origins as well as investigations into the possibility that HTLV-III may have achieved a different epidemiological stage in Africa.[12]

The second theory put forth to explain the heterosexual transmission of HIV in Africa focused on African sexual behavior. In brief, it was argued as early as 1985 that the heterosexual transmission of HIV in Africa was the result of higher levels of sexual promiscuity among Africans, or, in the current language of social science research on AIDS, "poly-partner sexual activities." The middle-class businessman or bureaucrat with a string of lovers; the truck driver with sexual contacts all across the African map; and, above all, the pervasive female prostitute, who was said to have literally hundreds of contacts each year—these people were identified as the main vectors of HIV transmission in Africa. Although the association of AIDS in Africa with sexual promiscuity was challenged by both African observers and others with broad knowledge of African societies and cultures, it nonetheless persisted and, like earlier stereotypes concerning black susceptibility to TB and syphilis, became the central focus of medical inquiries into the problem of AIDS.

Why, given all the social and economic factors that distinguish African populations from those in the West, did researchers choose to focus on sexual promiscuity? Officially, the conclusion was said to be based on medical evidence, including studies which indicated that Africans who had multiple sexual partners and other STDs were statistically at higher risk of being infected with HIV than those who did not. Yet evidence for this conclusion, as well as for the association of HIV infection with the years of peak sexual activity, was extremely limited prior to 1986. Therefore, other factors probably contributed to the development of this explanation.

One such factor appears to have been the association of AIDS in the West with the alleged sexual promiscuity of homosexuals. In essence, AIDS was defined as a sexually transmitted disease that was spread in the West within a population defined as sexually promiscuous. Its heterosexual spread in Africa therefore implied similar levels of promiscuity. More than one Western AIDS researcher, in fact, suggested that African heterosexuals had a pattern of promiscuity similar to that of promiscuous gay men in the United States and Europe (a conclusion that incorporated two discriminatory stereotypes).[13] More broadly, Western research on AIDS had already defined AIDS as a behavioral problem associated with aberrant life-styles.[14] There was thus a predisposition to look for "deviance" in an African setting.

Yet the role of sexual promiscuity in the spread of AIDS in Africa appears to have evolved in part out of prior assumptions about the sexuality of Africans. Thus, at a 1985 conference on AIDS held in the Central African Republic, Dr. Fakhri Assaad of the World Health Organization referred to the widespread pattern of "polygamy without wedding rings" in Africa. According to Assaad, this pattern resulted from the tendency of men to consider it a status symbol to have several wives or mistresses. He noted that, in reference to sexual and other cultural practices that might facilitate the transmission of HIV, that many of the practices had deep religious and traditional significance. In a similar fashion, researchers describing the sexual practices of patients suffering from "Slim Disease" in Uganda in 1985 observed that, although their subjects denied overt promiscuous behavior, they were "by western standards heterosexually promiscuous."[15] These researchers based their conclusion on the testimony of ten HIV-positive truck drivers who admitted to engaging in homosexual behavior. Labeling homosexual behavior as promiscuous by Western standards may have been consistent with the dominant view of Western society. Yet surely the issue in this case was not promiscuity but the fact that these subjects engaged in a known risk behavior. Nonetheless, it was not the homosexual behavior per se that was presented as the risk behavior, but the subjects' promiscuity.

Yet another example of this tendency to view Africans as sexually promiscuous can be found in a study that compared HIV infection among prostitutes and female controls in Rwanda. Commenting on their sampling procedures, the authors of this study noted, "Matching of the female controls was not extended to marital status since, *for the age group studied, celibacy [single status] in women is unusual in Central Africa and commonly associated with prostitution*" (emphasis added), a conclusion for which the authors presented not a shred of evidence.[16]

The parallel between these attitudes and those of early medical personnel faced with an epidemic of syphilis in East Africa, described above, along with the absence of any reliable data supporting these conclusions, forces us to ask whether the attitudes of medical researchers toward

AIDS in Africa did not also have their basis in a deeply imbedded image or trope which continues to shape Western medical and popular thought about African sexuality.

In a similar vein, it has been suggested that other cultural practices—such as scarification, the therapeutic use of razors, and female circumcision—might also play a role in the spread of HIV. Like sexual promiscuity, these risk behaviors were seen as culturally determined.

THE ROLE OF ANTHROPOLOGISTS

Having constructed AIDS as a behavioral problem resulting from particular culturally sanctioned practices, AIDS researchers turned to anthropologists for information on these practices. One might expect that social scientists with extensive African experience would have challenged the sexual stereotypes developed by medical researchers. Such challenges did not, however, occur to any great degree. Although recent social science research has questioned some of the behavioral assumptions underlying AIDS research in Africa, the activities of those social scientists who were most closely linked to the AIDS inquiry in its early stages tended to reinforce these assumptions.

Probably the main reason why anthropologists failed to challenge the dominant paradigm in AIDS research had to do with the conditions under which social scientists were brought into the AIDS inquiry. Instead of engaging in an open-ended dialogue with social scientists, assessing available data, and discussing how research methods and agendas might be modified to fit more closely with the contours of African experience, the medical research community expected the social scientist to adhere to the dominant behavioral model. Specifically, they asked anthropologists and other social scientists to provide information about the "risk behaviors" that might facilitate the transmission of AIDS. In other words, what were the practices, customs, or patterns of social intercourse that provided opportunities for HIV transmission? Constructed in this way, the question immediately narrowed the range of sociological data relevant for the discussion. The question became not "What is the social context within which HIV transmission occurs in Africa?" but, rather, "What are the patterns of behavior which are placing Africans at risk of infection?" While the first construction would have allowed for open-ended discussion of a wide range of social, political, and economic conditions that might be affecting health levels in Africa, the latter formulation quickly narrowed discussion to an inquiry into the "customs of the natives." At the same time, it placed responsibility for transmission on the actors themselves in a not too subtle form of victim blaming.

The result of this emphasis on "risk behaviors" was that anthropologists found themselves being asked to dig through the ethnographic record on African cultures in order to identify possible patterns of behavior that might facilitate HIV transmission. This exercise resulted in conferences, workshops, and seminars in which the medical community was presented with an array of information that was often excised from its social or economic context and presented in much the same way as ethnographic artifacts are presented in natural history museums. Descriptions and pictures of scarification taken among the Nubia in the 1940s and 1950s were displayed as examples of possible "risk behaviors" involving blood transfers. From the broad array of data on African sexual practices imbedded in the ethnographic record of Africa, data revealing a wide range of patterns and extreme variation with regard to sexual permissiveness anthropologists presented only those cases that constituted possible "risk behaviors." Take, for example, the following description of "risk behavior" reported in a survey on "Social Factors in the Transmission and Control of AIDS in Africa" commissioned by the United States Agency for International Development (USAID):

> There is a widespread fear of impotence [in Africa]. Our readings mention instances where an older man might ask a younger man to impregnate his wife. The Gwembe Tonga of Zambia use euphemistic invitation in these circumstances—"go and cut wood for me, my friend." . . . This illuminates our understanding of the perception of sexuality in *certain traditional African settings* but also indicates another—though limited—instance of a possible route for spreading AIDS through increasing the number of sexual partners.[17]

The same report contains a lengthy description of ritual sexual intercourse involving the widows of deceased men among the Giriama of Kenya. The authors follow the description with the observation "Clearly if the widow's deceased spouse was an AIDS victim then this custom will contribute to the spread of the disease."

In a similar vein, Daniel Hrdy, who is trained in both medicine and anthropology, wrote in an article on cultural practices relating to HIV transmission in Africa, "Although generalizations are difficult, most traditional African societies are promiscuous by Western standards. Promiscuity occurs both premaritally and postmaritally. For instance, in the Lese of Zaire, there is a period following puberty and before marriage when sexual relations between young men and a number of women is virtually sanctioned by the society."[18] This article was circulated in advance to the 300 or so participants who attended a conference on Anthropological Perspectives on AIDS (sponsored by the U.S. Agency for International Development and the National Institute of Allergy and Infectious Diseases), presumably because the organizers viewed it as a model of the types of data they hoped would be presented at the conference.

These behaviors may very well occur and may be potential avenues for HIV transmission. Reports of this type—by concentrating on "risk behaviors"—exclude from discussion broader patterns of everyday sexual activity, which in many cases are both less exotic and more monogamous. Moreover, they reinforce, perhaps unintentionally, the impression that sexual promiscuity is culturally determined. For example, Edward Green, in a recent article on the role of behavioral scientists in African AIDS research, noted, "Changes in behavior which promote the spread of AIDS will go against social and cultural norms and values in Africa and against deeply ingrained behavioral patterns." Similarly, Francis Conant, writing in the same volume, concluded, "In dealing with AIDS we are not just dealing with sex; we are dealing with life-ways and complex cultural patterns."[19]

Some of the contributions by anthropologists have been of such questionable relevance to the issue of HIV transmission as to border on being salacious. Take, for example, Hrdy's extensive account of female circumcision.[20] After spending a page describing various patterns of female circumcision in detail, he concludes that there is hardly any correlation between areas in which it is practiced and the distribution of HIV infection, leaving the reader to question the need for the descriptive detail. This pattern of selective reporting only reinforced the popular image of African promiscuity and at the same time strengthened the assumption that the heterosexual epidemic of AIDS in Africa was simply a product of the peculiarities of African behavior.

Remarkably, some of these same anthropologists cautioned us not to make generalizations about African sexual behavior and suggested that the problem was not generalized sexual promiscuity but "urbanization": "Away from the social constraints imposed by commitments and obligations to a network of kin, there is the opportunity to engage in behaviors, including poly-partner sexual activities, that would be difficult to undertake in the home village due to social constraints."[21] In a similar fashion, Hrdy concluded: "As people leave rural villages and migrate to urban areas, the general level of promiscuity usually increases. This increase may be attributable in part to the relaxation of traditional village values but appears to be due primarily to the destitution of poor migrant women, who may become prostitutes, and to the greater mobility and rootlessness of young male migrants and soldiers."[22] In short, urban promiscuity was the product of the loss of "traditional restraints." The image of the "detribalized" African, the bane of colonial urban authorities, was a central image in earlier discussions of black susceptibility to TB and syphilis. This image, which was fairly well excised from social science discussions in the 1970s, was being resurrected to explain the frequency of heterosexual transmission of HIV and Africans in the 1980s. This explanation both distinguished Africans from the West and placed responsibility for AIDS on the African. Moreover, given the behavioral thrust of the explanation, the recommended response was finding ways to modify urban sexual behavior. "An understanding of the patterns of population movement will help us to identify high-risk mobile populations and to focus educational resources before the virus is established in those populations."[23] While this stress on behavioral modification may not have been as manifestly self-serving as the above-described efforts of medical authorities working with TB to see overcrowding and malnutrition as the result of African ignorance, it shared a similar disregard for the root causes of African sexual patterns within an urban environment.

THE POLITICAL ECONOMY OF AFRICAN PROMISCUITY

None of this is to deny that AIDS is transmitted heterosexually or that multiple sexual partners may in fact be a common pattern within the rapidly growing urban centers of Africa. However, explanations that viewed this pattern as either a cultural phenomenon or as a product of declining social constraints ignored the context within which urbanization is occuring in Africa. At the same time, by focusing attention on sexual promiscuity and other cultural behaviors, these explanations have deflected attention from other cofactors that may be as important for the heterosexual transmission of AIDS in Africa as frequency of sexual contacts. In addition, concerns about African sexual behavior limit efforts to explore other avenues of HIV transmission.

There is every reason to believe that, whatever cultural attitudes shape African sexuality, the tendency to have multiple sexual partners has been encouraged by the separation of households. This separation has resulted from patterns of labor migration involving rural households, which often must send one or more of their members to seek wage employment in urban or industrial centers, including plantations and other large-scale agricultural projects. Labor migration, in turn, is the result of specific historical patterns of development in many parts of Africa—especially parts of Eastern Zaire, Tanzania, Rwanda, Uganda, Zambia, and Kenya. These areas all have large populations of impoverished rural households without access to land or labor and with few opportunities for acquiring income within the rural economy. As Hrdy rightfully notes, the numbers of men and women seeking employment in urban and industrial centers have increased dramatically since the early 1970s. What he does not indicate is why they have increased. Clearly, a major reason is that declining commodity prices and the increasing cost of agricultural inputs have made small-scale agricultural production unprofitable. The African small holder in many areas of East and Central Africa cannot make a living on the land other than on outgrower schemes, which are often highly exploitive in their treatment of growers. For these impoverished households, survival depends on access to some form of nonagricultural income, primarily wages. Yet employment opportunities are limited, in part because of the capital-intensive nature of many industries in Africa, and wages are often low, a product of lobbying efforts on the part of employers to ensure profits. All this has led to the creation of a class of semiproletarianized men and women, who work in urban and industrial settings but cannot afford to support their families there, and thus to the almost continual separation of rural households. For both men and women this existence fosters the development of "multiple sexual partners": Women who cannot find other employment often must work full or part time as prostitutes in urban and industrial settings; women left alone at home for long periods of time may take on "lovers"; and men may take on second "wives" near their place of employment.

This pattern of multiple sexual partners has undoubtedly also resulted from the political disruption of family life generated by warfare in places such as Mozambique, Angola, Burundi, and Uganda. Not only are families torn apart by these experiences, but the rape of rural women by marauding guerrilla armies must represent a particularly brutal form of "sexual poly-partnerism," which has little to do with cultural norms. Again, as with the impoverishment and disruption of rural households described above, it is important to understand the forces that have generated these wars, including the foreign governments that continue to support one side or the other to serve their own political ends.

It is important to understand that the pattern of multiple sexual partners is shaped by strong social, economic, and political pressures, and not simply by cultural norms. The presence of such forces will limit the success of efforts to control the spread of HIV through sex education, just as these factors have limited efforts to control population growth in Africa.

The parallel between AIDS prevention and birth control is in fact highly relevant. One of the principal obstacles to the success of population control programs in Africa and elsewhere in the developing world has been the economic pressures on parents to produce large families. These pressures, like those leading to the separation of households, have resulted from particular patterns of development that have created high demands for family labor. As long as this demand continues, unprotected sexual activity is going to occur with considerable frequency. For sexual activity is not simply about pleasure. It is also about social reproduction. If efforts to control the spread of HIV infection do not include policies that deal with the underlying causes of both family separation and the high demand for family labor, we may be fighting an uphill battle in trying to reduce the heterosexual transmission of AIDS in Africa through behavioral modification and condom use.

THE IMPACT OF MEDICAL PARADIGMS ON AIDS RESEARCH IN AFRICA

The early contributions of social scientists to our understanding of the epidemiology of AIDS in Africa, therefore, were not very helpful. Instead of providing information that might have encouraged medical researchers to develop a broader perspective on the social and economic factors shaping the AIDS epidemic, social scientists contributed to a narrowing of research and to the development of a medical model centered on the problem of African sexuality. This paradigm has prevented researchers from exploring factors that may be of equal or greater importance in the transmission and progression of AIDS but which are not suggested by the paradigm. This, we believe, has resulted in a premature closure of African AIDS research. Two of these understudied areas are the role of high levels of background infection and malnutrition, and unsterilized needle use in the transmission and progression of HIV.

THE ROLE OF BACKGROUND INFECTIONS AND MALNUTRITION IN AIDS

A number of studies have indicated a positive correlation between HIV seropositivity and the presence of other immunosuppressant conditions, such as malnutrition, tuberculosis, malaria, or trypanosomiasis.[24] Most of these studies assumed that these other conditions have followed on immune suppression caused by HIV infection. Yet a few studies suggest that these immune-suppressant conditions may have preceded HIV infection and facilitated its transmission. Lamoureaux and his colleagues, for example, noted the high incidence of TB in association with HIV infection among Haitians and Africans and evidence that in many cases infection with *Micobacterium tuberculosis* appears to have preceded HIV infection. They concluded:

> We feel that the prevalence and persistence of *M. tuberculosis* infection in Africans and Haitians, along with the concomitant increase, due to the infection, in CD4+ lymphocytes and macrophages, which are the target cells of HIV, as well as the frequent provocation of an immunosuppressed state in such TB-bacillus-infected individuals, probably represents a common factor predisposing these two populations to infection with HIV when exposed to the virus.[25]

Similarly, Thomas Quinn and his colleagues reported that "the immune systems of African heterosexuals, similar to those of US homosexual men, are in a chronically activated state associated with chronic viral and parasitic antigenic exposure, *which may cause them to be particularly susceptible to HIV infection or disease progression*" (emphasis added). The authors noted in addition:

> Our serological studies, as well as others, demonstrate that Africans are frequently exposed, due to hygienic conditions and other factors, to a wide variety of viruses, including CMV, EBV, hepatitis B virus and HSV, all of which are known to modulate the immune system. . . . Furthermore Africans in the present study are at additional risk for immunological alterations since they are frequently afflicted with a wide variety of diseases, such as malaria, trypanosomiasis, and filariasis, that are known to have a major effect on the immune system. The frequent exposure to these multiple microbial agents could act collectively or individually to result in immunological modulations rendering a host more susceptible to HIV infection or by influencing disease progression by increased viral replication and cytolysis of T4-positive cells.[26]

Quinn and his associates concluded: "Prospective studies are warranted in different population groups to examine the specific impact of these viral, bacterial, and parasitic infections and other antigenic stimuli on the susceptibility and development of HIV disease."

Unfortunately, such studies are extremely difficult to conduct, and to date none have been reported, although in NIAID's new International Collaboration in AIDS Research program, such studies will be encouraged.

Other studies have suggested that the infectivity of HIV-infected individuals may increase with disease progression. If declining immune function is in turn accelerated by the presence of concurrent infections or malnutrition, then the risk of transmitting infection, through heterosexual contact or otherwise, may be higher in Africans infected with HIV than in other HIV-infected persons who are not subject to the same levels of background infection.[27]

The one predisposing medical condition that has been examined in considerable detail is the role of genital ulcer diseases (GUDs), which are seen as disrupting genital epitheliums and thereby facilitating the sexual transmission of HIV.[28] Unfortunately, these studies have not controlled for the possibility that HIV is being transmitted by infected needles in the STD clinics where men and women with GUD go for treatment, rather than directly through sexual intercourse. Thus, the relationship between HIV transmission and genital ulcers remains clouded (see below for further discussion of the problem of needle transmission). We should note here that the high degree of attention given to GUDs, in contrast to the relative lack of attention to other infectious diseases that might facilitate HIV transmission, is consistent with our argument that AIDS research in Africa has been narrowly focused on the problem of sexual behavior. In this regard it is interesting to note a recent *New York Times* article reporting the conclusions of AIDS researchers about the spread of AIDS. These researchers have concluded that there is considerable variation in the risk of HIV infection as the result of heterosexual contact. This risk does not appear to be related to frequency of unguarded contacts. Instead, it is evidently related to one of a number of possible cofactors. With the exception of levels of HIV infection, all the cofactors being considered are directly related to sexual contact.[29] Presumably no attention is being given to nonsexual factors such as those suggested here.

In short, the susceptibility of Africans to HIV and the facility with which it is transmitted heterosexually may be a direct result of the high background levels of infection and malnutrition and other immunosuppressant conditions that exist in most African countries, and not simply a question of frequent sexual contacts or other "cultural practices."

If background infections do facilitate the transmission of HIV, then it seems likely that the population at greatest risk is not the urban middle class, who appear frequently in AIDS statistics, but the urban poor, who possess higher background levels of infection and malnutrition as a result of their impoverishment and lack of access to adequate medical care. Unfortunately, few studies have accounted for class, and those that have are inconclusive.[30]

If it is found that malnutrition and concurrent diseases that suppress the immune system predispose Africans to AIDS infection, and if HIV is transmitted through heterosexual contact, then the potential risk group may be very large indeed, and certainly is not limited to prostitutes, truck drivers, and bureaucrats. The risk group surely will include the rural families from which infected urban workers come and to which they eventually return. In this regard, one would expect to find high prevalence rates in the areas that have traditionally served as labor reserves for the cities which are currently centers for AIDS infection—for example, the Songea area of Tanzania; the Kwango region of Zaire; and areas of northeast Zambia that serve as labor reserves for the copper belt. These areas experience high rates of migration and are thus more likely to be exposed to AIDS infection emanating in the cities than other regions. They are also by definition impoverished regions and thus contain a population that may be particularly vulnerable to AIDS transmission.

Northeast Zambia is an interesting case. For it is not only a labor reserve area but also part of the so-called matrilineal belt of Africa. Hrdy, Brokensha, and Good have suggested that the rising incidence of AIDS in this area may be related to patterns of sexual promiscuity associated with matrilineal descent.[31] For example, Hrdy notes that "in the so-called 'matrilineal belt' centered in south-central Africa, there is an especially high degree of adolescent promiscuity and uncertainty about paternity." He goes on to describe inheritance patterns and concludes that "matrilineal inheritance . . . may reduce societal pressure to prevent promiscuity; matrilineal societies are often promiscuous societies." Whether or not this assertion is correct, linking matrilineality with HIV transmission represents a clear case of decontextualization, which ignores the wider social and economic conditions associated with participation in a labor reserve economy. It is thus another example of how, in their quest for "risk behaviors," certain anthropologists have contributed to the decontextualization of African lives and to the narrowing of AIDS research. Clearly, the two explanations call for very different responses. Knowing which one is correct is therefore of considerable importance.

NEEDLE USE: AN ALTERNATIVE MODEL

The second area of inquiry that appears to have been obscured as a result of the medical research community's fixation on African sexuality is the role of injections and transfusions in the spread of HIV. High levels of background infection are associated in Africa with high levels of needle use in a range of therapeutic settings, which may or may not observe adequate sterilization procedures. Where sterilization is not employed, there is a risk of HIV transmission. Although this area of risk has been recognized, it has been given inadequate attention.

In two control studies of infants and children in Kinshasa, Mann and his colleagues correlated HIV seropositivity with a history of frequent previous injections: "The greater number of injections previously received by seropositive children of seronegative mothers than by seropositive children of seropositive mothers (who presumably have similar HIV burdens) strengthens the argument that these injections represent an important route of exposure to HIV, rather than reflecting medical needs for HIV-associated illness."[32] The authors noted that all children and infants in Kinshasa are commonly given intramuscular injections and that there was a high expectation among mothers that injections are an essential part of any cure. "Injections are often administered in dispensaries which reuse needles and syringes yet may not adequately sterilize injection equipment. Furthermore injections are frequently given by untrained personnel or traditional healers." The seropositive infants and children in these studies also had a history of transfusions, which are commonly given to children who suffer from anemia due to malaria.

Children and infants are not the only segments of the African population who are at risk of transmission through injections and transfusions. The view that injections represent the most effective form of medical therapy is clearly widespread in Africa. And adults are just as vulnerable to this means of transmission as children. Of 500 cases studied by Quinn and his colleagues in Kinshasa, 80 percent had a history of prior injections. This was in fact the greatest risk associated with

AIDS in the study, though the authors noted that it was impossible to assess the significance of risk activities without information on control populations. Similarly, in a study of over 2,000 hospital workers, the only identifiable risk factors were hospitalization during the previous ten years, transfusion within the last ten years, and medical injection within the last three years.[33]

In this context it is worth noting that STD clinic attendees, who are reported to have high rates of HIV infection, also have higher than normal histories of injections. The number of such injections may in fact be remarkably high. It has been calculated that among prostitutes in Nairobi the mean time to reinfection after treatment was only twelve days.[34] Prostitutes and their customers may thus be repeatedly exposed to needles.

Melbye and his colleagues rejected the hypothesis that needles accounted for the high rates of HIV infection among the STD clinic attendees they studied in Lusaka, arguing that in the University Teaching Hospital's STD clinic, where they carried out their studies, "clinic needles are not *commonly* reused" (emphasis added).[35] In addition, they noted that the prevalence figures were as high for those STD clinic attendees who received injections as for those who did not. These arguments are not very convincing, in part because the researchers made no attempt to elicit information about treatment that these patients may have received from other clinics as well as from various indigenous healers, who may have been somewhat less careful about needle reuse. One might also imagine that clinic staff would have been more careful about sterilization in the presence of the AIDS researchers.

The association of hepatitis B infection with STD attendance also points toward a connection between injections and HIV transmission. Thus, Van de Perre and his associates, in a study of prostitutes drawn from an STD clinic in Butare, Rwanda, found that twenty-nine of thirty-three prostitutes were seropositive for HIV, as compared to four of thirty-three female controls; thirty-one of the prostitutes also had hepatitis B virus markers, as compared to only eighteen of the controls; and thirty-one of the subjects and thirteen of the controls tested positive for *Chlamydia trachoma*. While high prevalences of hepatitis B have also been reported among homosexual populations in the United States, its transmission among heterosexual populations has been more frequently associated with unsterilized needle use. This finding suggests that the subject population in this study may have been exposed to unsterilized needles more frequently than the controls and that this exposure may have accounted for their higher rates of HIV infection. Therefore, it is impossible to state with any certainty whether frequent sexual activity results directly in HIV transmission or only puts one at risk of exposure to other STDs and thereby at risk of being infected with HIV through exposure to unsterilized needles. The authors of the study, in fact, concluded: "This study suggests that HTLV-III has to be considered as an infectious agent transmitted among promiscuous Central African heterosexuals by sexual contact *and/or parenteral contact with unsterile needles used for STD treatments*" (emphasis added).[36]

The possible role of needle transmission among adults in STD clinic settings provides an alternative explanation for the commonly reported correlation between frequent prostitute contacts and HIV infection among African men, as well as the association between genital ulcers and HIV seropositivity. The studies that have shown a correlation between prostitute contact, genital ulcers, and HIV seropositivity in Africa have drawn their subject population from STD clinics and their control populations from among blood donors or medical staff populations.[37] As noted above, these studies have not controlled for the possibility that the chain of causation may involve contact with prostitutes, leading to STDs and genital ulcers, leading to clinic treatment and HIV infection through exposure to unclean needles. Prostitutes may be a major risk group for AIDS, but they need not be the primary vectors for HIV transmission that they are frequently made out to be. They may simply be a source for the transmission of STDs, which are a risk factor for HIV transmission through unsterile needle use or genital ulcers.[38] Clearly, studies need to be done which control for the possibility that needles may be a primary route of transmission.

If needle use is a significant means of HIV transmission, we need to examine why sterilization does not occur. Clearly, one of the reasons is that injections are performed by indigenous therapists who are unaware of the risks involved in reusing needles without sterilization. Yet lack of sterilization also occurs in government-run clinics. We should not conclude that the failure to sterilize needles is necessarily a product of laziness or ignorance on the part of African medical personnel, lest we construct another cultural stereotype to explain the spread of AIDS in Africa. Given limited medical budgets (averaging five dollars per capita) and shortages in foreign exchange in most African countries (a product of the declining value of African exports on world commodity markets and currency devaluations instigated by the International Monetary Fund), disposable needles, sterilizers, and even the chemicals needed for sterilization are often in short supply. The energy costs involved in running sterilizers, even where they exist, may also limit the sterilization of needles.

Warfare is also contributing to the reuse of needles in many countries, such as Mozambique, Uganda, and Angola, by disrupting electrical power supplies and urban and rural health services. In Mozambique, for example, Renamo "terrorists" frequently destroy power lines to the city of Beira. Until the recent acquisition of generators by the city, these actions disrupted needle sterilization within the city hospital. The destruction of rural clinics and medical equipment also increases pressure to reuse needles.

In short, as the World Health Organization has advocated, we need to examine the political economy of health care, and not simply the incidence of improper needle use.[39] In a similar vein, the role of transfusions in transmitting HIV needs to be viewed within the context of a lack of financial resources to properly screen donated blood and an extremely high incidence of trauma injuries requiring blood transfusions associated with warfare and automobile accidents.

AGE DISTRIBUTION STUDIES: A CRITIQUE

Data on the age distribution of both AIDS cases and seropositivity have been used to support the argument that injections do not contribute materially to the transmission of HIV in Africa. Evidence collected on the distribution of 500 AIDS cases in Kinshasa is presented in figures 6 and 7.

Commenting on this distribution, Quinn and his associates conclude, "The sex and age distribution of 500 AIDS cases reflect patterns seen in other sexually transmitted diseases both in developed and developing countries in which incidence and morbidity rates are higher among younger women."[40] On the last point, Peter Piot recently suggested at an AIDS conference in Washington that older men may be having sex with younger women.

These statements imply that the age-sex distribution of AIDS cases supports the assumption that AIDS is being transmitted through heterosexual contact. Yet if one looks at the age-sex distribution of tuberculosis, one sees a similar pattern. Surely no one would argue that TB is a sexually transmitted disease. As is now recognized, women in their childbearing years have a higher risk of contracting TB because of a generalized lowered resistance.[41] Conversely, children in the age range

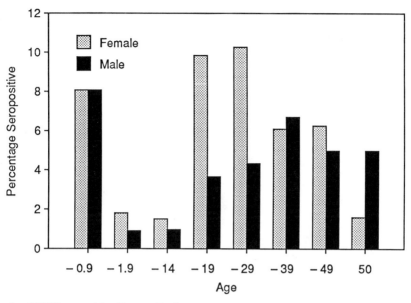

6. HIV Seropositive Rates, Kinshasa, 1984–1985

SOURCE: T. Quinn et al., "AIDS in Africa: An Epidemiological Paradigm," *Science* 234 (1984): 955–63.

from four to fourteen, for reasons that are not altogether clear, have a higher level of resistance to a number of diseases, including TB. This phenomenon may in fact occur in AIDS. Thus, several studies recently reported in the *New York Times* noted that children in their teens infected with HIV show fewer signs of a declining immune system than similarly infected adults. Dr. James Goedert of the National Cancer Institute followed up eighty-nine patients from a hemophilia center, all of whom were infected with HIV. After seven years 35 percent of the adults had symptoms of AIDS, whereas only 10 percent of those infected as children and teenagers had AIDS symptoms. Two other studies reported similar findings. Dr. Goedert concluded that "AIDS could resemble chicken pox, measles or other diseases that are more severe in adults than in children and adolescents."[42] If this is the case, then the low incidence of AIDS in the four-to-fourteen age range may reflect resistance to viral replication and AIDS rather than an absence of infection. In other words, the age distribution of AIDS cases in Africa need not support the hypothesis that AIDS is transmitted primarily through heterosexual contacts. Why, then, did Quinn and his associates choose

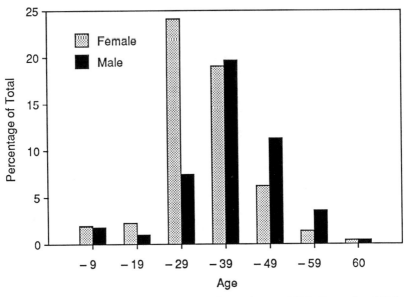

7. Distribution of 500 AIDS Cases, Kinshasa, August 1985–December 1985

SOURCE: T. Quinn et al., "AIDS in Africa: An Epidemiological Paradigm," *Science* 234 (1984): 955–63.

"other sexually transmitted diseases," rather than other infectious diseases, as their comparison?

The possibility that young children are resistant to HIV progression raises an additional issue. That is, in many parts of Africa, all children under five are vaccinated at the same time—often with unsterilized needles that are reused. Since this practice is widely recognized as a potential avenue for the transmission of HIV, one would expect to find more AIDS cases in young children. But few such cases have been found. This lack of cases may, as suggested above, be related to the children's resistance to disease progression rather than to an absence of infection. As a result, the cases acquired through this route would show up in the young-adult population.

Medical researchers will immediately object to this explanation on the ground that seropositivity data appear to reveal the same pattern of age and sex distribution. In other words, it is not just that fewer cases appear among children in the four-to-fourteen age range; they also appear to be infected less. This finding appears to support the heterosexual contact model and to call into question the importance of other forms of transmission, and particularly injections. Thus, Robert Biggar in a recent review of epidemiological data on AIDS concludes: "The results of serosurveys using accurate tests have shown that HIV infection in central Africa is largely heterosexually transmitted. Evidence supporting this includes ... the great concentration of HIV-infected persons in the years of greatest sexual activity (15–65 years old) with the peak age-specific prevalence being during the years of peak sexual activity (25–29 years for women; 30–34 years old for men)."[43]

How reasonable is this interpretation? First of all, it must be noted that there is little reliable cross-sectional data on the age-sex distribution of HIV seropositivity or AIDS cases in Africa. In fact, until recently statements about the age distribution of seropositivity were based on a small number of prevalence studies conducted in hospital or clinic settings involving the use of what have often been questionable sampling methods. The first study to present age-specific seroprevalence data using reliable screening methods, and the one that is cited by Biggar and others, was conducted by Melbye and his associates at the University Teaching Hospital in Lusaka, Zambia, in August 1985.[44] The 1,078 subjects in the study included inpatients and outpatients, blood donors, and medical staff. The study found that high levels of HIV seropositivity occurred in women and men between twenty and sixty years of age, with none of subjects under fifteen or over seventy being seropositive. The investigators concluded: "Our findings strongly suggest that heterosexual transmission is an important route of HIV infection in Africa. Seropositivity was restricted to subjects who were in their sexually most active years of life."[45]

Yet even a cursory examination of the data used in this study quickly reveals a significant problem in the sampling method employed. While the total sample consisted of 1,078 subjects, the "under fifteen years" subgroup included only 12 subjects, all of whom were surgery patients between ten and fifteen years of age. The "over sixty" group consisted of 47 subjects, and only 21 subjects were over seventy years of age. In effect, 97 percent of the sample fell between fifteen and seventy years of age; 94 percent, between fifteen and sixty. Similarly, if one looks just at the blood donors and hospital staff, 94 percent of the sample fell between fifteen and fifty years of age. The small sample size for the populations on either side of this age group, and particularly in the "under fifteen" age group, makes any conclusions about the distribution of seropositivity among the wider population from which this sample was drawn meaningless—especially when one realizes that more than 50 percent of the populations of most African countries are under fifteen years of age! In other words, the sample was not representative of the population from which it was drawn.

There is the additional problem created by the use of a hospital population who may have a range of risk factors, including injection and transfusion histories. Without knowing how these risk factors are distributed through the different age groups, one cannot know whether age or the frequency of particular risk factors is being reflected in the age distribution pattern.

It is unclear whether the same problems apply to later sources of prevalence data that are said to support the sexual transmission paradigm. A study of over 5,000 "healthy persons" living in Kinshasa who were tested between 1984 and 1985 revealed a similar distribution of HIV infection. The results were reported by Quinn and his associates in 1986.[46] The report, however, provided no details on how the sample was collected and made no reference to earlier reports that describe the methods involved. A more recent study, conducted in the Central African Republic and employing random sampling, reported an absence of antibodies to HIV in children four to fifteen years of age. The investigators warned, however, that more surveys were needed to confirm this finding because the sample for this age group was nonrepresentative.[47]

Even assuming that the distribution of HIV infection in the sample population in these studies accurately reflects its distribution in the underlying population, what does this finding indicate? Or, put another way, could the high prevalence of HIV among sexually active subjects and the relatively low prevalence among children reflect the presence of factors other than levels of sexual activity? For example, if the transmission of HIV is facilitated by the presence of preexisting immunosuppresant infections, and if children between the ages of four and fifteen are more resistant to such infections than either infants or adults, the four-to-fifteen age group would have a lower prevalence of HIV than other age groups regardless of how the infection is transmitted. Alternatively, their increased resistance to other infectious diseases may reduce their exposure to risk of infection through needles and/or transfusions. In short, age distribution data, even if correct, need not indicate that sex is the only avenue of HIV transmission in Africa.

These possibilities are admittedly speculative. Moreover, they run counter to the often-quoted instruction given to all medical students: "When you hear hoofbeats, think of horses, not zebras." AIDS, however, is a relatively new disease, about which there is a great deal more to be learned. Thinking of horses, while reasonable in a diagnostic setting, may prevent medical researchers in Africa from seeing the entire range of factors at play in the epidemiology of AIDS in Africa. In any case, in Africa one can just as easily come across a zebra as a horse.

CONCLUSION

The point in all this is that assumptions about the importance of sexual promiscuity in the transmission of HIV in Africa were initially based on limited, and in some cases methodologically questionable, data. These assumptions, nonetheless, shaped both the questions that AIDS researchers asked and the way that they interpreted data. This narrowing of research, in turn, discouraged serious consideration of the role of alternative avenues of transmission, such as injections, or of the role of possible cofactors, such as high background levels of infection and malnutrition and associated problems of poverty and maldevelopment, which may be as important in the heterosexual transmission of HIV as the frequency of sexual contacts.

We are, in fact, much further from understanding the epidemiology of AIDS in Africa than some medical researchers, development officers, and social scientists would have us believe. It is clear that heterosexual transmission of HIV occurs in Africa, but how or why it occurs has not been demonstrated. AIDS, like Burkett's lymphoma, may yet prove to have a complex etiology involving a combination of political and economic forces associated with underdevelopment in Africa. These forces have brought together particularly susceptible populations—populations subject to high background levels of viral, parasitic, and bacterial infections—in a social setting marked by high levels of familial separation and multiple sexual partners. These conditions, in turn, have contributed to the spread of other STDs, which in turn have created a high risk of exposure to HIV via genital ulcers and/or infected needles.

The medical research community and the social science community working with it must develop research agendas that will illuminate these complex interactions, instead of obscuring them through a precipitous move to find quick answers that can be easily translated into AIDS containment programs. The early history of Western research on TB and syphilis should serve as a warning that, if we continue to look for easy solutions, those solutions may have a limited impact and, at the same time, our understanding of the wider epidemiology of AIDS may be

diminished. Before we spend millions on the type of behavior modification model of intervention now being developed, we must have a higher
degree of certainty about how HIV is being transmitted and what the
real risk factors are, as well as knowledge of the social and economic
context within which risk behaviors are set. If primary risk factors are
poverty and unemployment, our proposed interventions must address
the causes of these conditions. We must not allow AIDS to become one
more symptom for which the West finds a cure without addressing the
underlying causes of this and many other health problems. At the very
least, studies that explore other cofactors and avenues of transmission
need to parallel efforts to understand and prevent the sexual transmission of HIV.

Any attempt to initiate a more comprehensive approach to AIDS research in Africa requires that medical researchers and social scientists
develop a more productive working relationship. Such a relationship
will necessitate adjustments on both sides. Social scientists need to resist
attempts to limit their input to collecting and presenting cultural artifacts; they need to be critical of colleagues who continue to accept this
limited role. If the conferences and workshops at which social scientists
and medical researchers are brought together are to be productive, their
agendas must be expanded to address broader issues of African social
and economic life and not simply the "sexual life of the natives" and
other forms of risk behaviors. At the same time, any attempt to open
up the agenda must be sensitive to the medical research community's
need for questions and hypotheses that take account of the existing
epidemiological data and that can be empirically tested.

For their part, medical researchers need to take a more open view of
how the social science community can contribute to epidemiological
research on AIDS in Africa. They need to recognize that AIDS research
in Africa can be illuminated by a more fundamental knowledge and
understanding of the contours of African social and economic life, which
involves more than a cataloging of risk behaviors. Medical researchers,
like social scientists, also need to be more openly critical of their own
colleagues. Research based on unrepresentative samples or faulty sampling methods need to be challenged. Peer review procedures need to be
uniform, so that conclusions presented on AIDS in Lusaka are viewed
as critically as conclusions made about AIDS in New York City. The
medical community also needs to be more forthright and open about
the limits of our present knowledge about the epidemiology of AIDS in
Africa. Too many studies have taken an authoritatitve tone that is not

warranted by the data available and, in doing so, have encouraged premature closure of African AIDS research.

NOTES

A different version of this essay is forthcoming in *Social Science and Medicine* and is reprinted with the editor's permission.

1. In this regard, of course, Western medical research on AIDS in Africa also resembles the earlier development of medical ideas about diseases in Europe and the United States. Thus, Charles Rosenberg notes in his history of cholera in nineteenth-century America, "A disease is no absolute physical entity but a complex intellectual construct, an amalgam of biological state and social definition" (Charles Rosenberg, *The Cholera Years* [Chicago: University of Chicago Press, 1962], p. 5). More recently Susan Sontag and Sander Gilman have observed that a number of metaphors have been embedded in the medical construction of AIDS in the West.

2. R. Packard, "Tuberculosis and Industrial Health Policy on the Witwatersrand, 1902–1932," *Journal of Southern African Studies* 13 (1987): 187–209.

3. N. Fendell, "Public Health and Urbanization in Africa," *Public Health Reports* 78 (1963): 574.

4. Marc Dawson, "Socio-economic and Epidemiological Change in Kenya: 1880–1925," Ph.D. diss., University of Wisconsin-Madison, 1983, pp. 211–18.

5. Quoted in Dawson, p. 212.

6. Quoted in Dawson, p. 213.

7. Quoted in Dawson, p. 230.

8. Sander Gilman, *Difference and Pathology: Stereo Types of Sexuality, Race and Madness* (Ithaca, N.Y.: Cornell University Press, 1985); and *Disease and Representation: Images of Illness from Madness to AIDS* (Ithaca, N.Y.: Cornell University Press, 1988).

9. See, for example, Peter Piot et al., "AIDS in a Heterosexual Population in Zaire," *Lancet* 1, no. 8394 (July 14, 1984): 67.

10. R. C. Gallo, "The AIDS Virus," *Scientific American*, January 1987, pp. 39–48; P. J. Kanki, J. Avroy, and M. Essex, "Isolation of T-Lymphotropic Retrovirus Related to HTLV-III/LAV from Wild African Green Monkeys," *Science* 230 (1985): 951–54.

11. For a fascinating account of this debate from an African perspective, see C. Chirimuuta and J. Chirimuuta, *Aids, Africa and Racism* (Trenton, N.J.: Africa World Press, 1989).

12. For one notable exception to this pattern, see N. Nzilambi et al., "The Prevalence of Infection with Immunodeficiency Virus over a 10-Year Period in Rural Zaire," *New England Journal of Medicine* 318 (September 27, 1986): 707–9. This question deserves more research.

13. Peter Piot et al., "Heterosexual Transmission of HIV," *AIDS* 1 (1987):

199–206. A similar statement is attributed to N. Clumeck, a Belgian AIDS researcher who was apparently one of the earliest and strongest proponents of the sexual promiscuity theory (Report on the Second International Symposium on AIDS in Africa, reported in *Washington Post*, October 10, 1987).

14. See Gilman, *Disease and Representation*, for a discussion of the early construction of AIDS in the West as a disease associated with deviancy.

15. D. Serwadda et al., "Slim Disease: A New Disease in Uganda and Its Association with HTLV-III Infection, "*Lancet* 2, no. 8460 (October 19, 1985): 849–52.

16. P. Van de Perre et al., "Female Prostitutes: A Risk Group for Infection with Human T-Cell Lymphotropic Virus Type III," *Lancet* 2 (September 7, 1985): 524.

17. David Brokensha et al., "Social Factors in the Transmission of AIDS in Africa," report prepared for the Directorate for Health, Bureau for Science and Technology, Agency for International Development, 1987.

18. Daniel B. Hrdy, "Cultural Practices Contributing to the Transmission of Human Immunodeficiency Virus in Africa," *Reviews of Infectious Diseases* 9 (November–December 1987): 1109–19, at p. 1112.

19. E. Green, "AIDS in Africa: An Agenda for Behavioral Scientists," and Francis Conant, "Evaluating Social Science Data Relating to AIDS," in *AIDS in Africa*, ed. R. Rockwell and N. Miller (Lewiston, N.Y.: Edwin Mellen Press, 1988) pp. 176, 198.

20. Hrdy, "Cultural Practices."

21. Brokensha et al., "Social Factors in the Transmission of AIDS," p. 12.

22. Hrdy, "Cultural Practices," p. 1112.

23. Brokensha et al., "Social Factors in the Transmission of AIDS," p. 11.

24. J. M. Mann et al., "Human Immunodeficiency Virus Seroprevalence in Pediatric Patients 2 to 14 Months of Age at Mama Yemo Hospital, Kinshasa, Zaire," *Pediatrics* 78 (1987): 673–77; J. L. Lesbordes et al., "Malnutrition and HIV Infection in Children in the Central African Republic" [letter], *Lancet* 2, no. 8502 (August 9, 1986): 337–38. For a review of data on the relationship between nutrition, immunity, and infection, see R. K. Chandra, "Nutrition, Immunity and Infection: Present Knowledge and Future Directions," *Lancet* 1, no. 8325 (March 26, 1983): 688–91; J. Mann et al., "Association between HTLV-III/LAV Infection and Tuberculosis in Zaire," *Journal of the American Medical Association* 256 (July, 18, 1986): 346; William Legg et al., "Association of Tuberculosis and HIV Infection in Zimbabwe," paper presented at the Fifth International Conference on AIDS, Montreal, June 8, 1989.

25. G. Lamoureaux et al., "Is Prior Mycobacterial Infection a Common Predisposing Factor to AIDS in Haitians and Africans?" *Annales Institut Pasteur/Immunologie* 138 (1987): 521–29.

26. T. C. Quinn et al., "Serologic and Immunologic Studies in Patients with AIDS in North America and Africa: The Potential Role of Infectious Agents as Co-factors in Human Immunodeficiency Virus Infection," *Journal of the American Medical Association* 257 (1987): 2617–21.

27. Linda Jackson, "Bioanthropological Perspectives on Endemic Virus versus Epidemic HIV-Infections and AIDS in Tropical Africa," unpublished paper.

Jackson suggests that the progression of HIV infections may also be facilitated by the widespread use in an unsupervised setting of antibiotics, antimalarials (especially quinine compounds), and antihelminiths, which can increase levels of chemical immunosuppression and thereby magnify the clinical response to HIV exposure.

28. Robert Ryder et al., "Extramarital Prostitute Sex and Genital Ulcer Disease (GUD) Are Important HIV Risk Factors in 7068 Male Kinshasa Factory Workers and Their 4548 Wives," and Marie Lana et al., "High Prevalence and Incidence of HIV and Other Sexually Transmitted Diseases (STD) among 801 Kinshasa Prostitutes," papers presented at the Fifth International Conference on AIDS, Montreal, June 5, 1989.

29. Elizabeth Rosenthal, "The Spread of AIDS: The Mystery Unravels," *New York Times*, August 28, 1990, p. C1.

30. For example, Biggar's research in eastern Zaire suggested that there may be a socioeconomic gradient for HIV seropositivity, with seropositivity rates being highest among the poorest agricultural workers he surveyed (R. J. Biggar et al., "Seroepidemiology of HTLV-III Antibodies in a Remote Population in Zaire," *British Medical Journal* 290 (1985): 810). Joan Kreiss and her colleagues, in their study of Nairobi prostitutes, noted that seropositivity was significantly lower in upper-class (33 percent positive) than in lower-class prostitutes (66 percent seropositive) (J. K. Kreiss et al., "Aids Virus Infection in Nairobi Prostitutes," *New England Journal of Medicine* 314, no. 7 (February 13, 1986): 414–418). The authors, however, make little effort to explore the constellation of factors that might be associated with "low status," limiting their research instead to the presence or absence of risk behaviors or exposures, such as scarification, transfusions, the presence of STDs, and, most important, the frequency of sexual contacts. Factors such as malnutrition and the presence of other immunosuppressant diseases, which may facilitate the transmission of HIV, were not explored. The study did measure immune levels (T-cell helper/ suppressor ratios) and compared those of the seropositives against those of the seronegatives. They did not, however, measure, or at least did not report, the comparative immune levels of high- versus low-class prostitutes. On the other hand, M. Melbye and his colleagues found a positive correlation between high education and occupational levels and HIV seropositivity (M. Melbye et al., "Evidence for Heterosexual Transmission and Clinical Manifestations of HIV Infection and Related Conditions in Lusaka, Zambia," *Lancet* 2, no. 8516 (November 15, 1986): 1113–15). Clearly, more studies that control for social class are needed.

31. Hrdy, "Cultural Practices," p. 1112; Brokensha et al., "Social Factors in the Transmission of AIDS"; Charles Good, presentation at the Conference on Anthropological Perspectives on AIDS in Africa, January 7, 1988.

32. J. M. Mann et al., "Risk Factors for Human Immunodeficiency Virus Seropositivity among Children 1–24 Months Old in Kinshasa, Zaire," *Lancet* no. 8508 (1986): 676.

33. T. Quinn et al., "AIDS in Africa: An Epidemiological Paradigm," *Science* 234 (1986): 955–63.

34. L. J. D'Costa et al., "Prostitutes Are a Major Reservoir of Sexually

Transmitted Diseases in Nairobi, Kenya," *Sexually Transmitted Diseases* 12 (1985): 64–67.

35. Melbye et al., "Evidence for Heterosexual Transmission," p. 1115.

36. P. van de Perre, "Seroepidemiological Study of Sexually Transmitted Diseases and Hepatitis B in African Promiscuous Heterosexuals in Relation to HTLV-III Infections," *European Journal of Epidemiology* 3, no. 1 (1987): 4–8, at p. 8.

37. Ryder and colleagues ("Extramarital Prostitute Sex and Genital Ulcer Disease") drew their sample population from outside clinic settings. However, they did not control for the possibility of needle transmission.

38. J. A. De Hovitz, "A Perspective on the Heterosexual Transmission of the Acquired Immunodeficiency Syndrome," *New York State Journal of Medicine* 86 (1986): 117–18.

39. World Health Organization, Special Programme on Africa, *Strategies and Structure: Project Needs*, vol. 2 (Geneva: WHO, 1987), pp. 3–4.

40. Quinn et al., "AIDS in Africa," p. 957.

41. This susceptibility suggests that we need to be careful in extrapolating general levels of HIV infection from prevalence surveys using pregnant women.

42. Gina Kolata, "AIDS Symptoms Found Slowed in Teen-Agers," *New York Times*, April 3, 1988, p. 25. Dr. Goedert reported at the International AIDS Conference in Stockholm in 1988 that children between the ages of two and eighteen had a 12 percent risk of developing AIDS eight years after infection, whereas adults eighteen to thirty-four had a 26 percent chance of doing so (G. Kolata, "Studies Link Age to AIDS Development," *New York Times*, May 21, 1989, p. 34).

43. R. J. Biggar, "Overview: Africa, AIDS and Epidemiology," in *AIDS in Africa*, ed. Rockwell and Miller, p. 3.

44. Melbye et al, "Evidence for Heterosexual Transmission," p. 1115.

45. Ibid.

46. Quinn et al., "AIDS in Africa," p. 958.

47. M. Merlin et al., " Epidemiology of HIV1 Infection among Randomized Representative Central African Populations," *Annales Institut Pasteur/Virologie* 138 (1987): 503–10.

AIDS and HIV Infection in the Third World: A First World Chronicle

Paula A. Treichler

Understanding the AIDS epidemic as a medical phenomenon involves understanding it as a cultural phenomenon. Yet excessively positivist or commonsensical notions of "culture" may limit our ability to recognize that AIDS is also a complex and contradictory *construction* of culture. This is particularly true of AIDS in developing countries. AIDS in the developed world (the "First World" and, to a lesser extent, the "Second World") is now routinely characterized as a social as well as a medical epidemic, as a challenge to conflicting values, and as an unprecedentedly complex cultural phenomenon; in contrast, AIDS in the developing world—the "Third World"—is believed to lead a much simpler life.[1] Even when these cultures themselves are seen as mysterious, AIDS is seen as a scientifically understood infectious disease that, without our help, will devastate whole countries, whose passive citizens struggle against it in vain.

This vision is well intentioned and perhaps even necessary to marshal external resources. But it obscures the fact that diverse interests are articulated around AIDS in the developing world in ways that are socially and culturally localized and specific. Deeply entrenched institutional agendas and cultural precedents in the First World prevent us from hearing the story of AIDS in the Third World as a complex narrative. One consequence of this inadvertent cultural imperialism is that very simple generalizations about the epidemic may be accepted as "the truth about AIDS," with few efforts made to unravel their diverse and often contradictory claims.

This essay does not seek to determine "the truth about AIDS." Rather, I look closely at how selected First and Third World publications attempt to chronicle and conceptualize the epidemic. I begin with a discussion of AIDS in Haiti, to show a typical discursive construction of "Third World AIDS." I then contrast the familiar statistical chronicle of the global epidemic with other accounts, suggesting how differing conceptualizations, different "truths," work to promote differing material consequences. Contradictory accounts of the epidemic in Kenya, for example, suggest the value of listening carefully to contradictions; selecting too readily a given account as the definitive truth short-circuits efforts to better understand how truth is situated—and how it is produced, legitimated, sustained, and interpreted. I conclude that understanding the discursive production of the AIDS crisis—the production, that is, of these differing narratives—is a necessary if not sufficient part of addressing its conceptual and material complexity. In turn, such understanding provides crucial grounding for genuine cooperation between the developed and the developing worlds.

A U.S. DOCTOR UNMASKS TRUTH IN HAITI: THIRD WORLD AIDS IN FIRST WORLD MEDIA

We had come near the end of a long line of anthropologists working in these remote villages. . . . Coming at the end gave us certain advantages. . . . But as time passed we became aware that we had also inherited serious problems. The !Kung had been observing anthropologists for almost six years and had learned quite a bit about them. Precedents had been set that the !Kung expected us to follow.

Shostak, *Nisa*[2]

The very activity of ethnographic *writing*—seen as inscription or textualization—enacts a redemptive Western allegory.

Clifford, "Allegory"[3]

All accounts of the AIDS epidemic in the Third World, whether they are medical reports, patient testimony, media observations, investigative journalism, World Health Organization news bulletins, or government reports, are at some level linguistic constructions. These diverse representations of AIDS in the Third World draw their authority from many sources, including the credentials and persuasive powers of individual authors, consistency with accepted beliefs and knowledge about AIDS and about the Third World, compatibility with our own social and political perspectives, and resonance with familiar traditions of discourse. Though often covert, the influence of discourse is powerful and pervasive in establishing and legitimating a given representation.

Discourse about AIDS, for example, draws on widely accepted narratives of past epidemics. Though these histories may be employed to supply a variety of arguments and moral conclusions about today's epidemic, they share the premise that any infectious disease is a knowable biological phenomenon whose strange and seemingly contradictory aspects are ultimately illusory: decoded by experts, its mysteries will one by one become controllable material realities. Discourse about AIDS in the Third World shares but exaggerates this premise, first equating the Third World (especially Africa, "the dark continent") with the savage, the alien, or the incomprehensible, then asserting the importance and achievability of reason and control. Though these two features may initially seem to be in conflict, they exist in fact in a relationship of discursive symbiosis: the metaphors of mystery and otherness produce the desire for control, which is in turn fulfilled and justified by the metaphors of otherness and mystery.[4]

A highly visible story, for example, was written for *Life* magazine by the physician-author Richard Selzer, who visited Haiti in the mid-1980s in an effort to learn the truth about AIDS behind the government's apparent attempts to downplay its prevalence.[5] The metaphor of the article's title, "A Mask on the Face of Death," invokes the government's denials in the language of exotic tropical rituals such as carnival and voodoo. The subtitle is "As AIDS Ravages Haiti, a U.S. Doctor Finds a Taboo against Truth"; although these probably are not Selzer's words, they suggest to the reader not only that official denials mask the brutality of the epidemic but also that Selzer, the expert medical observer, can perceive the reality beneath the mask. Selzer's article is in the tradition of the privileged First World informant of conventional anthropological, ethnographic, and travel literature—the stranger in a strange land, whose representation of AIDS in the Third World is legitimated by its claim to be an objective, scientific account of phenomena observed or experienced firsthand. As Mary Louise Pratt has observed, travel writing has provided ethnographic description with a discursive legacy, despite the ethnographer's desire to repudiate it; both, in turn, permeate representations in other genres.[6] Thus, Selzer's article opens with the conventional arrival scene of this dual legacy: "It is 10 o'clock at night as we drive up to the Copacabana, a dilapidated brothel on the rue Dessalines in the red-light district of Port-au-Prince" (p. 59). Outside the bar Selzer is importuned by men and women offering a variety of sexual pleasures; inside, he interviews three female prostitutes from the Dominican Republic who describe AIDS as an economic problem for them, not a health problem. The direct interrogation of the native informant is another staple of privileged observer accounts; in AIDS narratives it is often prostitutes who are interviewed, and they always seem to be wearing red.[7] The following day, Selzer talks with physicians and examines a large number of patients with apparent HIV-related illnesses for whom little in the way of treatment is available.

Selzer is carefully nonjudgmental with respect to street life and indeed speculates that the virus may have entered Haiti as an accidental feature of First World exploitation: "Could it have come from the American and Canadian homosexual tourists, and, yes, even some U.S. diplomats who have traveled to the island to have sex with impoverished Haitian men all too willing to sell themselves to feed their families? Throughout the international gay community Haiti was known as a good place to go for sex" (p. 64). Selzer pursues this characterization of Haiti as sexual victim ravaged by Western capitalists. Acting on "a private tip from an official at the Ministry of Tourism," Selzer and guide drive to a once luxurious hotel fifty miles from Port-au-Prince that was a prime vacation spot for gay men. Because the two Frenchmen who own the hotel are out of the country, Selzer and his guide are shown around by a staff member, a man about thirty who clearly

> is desperately ill. Tottering, short of breath, he shows us about the empty hotel. The furnishings are opulent and extreme—tiger skins on the wall, a live leopard in the garden, a bedroom containing a giant bathtub with gold faucets. Is it the heat of the day or the heat of my imagination that makes these walls echo with the painful cries of pederasty? (p. 64)

Ill at ease among the tiger skins of a hotel in Haiti, the Western travel writer goes to work on "Third World AIDS." Ultimately, for Selzer, AIDS in Haiti is an unambiguous mor(t)ality tale about the evils of sexual excess: as northern homosexual men ravaged Haitian boys, so does AIDS ravage Haiti. Nostalgia for the observed culture's original innocence gives way to regret at its exploitation by decadent foreigners and speculation about the deadly effects of exotic customs and sexual practices. Selzer's account therefore tells us something about his concrete daily activities, his heated imagination, and his strategies for transforming selected experiences into prose, but his desire to bring the country's plight to world attention is as much about language as about AIDS in Haiti.

The status of Selzer's article as a firsthand report of observed phenomena does not rest on our firsthand knowledge about AIDS, the Third World, or Haiti. In certain concrete ways, just as cinematic convention represents scenes viewed through binoculars as two intersecting circles, Western AIDS discourse transforms a culture so that it ceases to recognize itself but paradoxically becomes recognizable in the West. What is needed is to sort out the multiple voices, texts, and subtexts of the AIDS epidemic—which has in part evolved, as Jan Zita Grover puts it, as a "creature of language."[8]

Several elements of Selzer's account of AIDS in Haiti are now virtually obligatory in First World chronicles of Third World AIDS. First, the opening arrival scene, as I have noted, situates the First World observer in relation to the Third World culture—a culture that, in AIDS chronicles, almost always belongs to the fallen world of postcolonial development. Indeed, the term *Third World* grew out of the perceived confrontation between capitalist and communist interests and hence presupposes an analysis dependent on such concepts as colonialism, industrialization, modernity, and development. Second, the statistics provided by Haitian physicians function in at least two ways: to anchor in objective fact Selzer's more personal observations about the prevalence of AIDS, and to demonstrate the specialized knowledge of expert native informants whose on-the-scene experience equips them to reveal the truth behind the official mask. (In Selzer's story the inside informants assert that AIDS is more widespread than officials admit; but in other AIDS stories insiders also function to accuse the government and the media of exaggerating the AIDS crisis for political gains.) Another element is provided by "the reigning American pastor," a nonnative informant whose unreliability as a cultural informant is demonstrated by his moralistic condemnation of voodoo—a system of practices believed by some to facilitate the spread of HIV. Voodoo, he tells Selzer, is "a demonic religion, a cancer on Haiti" that is "worse than AIDS" (p. 62). In positioning himself against his fellow American, "a tall, handsome Midwesterner with an ecclesiastical smile," Selzer secures his own reliability, much as ethnographers quote descriptions of a given culture by earlier travel writers to repudiate the bias of such unscientific observations. Selzer's visits to health care settings constitute another element, revealing a devastated health care system—part of the economic fallen world that parallels his image elsewhere of Haiti as the victim of First World sexual exploitation. A further familiar feature of AIDS stories is "the view from the street," represented by Selzer's talk with the three healthy Dominican prostitutes. Their remarks seem designed to underscore the ignorance and dangerous false security engendered by the government's official silence. One of them, Carmen, scoffs at Selzer's suggestion that prostitutes as a population are sick with AIDS:

> "AIDS!" Her lips curl about the syllable. "There is no such thing. It is a false disease invented by the American government to take advantage of the poor countries. The American President hates poor people, so now he makes up AIDS to take away the little we have." The others nod vehemently. (p. 60)

The notion that AIDS is an American invention is, like so-called conspiracy theories, a recurrent element of the international AIDS story. It is one not easily incorporated within a Western positivist frame—in part, perhaps, because it often reveals an underlying narrative about colonialism in a postcolonial world. The West accordingly attributes such theories to ignorance, state propaganda, or psychological denial; or it interprets them as some new global version of an urban legend, like alligators in the New York City sewer system.[9]

But Carmen's theory of AIDS invokes two further narratives that reinforce the notion of a global economy changing in ways the West cannot fully control. One is a tale of postmodern scholarship about the difficulty of finding good native informants these days. As Shostak's introduction to her ethnographic study *Nisa* makes clear, native informants are quite likely to be already wise in the ways of Western inquisitors. Discussing *Nisa*, Pratt convincingly argues that Shostak is nevertheless able ultimately to transcend the "degraded" ethnographic culture of too-knowing informants and achieve a redemptive resolution for her story. Selzer's framing of Carmen accomplishes something similar, together with a second narrative, to which I have already alluded, concerning the construction of the subject in a fallen world. Pratt suggests that ethnographic characterizations of the !Kung changed in the course of foreign colonization. Precolonial ethnographers rendered them as sly, bloodthirsty, untrustworthy, appetitive, manipulative; after colonization they came to be represented as helpful, friendly, innocent, good, and vulnerable. Carmen's speech takes place at a pivotal moment in the global AIDS drama, and this context encourages us to hear her emphatic denial of AIDS as a prelude to tragedy—perhaps as we would hear Violetta in the first act of *La Traviata*.[10]

Selzer finally sums up: "This evening I leave Haiti. For two weeks I have fastened myself to this lovely fragile land like an ear pressed to the ground. It is a country to break a traveler's heart. . . . Perhaps one day the plague will be rendered in poetry, music, painting. But not now, not now" (p. 64). Here the stance of physician as ethnographer is clearer, the physician's ear pressed to the body of Haiti as he might press it to the body of a patient. But though the diagnosis is grim, the language is utopian: the First World AIDS narrative successfully repels the various threats of postmodern disruption to deliver a message of transcendent, universal humanism.

What are we to make of this? I am not suggesting that Selzer's account is not "true," or that we should exonerate the government of Haiti on its AIDS policies. I wish rather to point out how narrative conventions establish and sustain our *sense* of what is true. Visual representations reinforce the illusion of truth, in part because they reproduce familiar representations of the Third World and reinforce what we think we already know about AIDS in those regions. Thus, the color photographs in Selzer's *Life* story show us frail, wasting bodies in gloomy clinics; small children in rickety cribs; the prostitutes in red. One of the Dominican prostitutes, for example, is glamorously photographed, the full skirt of her red dress fanned out across a bed. Similarly, an April 1988 news account of the fear of AIDS in Mombasa, Kenya, reports an exchange between a U.S. sailor and a prostitute, a "23-year-old Ugandan woman in red shorts"; and a *Newsweek* photograph of a woman in red leggings and a skirt is captioned: " 'Avoid promiscuity': Prostitute with men in Zaire." Photographs in a 1986 *Newsweek* story on AIDS in Africa depict the "Third Worldness" of its health care system: in Tanzania a man with AIDS lies hospitalized on a plain cot with none of the high-tech paraphernalia of U.S. representations; a widely reprinted photograph shows six "emaciated patients in a Uganda AIDS ward," two in cots, four on mats on the the floor; rarely are physicians shown. A story on Brazil carries similar low-tech images. In contrast, publications originating in these countries do not omit technical images: African publications often show African scientists and physicians, and among the photographs in a 1987 story on AIDS in *Veja,* the Brazilian equivalent of *Newsweek,* are an enormous fully equipped modern hospital and masked and gowned physicians and nurses.[11]

A different problem occurs in a 1988 *National Geographic* story called "Uganda: Land beyond Sorrow." The story's portrait of unrelieved despair is oddly challenged by the magazine's characteristically stunning photographs. A young woman with AIDS in a long, flowing dress, for example, stands supported by her mother, who is wearing vivid pink; the caption tells us that the woman, Jane Namirimu, is pregnant and already too weak to stand alone. Yet the beauty of the composition, even the adjacent photograph of her grave taken when the photographer returned three months later, transforms the text's bleak assertions into an almost utopian narrative of elegiac fatefulness in which aesthetic universality redeems individual suffering.[12]

A final problem is the literal appropriation of images. J. B. Diederich's photographs for the Selzer story were at least original for *Life;* but some AIDS photographs are familiar not simply because they invoke a familiar tradition but because precisely the same images circulate among diverse publications. In one of Diederich's photographs, a large, striking study in brown and white, an emaciated Haitian woman in a white dress sits gracefully on a wooden bench and looks out at the camera. The caption reads, "Tuberculosis is but one of the wasting infections of what Haitians call *maladi-a.*" Selzer's article does not define *maladi-a* or tell us whether tuberculosis is counted in Haiti as a disease that signals AIDS or is, like AIDS, simply one of many wasting diseases; nor is it clear that the woman in the photograph has actually been diagnosed with AIDS. But reproduced months later in the Canadian newsmagazine *Macleans,* the identical photo, no longer ambiguous, is captioned "Haitian AIDS victim: a former playground for holidayers."[13]

Hence, our understanding of the situation in Haiti is based on a series of filtering devices, a layering of representational elements, narrative voices, and replicating images. These mediating processes are not, of course, a simple function of high-tech Western representation. Firsthand experience is not unmediated either, so one cannot get off a plane in Port-au-Prince or Nairobi, look around, and determine who is correct. Within these countries there are also differing constructions: there are people who agree with the Western media's account that AIDS is devastating the whole region; there are people like Carmen, who believe the disease is largely imaginary, the latest Western trick to reduce the Third World's population in the wake of failed birth control strategies in the past; there are others, including scientific investigators, who believe the disease exists but is a "white man's disease"; and there are still others who point to serious flaws in most existing data about the prevalence, incidence, epidemiology, chronology, and social history of AIDS and HIV infection in the Third World.[14]

Discrepancies between doomsday predictions by the Western media and official denials by Third World governments introduce another complicating factor: every state has a "social imaginary," something it dreams itself to be, and its explicit declarations and official statistics are likely to be pervaded by this implicit social dream.[15] The dream of controlling the AIDS epidemic—whether controlling the blood supply, statistical and epidemiological knowledge, media coverage, biotechnology, or moral and sexual behavior—may well declare itself in a Western tongue. The photograph of the Brazilian hospital may accurately document the existence in Brazil of sophisticated medical capabilities. But as a representation of "the AIDS epidemic," it may be as bogus as the "Haitian AIDS victim." Symbiosis is self-perpetuating: while Third World representations function as elegiac icons that can be seamlessly decontextualized and appropriated by the First World narrative voice, the Third World media, dependent in varying degrees on First World sources and technology, recontextualize these images as their own. As Edward Said argues, modern representation in the decolonized world depends increasingly on a concentration of media power in metropolitan centers; this contributes to the monolithic nature of Third World representations, which are in turn a major source of information about Third World populations not only for the "outside world" but also for those populations themselves.[16]

There is, however, another way of confronting the epidemic. If we relinquish the compulsion to separate true representations of AIDS from false ones and concentrate instead on representation and discursive production, we can begin to sort out how particular versions of truth are produced and sustained, and what cultural work they do in given contexts. Such an approach illuminates the construction of AIDS as a complex narrative and raises questions not so much about truth as about power and representation. Richard Selzer's essay on AIDS in Haiti provides useful information—not necessarily about the true nature of AIDS in the Third World but about the power of individual authors and Western mass print media to produce and transmit particular representations of AIDS according to certain conventions and, in doing so, to sustain their acceptance as true.[17] This is what Michel Foucault refers to as a regime of truth.[18] Other forms of representation, drawing on different conventions, different rules, may make claims to truth in different ways.

THE COUNTRY AND THE CITY: DREAMS OF THIRD WORLD AIDS

It is not impossible that in the future, as in the past,
effective steps in the prevention of disease will be motivated by an emotional revolt against some of the inadequacies of the modern world. . . . Knowledge and
power may arise from dreams as well as from facts and
logic.

> Dubos, *Mirage of Health* [19]

A regime of truth is that circular relation which truth
has to the systems of power that produce and sustain
it, and to the effects of power which it induces and
which redirect it.

> Tagg, *Burden of Representation* [20]

You'd be surprised: They're all individual countries.

> Ronald Reagan [21]

"The statistical mode of analysis," argued Raymond Williams in
The Country and the City, was "devised in response to the impossibility
of understanding contemporary society from experience." Characterizing preindustrial English society as knowable through experience (if only
partially so), Williams contrasted this "knowable community" with the
"new sense of the darkly unknowable" produced by urbanization and
industrialization. The metaphor of darkness was routinely invoked in
discussions of the rise of cities: the East End, for instance, was called
"Darkest London." Statistical analysis was one of the new forms of
knowledge "devised to penetrate what was rightly perceived to be to a
large extent obscure." [22]

Given this historical mission, it is not surprising that statistical analysis is widely seen as a powerful way to understand the latest incarnation
of the "darkly unknowable": AIDS in the Third World. Statistical data,
at the least, are seen as the necessary foundation for other knowledge.
The ability to produce statistical information is used to measure a nation's degree of development, predict its ability to cope with the AIDS
crisis, and in some cases determine its eligibility for external aid. [23] Even
if a country cannot produce its own statistics internally, it can demonstrate its ability to cope by cooperating with external studies. [24] But more
obviously, the international discourse on AIDS and HIV infection in the

Third World is shaped on a day-to-day basis by statistical findings and projections. Once numbers are generated and publicized, they take on a life of their own. Because they may generate calls for action (and therefore time, money, and organization), AIDS estimates may be initially resisted. But though specific numbers may be questioned and even denounced in given instances, the use of numbers as a fundamental measure of the reality of AIDS is not.

Data with regard to AIDS/HIV in Third World countries are regularly generated by several sources, including the U.S. Public Health Service Centers for Disease Control (CDC) and the World Health Organization's (WHO) Global AIDS Program (GPA); the GPA's AIDS Surveillance Unit is widely regarded as a legitimate producer, synthesizer, and interpreter of international numbers. By January 31, 1989, the number of countries reporting to the GPA was 177, of which 144 had reported one or more cases of AIDS (up from 175 and 138 in three months): a total of 139,886 cases worldwide had been reported to WHO, though WHO considers a more realistic total to be 250,000 to 500,000; WHO estimates that 5 million are infected worldwide, with a million or more infected in Africa alone. These totals mean that at least one new case of AIDS is being reported somewhere in the world every minute, or 60 new cases every hour and 1,440 each day. Projections about the worldwide distribution and future prospects of AIDS and HIV infection led Jonathan Mann, then director of the GPA, to conclude that "the global situation will get much worse before it can be brought under control." [25]

WHO did not officially acknowledge AIDS as a global health problem until late 1986—some five years into the epidemic for some countries. By the end of 1987, however, WHO's surveillance reports and seroprevalence data were sufficient to suggest three broad global patterns of AIDS: [26] *Pattern I,* typical of industrialized countries with large numbers of reported cases (the "First World," roughly, including the United States, Canada, Western Europe, Australia, and New Zealand), is characterized by the initial appearance of HIV infection in the late 1970s; rapid spread primarily among gay men, bisexual men, and IV drug users in urban coastal centers; and recipients of blood products. HIV infection and illness are at present slowly increasing in the heterosexual population but at highly variable rates, with perinatal transmission (from mother to infant) likewise increasing but not uniformly widespread; infection in the overall population is estimated to be less than 1 percent. In *Pattern II* countries (typically in sub-Saharan central

Africa, the Caribbean, and Latin America), HIV infection may have appeared in the late 1970s but was not widely identified as AIDS-related until 1983; heterosexual transmission is the norm, with males and females often equally infected and perinatal transmission therefore common; transmission via gay sexual contact or IV drug use is believed to be low or absent. A *Pattern III* profile is attributed to the Second World countries of the Soviet bloc as well as to much of North Africa, the Middle East, Asia, and the Pacific (excluding Australia and New Zealand): HIV is judged to have appeared in the early to mid-1980s, and only a small numbers of cases have been identified, primarily in people who have traveled to and engaged in some form of high-risk involvement with infected persons in Pattern I or II areas.[27]

What will be the material effects of the global epidemic? Again we can identify a widely accepted set of predictions. In developed countries such as the United States, where 13 percent of the gross national product is spent on health care, AIDS and HIV-related illnesses are already straining the health care system; in many developing countries, where annual expenditures on health care are often less than five dollars per person and inadequate even for current needs, future prospects are grim. The epidemic will almost certainly jeopardize the World Health Organization's ambitious global goal of Health for All by the Year 2000. Further, despite the widespread stereotype of people with AIDS as the disadvantaged of society, the twenty-to-forty age group is the most vulnerable worldwide—the age group most central to the labor force, to childbearing, to caring for the dependent young and old, and, ironically, to marshaling and managing the resources for addressing the AIDS epidemic.[28] Synthesizing many studies on AIDS in Africa, Miller and Rockwell spell out in further detail the demographic, economic, and medical consequences of the epidemic. Education and prevention, they point out, still the best resources for controlling the spread of the virus, are difficult enough in media-rich Western countries; the task of communicating complex health messages to the diverse populations and geographical sites of Third World countries is formidable.[29] These predictions have combined to bring about widespread international agreement about the significance of the epidemic; and as experience increasingly documents the futility of closing boundaries to the virus, so also are global leaders coming to agree with the WHO doctrine that "AIDS cannot be stopped in any country until it is stopped in all countries."[30]

The power and centrality of numbers to these constructions of AIDS are obvious. Without the sophistication and authority of statistical methods, the epidemic as a global issue could not have been articulated at all. Yet while this First World numerical chronicle of global AIDS may appear to be unfolding smoothly as our knowledge grows, in fact it is problematic. Consider the following judgments about Africa, all published in 1988:

1.   "The continent hardest hit by the AIDS pandemic is Africa where all three infection patterns can be found." (WHO)

2.   "Medical experts consider the epidemic an accelerating catastrophe that, in the words of one, 'will make the Ethiopian famine look like a picnic.' " (Congressional Research Service)

3.   In many of the urban centers of Congo, Rwanda, Tanzania, Uganda, Zaire, and Zambia, "from 5 to 20 percent of the sexually active age-group has already been infected with HIV. Rates of infection among some prostitute groups range from 27 percent in Kinshasa, Zaire, to 66 percent in Nairobi, Kenya, and 88 percent in Butare, Rwanda. Close to half of all patients in the medical wards of hospitals in those cities are currently infected with HIV. By the early 1990s the total adult mortality rate in these urban areas will have been doubled or tripled by AIDS." (WHO)

4.   "A *Newsweek* cover story claimed one Rakai village [in Uganda] had seven discos and 'sex orgies.' In reality it has 20 mud huts, a handful of fishing boats, and no electricity." *(The Guardian)*

5.   "The tale of AIDS in Africa is not one of widespread devastation and the collapse of nations. There are 53 countries in Africa and AIDS exists substantially in only a few of them." *(Washington Post)*

6.   "Like the tenacious theories put forward as explanations for the heterosexual spread of HIV in Africa, the whole AIDS pandemic is shrouded in mystery and uncertainty. There is no reliable information on AIDS and by the time one message has percolated its way down to the general population, it is out of date and a new one is already on its way to replace it." *(West Africa)* [31]

Given the statistics cited above, how can it be that the most fundamental meaning of the narrative remains contested?

Several sources of confusion and contradiction can be identified. Estimates of infection and actual cases of AIDS for entire populations may be derived from inadequate data: too few studies, studies of too small a sample size, nonrepresentative samples, and so on. Rates estimated for all Africans are often based on small studies in urban areas; studies of "prostitutes" may in fact classify all sexually active single women as prostitutes. Chronological claims (about when AIDS first appeared) are primarily based on flawed blood-testing procedures and other problems of diagnostic method. In Africa "underreporting" is taken for granted and estimates corrected upward; at the same time, the number of positive cases actually diagnosed may be too high or too low, depending on the procedure used. Research cited as evidence may be unpublished, based on conference papers unavailable for detailed scrutiny, or sloppily interpreted; and many published papers do not report important data. Moreover, interpretations of the epidemic may be based on divergent and not mutually understood paradigms and forms of evidence. Testing blood samples in a laboratory involves different practical operations and generates knowledge different from that produced by a clinician examining patients or a journalist interviewing people on the street. Experienced medical experts in Africa, who tend to make lower estimates of cases, claim that their knowledge is discounted as clinical and experiential by Western and European academic scientists.[32]

Rumor and fantasy play their part as well. Cultural practices are taken out of context, exaggerated, distorted, or invented. Voodoo continues to animate accounts of HIV in Haiti, with grizzly descriptions of Voodoo sorcerers biting off the heads of infected chickens and sucking the bloody stumps. African tales often involve the notorious African green monkey, whose photograph keeps circulating long after his role in AIDS has been discounted. Africans are said to have sexual contact with these monkeys, or eat them, or eat other animals they have infected (Haitian chickens?), or give their children dead monkeys as toys. Purporting to explain why HIV transmission is heterosexual in Africa, reports hypothesize radical differences between African and Western bodies based on physiological, behavioral, cultural, moral, and/or biological factors. As Sander Gilman has comprehensively documented, these rumors are tirelessly fueled by historically entrenched myths of the exotic.[33]

While increased international scientific dialogue has answered some questions about global AIDS and HIV, it has confirmed the difficulty of answering others and has underscored the need for thick description—complex, multileveled, multilayered research. Jay A. Levy's 1988 state-of-the-art collection on AIDS, for example, includes detailed review chapters on AIDS in Haiti and in Africa. Both demonstrate the diverse and very different clinical manifestations of HIV infection in those settings and emphasize the need for revised diagnostic and reporting systems. Treated at length in the Haiti chapter are the complex interaction of HIV infection with tuberculosis (alluded to by Selzer), while the Africa chapter reviews controversial origin questions as well as various explanations for the high rate of heterosexual transmission; both chapters emphasize remaining questions and the need for continuing investigation.[34]

The overwhelming difficulty of even characterizing the diversity of the epidemic, let alone containing it, suggests that statistical measures—numbers—may once again be functioning as Williams says they did in the late nineteenth century: to offer us the illusion of control. As these numbers are taken up and deployed for various urgent purposes, however, they may take on a life of their own and reinforce a view of HIV disease as an unmediated epidemiological phenomenon in which cultural differences (such as differences in sexual practices) can simply be factored into a universal equation. But the local interacts with the global, AIDS continually escapes the boundaries placed on it by positivist medical science, and its meanings mutate on a parallel with the virus itself. Added to the medical, epidemiological, social, economic, and educational challenges of the AIDS crisis is its inevitably political subtext. AIDS is not a precious national resource; it is something nobody wants. Wherever it appears, AIDS discourse quickly becomes political as it is articulated to preexisting local concerns. To begin to identify these concerns, it may be useful to retreat from the power of numbers and see what other forms of knowledge tell us.

In Africa analysis of AIDS must inevitably confront questions of decolonization, urbanization, modernization, poverty, endemic disease, and development: in Uganda, for example, the legacy of civil war is significant in assessing the AIDS situation, as is the influence of the church in discussions of health education; in Kenya, for the independent press at any rate, AIDS is used as an ongoing test of the central government's ability to acknowledge and resolve conflict.[35] In France Jamie Feldman found in interviews that for French AIDS researchers the AIDS epidemic "reveals the impact that France's colonial past and present African immigration have on French life."[36] In his ethnographic study of AIDS in urban Brazil, Richard Parker suggests that the epidemic needs to be linked to "the social and cultural construction of sexual ideology," or what he calls the "cultural grammar" of the Brazilian sexual universe.[37] In both the United States and Great Britain, AIDS intensifies stress on health care systems already in crisis. In South Africa apartheid is seen to reproduce itself in the government's public health campaign: a post-campaign survey of black attitudes in the Johannesburg area found that many believed there were "two totally different kinds of AIDS. The one that only affected blacks was acquired through sexual and ritual contact with baboons in central Africa. The other was acquired by sexual contact with homosexuals—white AIDS."[38] In Cuba mandatory HIV testing of the general population has identified a small number of infected people, who have been placed under indefinite quarantine. Placed in AIDS sanitoria, they receive air conditioning, color television, regular health checkups, and other amenities not generally available to the population at large. This treatment is variously interpreted by Western commentators as a manifestation of Cuba's progressive health care policies (one can certainly argue that Cuba is providing more support and resources for its infected citizens than many other countries) or as totalitarian and homophobic repression in a police state.[39]

These examples and others suggest that the reproduction in AIDS discourse of existing social divisions appears to be virtually universal, whether it is white or black AIDS, gay or straight AIDS, European or African AIDS, wet or hot AIDS, East or West German AIDS, central African or western African AIDS, foreign or native AIDS, guilty or innocent AIDS.[40] A First World/Third World dichotomy manifests itself in diverse ways. In Africa people with AIDS are sometimes described by those in their own countries as having sexual practices as strange as those of gay white men in San Francisco.[41] In Japan officials believed initially that transfusion-related HIV infection among Japanese would not be a threat thanks to procedures for sequestering the national blood supply; while this Japanese/foreign division remains an animating feature of AIDS discussion and policy, statistics make clear that it can no longer be considered a safeguard.[42] Richard Parker identifies a similar dichotomy in the Brazilian medical community's transition from conceptualizing AIDS as a "foreign import" to accepting it (from 1985 on) as a disease that has "taken root."[43] Great Britain's announcement that HIV-positive applications for visas from high-risk countries would be denied entry provoked accusations of racial imperialism when central African countries were classified as "high risk" but the United States was not.[44]

These divisions are, at least in part, produced by what Dubos calls the inadequacies of the modern world—that is, by a set of historically produced social arrangements. When AIDS in Africa or Brazil is termed "a disease of development," it is precisely the intractable social topography of recent history that is invoked, the problematic contours of development—environmental devastation, malnutrition, war, social upheaval, poverty, debt, endemic disease—now unavoidably illuminated and scrutinized in the international light of the AIDS crisis. As Rudolph Virchow wrote in 1948, "Epidemics correspond to large signs of warning which tell the true statesman that a disturbance has occurred in the development of his people which even a policy of unconcern can no longer overlook."[45]

Even the seemingly simple message to "use a condom" is actually a complicated drama that must incorporate competing scripts, play to hostile audiences, and ultimately raise as many questions as it answers. Already it has returned to the world stage such stock characters as the Ugly American who, in the guise of the U.S. Agency for International Development, distributed in central Africa condoms that were too small and inelastic.[46] But the larger point is that, as Brooke Grundfest Schoepf and her colleagues argue, the adoption of condoms involves "much more than a simple transfer of material culture."[47] Describing their experience with Project CONAISSIDA (an AIDS education and research program in Zaire), these researchers identify myriad ways that the condom question puts stress on the entire fabric of social relations. They point out, too, that the AIDS crisis is embedded in a continuing economic crisis that affects men and women differently: married women in plural households may take up prostitution as a means of economic existence when their husbands can under current conditions no longer support the traditional plural households. Women's groups with whom CONAISSIDA has contact express interest in information about AIDS, and about condoms; but they also articulate resistance to the view that information and condoms offer a total solution, emphasizing the role of deepening poverty and the need for income-generating activities for women to provide alternatives to multiple-partner sex.

A different sort of complication is raised in Africa by the important role of nongovernmental organizations (NGOs). While these organizations may be reluctant to shift their agendas for AIDS or to ally their already fragile causes with a yet more stigmatized one, they nevertheless often have excellent international and community networks. The International Family Planning Agency has prepared and distributed a well-received manual on AIDS for local as well as national use; such efforts are likely to bring about increased U.S. aid for family planning.[48] But as Schoepf and her colleagues point out,

> Ideological issues also need to be addressed. In Zaire nationalist sentiment currently links contraception and condom use to western population control strategies, which are viewed as a form of imperialism. Some husbands also

view contraception as an encouragement for wives' extramarital sexual relations. . . . These considerations suggest that it may be preferable to separate AIDS prevention from birth control efforts, rather than to place responsibilty for AIDS interventions within family planning programs.[49]

But fruitful acknowledgment of division is not accomplished by formula. To take one final example, the system of sexual classification that dominates discussions of AIDS internationally—heterosexual, homosexual, bisexual—is not universal. Criticisms of this system applied to AIDS discourse in Western industrialized countries are all the more valid in other cultures; for not only is sexuality complicated for individuals, with no fixed correspondence among the components of sexual desire, actual practice, self-perceived identity, and official definition; it is culturally complicated as well. Richard Parker argues that the hetero/homo/bi classification is seriously, conceptually, at odds with "the fluidity of sexual desire" in contemporary Brazil.[50] While the medical model's distinctions clearly exist in Brazilian society and are increasingly familiar as a result of media dissemination, they remain largely part of an elite discourse introduced to Brazil in the mid-twentieth century. The traditional classification relates sexual practices to gender *roles,* with both gender and sex constructed by a fundamental division between a masculine *atividade* (activity) and feminine *passividade* (passivity). Two males engaged in anal intercourse would be distinguished by who was the active masculine penetrator, who the passive feminine penetrated. Neither would necessarily perceive his behavior as "homosexual," nor would everyday language readily furnish him with the lexicon to do so. As Parker suggests, this different perception of same-sex behavior has obvious and dismaying implications for conventional notions of "risk group" identification and "safer sex" education.[51]

Parker's work, like other projects noted here, demonstrates the contributions of interpretive cultural analysis. The provisional nature of science is very difficult for policy and funding agencies to live with. Rather, there is pressure to produce a coherent narrative in which qualifications and ambiguities, if they must be mentioned, become simply routinized features of the story, to be quickly forgotten; problems of data are perceived to be mere temporary impediments to a refined and comprehensive analysis. Western medical science is conceived as a transhistorical, transcultural model of reality; when cultural differences among human communities are taken into account, they tend to be enlisted in the service of this reality, but their status remains utilitarian. This utilization may effectively accomplish specific goals: it is reported that some native practitioners (e.g., of voodoo) have successfully over-come men's traditional resistance to the use of condoms by describing AIDS as the work of an evil spirit who uses sexual desire and the virus as secret weapons; condoms provide a means to trick the spirit and escape its lethal designs.[52]

One can certainly support a global anti-AIDS strategy that mobilizes the scientific model of AIDS in culturally specific ways, yet acknowledge imperialist aspects of a strategy that valorizes itself as universal rather than culturally produced. As the foregoing examples suggest, ethnography and other forms of interpretive research are neither better nor less mediated than statistical approaches or other "objective" ways of knowing a culture, but they are different and produce unique insights. Nor are they incompatible with theoretical sophistication.

Research of this kind is not, however, the currency of the First World/ Third World transaction. Expert advising is now a major Third World industry: more than half of the $7–8 billion spent yearly on aid to Africa goes to European and North American professionals trained to provide expertise to the Third World.[53] Gathering information, report-ing facts, and advising the Third World are also mediated activities, permeated by history and convention. In *Blaming Others,* the Panos Institute's immensely useful 1988 sequel to and self-critique of its indis-pensable 1986 dossier *AIDS and the Third World,* Renée Sabatier ob-serves how ironic it is that in the information age, information should be such an elusive resource.[54] But a second irony explains the first. It is not, precisely, a question of obtaining and disseminating "information" but, rather, of acknowledging what information entails: acknowledging how language works in culture, how stories contradict one another, how narratives perform as well as inform, how information constructs reality. Cultural analysts in many fields are acknowledging the inevita-bility and indeed even the necessity of such multiple and contradictory stories. Yet, having recognized the theoretical complexity of commu-nication, we are pressing communication into a purely pragmatic role that subordinates complication and contradiction to unequivocal asser-tion and scientific harmony.

Different accounts of truth produce differing material consequences. Tracing the historical relationship between the "country" and the "city" and their evolution in English literature and social thought, Raymond Williams argues that in the course of nineteenth-century imperialism these two ideas became a model for the world, dividing not only the rural from the urban within a single state but the undeveloped world from the developed one. Underlying this model is the notion of universal industrialization, underdeveloped countries always on their way toward becoming developed, just as the poor man is always assumed to be striving to become rich. "All the 'country' will become 'city': that is the logic of its development."[55] Though this linear progression is largely a myth of late capitalism, that does not impede its deployment as an agenda item for the Third World.

For the new possibilities arising out of the AIDS epidemic, the "country" is a very fertile field. As of 1986, according to a reference work called *Emerging AIDS Markets,* 1,119 companies and other organizations are involved in AIDS-related activities: only 20 to 30 of them are based in Third World countries, but at least 200 of them are engaged in research on AIDS in Africa and other projects likely to entail the use of Third World populations as trial subjects in the development of diagnostic products and vaccines.[56] Recent reports about vaccine trials make explicit the need for test populations that are "pharmacologically virgin" and, further, are still becoming infected at high rates. Gay men and IV drug users in the First World do not fulfill these criteria, not only because infection is leveling off in the first group and pharmacological virginity is not characteristic of the second, but also because *any* First World population is too educated, too exposed to the media, and too likely to take steps (including alternative treatments) to avoid infection or reduce clinical illness. In the mind of the city, only the country can furnish the unspoiled virgin material that the market needs, the naive informant still too ignorant to contradict instructions.[57]

FIRST AND THIRD WORLD CHRONICLES

History is a legend, an invention of the present.
        Mudimbe, *Invention of Africa*[58]

The ethnographer's trials in working to know another people now become the reader's trials in making sense of the text.
        Pratt, "Fieldwork in Common Places"[59]

But there is always another story, and a continuing one in the AIDS epidemic involves the untrustworthiness of other stories—their sources, motives, data, presuppositions, methodology, and conclusions. In January 1985, for example, the Nairobi *Standard* publicly reported the presence of AIDS in Kenya for the first time in stories headlined "Killer disease in Kenya" and "Horror sex disease in Kakamenga."[60] Subsequent accounts in state-owned newspapers repudiated the report, claiming that the deaths were from skin cancer rather than AIDS, but Western press accounts speculated increasingly on the frightening implications of the presence of AIDS in central Africa. Then in November 1985 Lawrence K. Altman's multipart series on AIDS in Africa in the *New York Times* reported not only that the epidemic was spreading rapidly in Africa but also that prominent U.S. researchers were convinced the disease started there. Altman's opening sentence dramatically presented the thesis that was to become most controversial: "Tantalizing but sketchy clues pointing to Africa as the origin of AIDS have unleashed one of the bitterest disputes in the recent annals of medicine."[61] Altman went on to say that these "sketchy clues," including blood samples, "have led to what has now emerged as the prevailing thesis in American and European medical circles that the worldwide spread of acquired immune deficiency syndrome began in Central Africa, the home of several other recently recognized diseases."

But, as Altman conceded, not everyone accepts this designation of the virus's homeland: "The Africans vigorously disagree, and there is some criticism of the validity of the studies on which the theories are predicated. Indeed, controversial new results point both to and against AIDS originating in Africa, a fact that is fueling the international furor."[62]

Two effects in the West of the *Times* series were to establish AIDS in Africa as an important scientific question and to place Africa firmly on the national agenda for AIDS media coverage, culminating in the journalistic frenzy of late 1986, which represented Africa as "devastated" by AIDS and AIDS-related illnesses. In Africa the effect was different. When Altman's series began to run in the *International Herald Tribune* in November 1985, for example, outraged Kenyan officials confiscated the entire shipment. The African offensive against the "African origin" theory was launched with an editorial in *Medicus,* the official publication of the Kenya Medical Association, which hypothesized that tourists from around the world had introduced AIDS into Africa.[63]

At this point the Kenyan newsmagazine *Weekly Review,* published and edited in Nairobi by Hilary Ng'weno and widely considered one of the best newsmagazines in Africa, took on the responsibility of keeping the public informed about AIDS reports in the African and international press. In the face of increasingly vocal controversy and government silence, the magazine took the general position that developing adequate public health measures was more important than countering Western propaganda. Thus, the *Weekly Review* began providing summaries and analyses of scientific and press reports printed in the West, citing the numbers of AIDS patients reported in Zaire, Rwanda, Uganda, and Kenya. Although itself often critical of the Kenyan government's mode of responding to the AIDS epidemic, the *Weekly Review* has also been critical of Western reporting. What Africa needs, Ng'weno told the Panos Institute, is concrete assistance, not "a never ending siren recounting a litany of disasters about to engulf the continent."[64]

An insightful analysis of the AIDS situation in Kenya is provided by the political scientist Alfred J. Fortin. Although Fortin criticizes the actions of the African government, he is primarily critical of what he has elsewhere called the "aggressive bureaucratic and careerist politics" of the "development establishment"; unless development agencies remain under fire, he argues, the AIDS epidemic will allow them to reproduce the power relations of dominance and dependency already in place. In "The Politics of AIDS in Kenya," Fortin argues further that the dominance-dependency relationship of development guarantees English as the international language of AIDS discourse, a language that is necessarily "blind to the African world of meaning." He concludes that, despite Kenya's "comparatively well-developed medical infrastructure and working coterie of Western scientists, its efforts have fallen short of even the minimum requirements suggested by its statistics."[65]

However much the *Weekly Review* may itself be skeptical of "the development establishment" as well as Kenya's response to the AIDS epidemic, it does not buy Fortin's position either. Calling his paper "a hard-hitting and indictive, if lopsided, criticism of the Kenyan government, the ministry of health and the local press," the editor goes on to contest a number of points of Fortin's analysis—for example, Fortin's point about language:

> [Fortin's] paper questions the language of discourse at discussions on AIDS in Africa. It argues that Africans have chosen to use the Western language when talking about the disease and since the language is transplanted, Africa is dependent on the West for its meaning and its continued development. Since the language is not indigenous to Africa, Fortin says, hence it is "blind to the African world of meaning."
>
> Students of African history have long argued that most of the diseases prevalent in Africa today were first witnessed with the advent of the foreigners on the continent and most of the terminology used by the medical practitioners in Africa [is] also borrowed from the developed world.

African government and researchers have also been emphatic that the AIDS virus was first diagnosed in the United States and, therefore, it would follow automatically that the language used in reference to the disease should be that developed by those who diagnosed it first.[66]

As I understand it, Fortin's argument about discourse was intended to challenge—as Parker's is with regard to Brazil—the entire discursive formation of international AIDS discussions applied unthinkingly and hence in some sense imperialistically to diverse cultures; it is a position most discourse analysts would share. Ng'weno, however, rejects the corollary implication of this view: that English is somehow "foreign" to Kenya and Kenyan leaders. Though English is indeed a colonial legacy, it plays many roles in Kenyan activities today. Hence, Zairean philosopher V. Y. Mudimbe argues that Western discourse has contributed to but not monopolized what he calls "the invention of Africa"; rather, the objects of that discourse are also subjects who have produced an intricate interweaving of European and African commentary, rendering the notion of a "purely African discourse" an impossible dream.[67] At the same time, Ng'weno makes the political point that language marks nationality and origin: to use English with regard to AIDS helps sustain its identity as a Western disease. Ng'weno's position acknowledges the power of linguistic constructions of reality, and demands the right of Africans to participate in that construction process. This resistance to adopting AIDS, to giving it—in the words of the Altman story—a home, is reflected elsewhere in the *Weekly Review,* where supposedly indigenous African terms for AIDS and AIDS-related terms (like "slim disease" and "AIDS belt") are placed in quotation marks and often explicitly rejected; the term *magada,* cited by Fortin as the name for AIDS in Swahili, is never used in the *Review.*[68]

The juxtaposition of these two complex and interlocking analyses makes clear that the chronicle of AIDS in the Third World cannot be understood monolithically. It must be understood not only in terms of the "rich history and complex political chemistry" of each affected country but also as a heteroglossic series of conflicted, shifting, and contradictory positions.[69] Even "AIDS" and "the AIDS epidemic" and "HIV disease" must be understood this way. We are talking, after all, about an epidemic disease with more than forty distinct clinical manifestations, some of which consist of the absence of manifestation, some of which are unique to particular regions of the world, and some of which apparently have nothing to do with a deficiency of the immune system. When we talk about the Third World, we are talking about more than one hundred countries of the world. In Africa alone, we are talking about a continent four times as large as the United States, which has more than 50 countries, 900 ethnic groups, and 300 language families (Zambia alone has 74 languages). As Miller and Rockwell argue, it is absurd to talk about "the AIDS problem in Africa" except for specific and well-defined purposes.[70]

The international AIDS narrative is hence neither complete nor fully accessible. The present invents the past, but the present itself has not yet been invented; accordingly, this is a narrative necessarily in process, which we must read with all our critical faculties at work. A crisis serves as a point of articulation for multiple voices and interests, and the AIDS crisis in the Third World is no different. My goal has been to demonstrate that, as in the First World, (1) diverse interests are articulated around AIDS in ways that are socially and culturally localized and specific; (2) institutional forces and cultural precedents in the First World prevent us from hearing the story of AIDS in the Third World as a complex narrative; (3) understanding this complexity is a necessary if not sufficient condition for identifying the material and conceptual nature of the epidemic; and (4) such an identification is necessary to effectively mobilize resources and programs in a given country or region.

In the course of this essay, I have identified several analytic strategies through which we may explore these questions and tried to suggest areas of discourse where better understandings may be particularly valuable: the conventions of mass media stories; the discursive traditions and modes of representation that figure in the AIDS narrative of the sciences and social sciences (including tropes, stereotypes, linguistic structures, and pervasive metaphors); the emergence of a dominant international AIDS narrative and its role in the linguistic and professional management of the epidemic; the processes through which AIDS is conceptualized within given institutions for everyday use; and the very terms through which we identify what chronicle we think we are telling. The checks and balances provided by the warring voices at each of these multiple discursive points render it impossible to refuse contradiction— that is, to argue that any single unchallenged account of AIDS exists in the Third World, any more than it does in the First World.

To hear the story "AIDS in the Third World," we must confront familiar problems in the human sciences: How do we know what we know? What cultural work will we ask that knowledge to perform? What are our own stakes in the success or failure of that performance? How do we document history as it unfolds? In concrete terms, we certainly need to forsake, at least part of the time, the coherent AIDS narrative of the Western professional and technological agencies and listen instead to multiple sources about and within the Third World.[71] When we do so, we may find it less instructive to determine whether a given account is true or false than to identify the diverse rules and conventions that govern whether and where a particular account is received as true or false, by whom, and with what material consequences.

The performative work that such narrative structures do can be identified, challenged, recuperated, reassigned; it cannot be eradicated. Language about AIDS, illness, and epidemics is already informed with metaphor (*influenza* got its name because illnesses were believed to be under the *influence* of the stars; *infect* means "to contaminate," "to communicate," and "to stain or dye," a connotative web even the most vigilant housekeeping cannot sweep away). To believe that information and communication about AIDS will separate fact from fiction and reality from metaphor is to suppress the linguistic complexity of everyday life. Further, to inform is also to perform; to communicate is also to construct and interpret. Information does not simply exist; it issues from and in turn sustains a way of looking at and behaving toward the world; it shapes programmatic agendas and even guides capital investments.

Diverse voices, then, represent not diverse accounts of reality but significant points of articulation for ongoing social and cultural struggles. Further, once we adopt the view that reality is inevitably mediated, we become ourselves participants in the mediation process; such voices may then provide important models for challenging existing regimes of truth and disrupting their effects—in the Third World, as in the First.

NOTES

A different version of this essay was published in *Remaking History*, ed. Phil Mariani and Barbara Kruger (New York: Dia Art Foundation, 1989), pp. 31–86, and is reprinted with permission. Research for this project has been supported in part by grants from the National Council of Teachers of English and the University of Illinois at Urbana-Champaign Graduate College Research Board and by a fellowship at the Society for the Humanities, Cornell University. For comments, suggestions, and resources, I would like to thank K. Anthony Appiah, Awour Ayodo, Stacie Colwell, Paul Farmer, Elizabeth Fee, Daniel M. Fox, Gertrude Fraser, Colin Garrett, Ibulaimu Kakoma, Cary Nelson, Elisabeth Santos, and Simon Watney, as well as University of Illinois librarians John Littlewood (Documents) and Yvette Scheven (Africana).

The term *AIDS* in this essay refers to the AIDS epidemic as a broad social and cultural crisis; the terms *HIV disease* and *AIDS and HIV infection* are used interchangeably to mean the broad clinical spectrum of HIV-related conditions from symptomatic infection to the specific diseases presently used to define "AIDS" (I use *AIDS* to mean the inclusive medical spectrum only if this sense is clear in context).

1. For an excellent discussion of the vexing terms *First World, Third World,* and *Second World,* see Carl E. Pletsch, "The Three Worlds, or the Division of Social Scientific Labor, circa 1950 to 1975," *Comparative Studies in Society and History* 23, no. 4 (1981): 565–90. Pletsch argues that the notion of the Third World is bogus; indeed, he writes that, except for the political categories of left and right, "the scheme of three worlds is perhaps the most primitive system of classification in our social scientific discourse" (p. 566). I agree with Pletsch that as a framework for investigation this classification system yields studies in which non-Western civilizations—that is, the Second and Third Worlds—are "almost pure fantasies" (p. 566). Because it is these "fantasies" I am attempting to chronicle, I deliberately use the First World/Third World terminology in this essay, along with such alternative signifiers as *colonial, postcolonial, industrialized, developing,* and *poor.* See also my "AIDS, Homophobia, and Biomedical Discourse: An Epidemic of Signification," in *AIDS: Cultural Analysis/Cultural Activism,* ed. Douglas Crimp (Cambridge, Mass.: MIT Press, 1988), pp. 31–70.

2. Marjorie Shostak, *Nisa: The Life and Words of a !Kung Woman* (New York: Vintage, 1983), p. 26.

3. James Clifford, "On Ethnographic Allegory," in *Writing Culture,* ed. James Clifford and George E. Marcus (Berkeley: University of California Press, 1986), p. 99.

4. See Homi Bhabha, "The Other Question—the Stereotype and Colonial Discourse," *Screen* 24, no. 6 (November–December 1983): 18–36; and Chandra Talpade Mohanty, "Under Western Eyes: Feminist Scholarship and Colonial Discourses," *Boundary* 2 12, no. 3 and 13, no. 1 (Spring and Fall 1984): 333–58.

5. Richard Selzer, "A Mask on the Face of Death: As AIDS Ravages Haiti, a U.S. Doctor Finds a Taboo against Truth," *Life* 10 (August 1987): 58–64. Hereafter documented internally by page number.

6. Mary Louise Pratt, "Fieldwork in Common Places," in *Writing Culture,* ed. Clifford and Marcuse, pp. 27–50; see pp. 35–45 for discussion of arrival scenes. The Clifford and Marcus collection offers an extended reflection on relationships between anthropology, ethnography, and travel writing.

7. Photograph of "Mercedes" by J. B. Diederich for *Life* 10 (August 1987): 60; story on Mombasa by Tom Masland, "AIDS Threat Turns Shore Leave into Naval Exercise in Caution," *Chicago Tribune,* March 17, 1988, sec. 1, p. 13; *Newsweek* photo of prostitute, p. 46 in Rod Nordland, with Ray Wilkinson and Ruth Marshall, "Africa in the Plague Years," *Newsweek,* November 24, 1986, pp. 44–47.

8. Jan Zita Grover, "A Matter of Life and Death," *Women's Review of Books* 5, no. 6 (March 1988): 3. See also Simon Watney, "Missionary Posi-

tions: AIDS, 'Africa,' and Race," *Differences: A Journal of Feminist Cultural Studies* 1, no. 1 (1989): 83–100.

9. Conspiracy theories of AIDS are reviewed by Robert Lederer, "Origin and Spread of AIDS," *CovertAction*, no. 29 (1988): 52–67, and are reported regularly in the *New York Native*, a gay New York City weekly periodical. The function of conspiracy theories in postcolonial settings is discussed by Paul Farmer, "Sending Sickness: Sorcery, Politics, and Changing Concepts of AIDS in Rural Haiti," *Medical Anthropology Quarterly* 4, no. 1 (1990): 6–27; and Alma Gottleib, "Hot Blood, Vengeful Blood: AIDS and Blood Symbolism in Africa," paper presented at the conference on the Impact of AIDS on Maternal-Child Health Care Delivery in Africa, University of Illinois at Urbana, May 5, 1990.

10. A parallel shift in the course of the AIDS epidemic in the United States is clearly evident in representations of gay men, as illness and death transform a threatening and alien community into a vulnerable one. Pratt (in "Fieldwork in Common Places," pp. 44–50) discusses redemptive endings. Working against them is the ethnographic paradox that the Other becomes worldly-wise through contact with "modern civilization"—often in the guise of ethnographers themselves. In Selzer's encounter, the fact that he pays the prostitutes to talk to him parallels the further irony of ethnographic research in which the privileged investigator enters into a commodity exchange with the native informant—an exchange which, as Pratt puts it, turns the "anthropologist preserver-of-the-culture" into an "interventionist corrupter-of-the-culture."

11. See photographs in Nordland et al., "Africa in the Plague Years," and Kenneth M. Pierce, "Nowhere to Run, Nowhere to Hide," *Time*, September 1, 1986, p. 36. Images of AIDS in Brazilian magazines like *Veja*, first brought to my attention by Elisabeth Santos, are further analyzed in Haydée Seijo-Maldonado and Christine A. Horak, "AIDS in Latin American Newsmagazines: A Contest for Meaning," unpublished manuscript, 1991. Odd linkages among photographs, captions, and text do not only occur in Third World contexts, of course. A story on AIDS in the Canadian journal *Macleans,* for example, includes a photograph of pedestrians on a crowded Toronto city street; shot from behind so that the pedestrians are moving away from the camera, the photo appears to illustrate the caption: "Toronto sidewalk traffic: Growing fear on AIDS virus spreads to general public" (*Macleans,* August 24, 1987, p. 31).

12. Robert Caputo, "Uganda: Land beyond Sorrow," *National Geographic* 173, no. 4 (April 1988): 468–74; the Caputo photo of Jane Namirimu and her mother is on p. 470. Pratt (in "Fieldwork in Common Places," p. 40 and p. 45) discusses respectively the fallen postcolonial world of ethnographic writing and the trope of utopian universality.

13. Selzer, "Mask on the Face of Death," p. 63. The Diederich photograph is reprinted in *Macleans,* August 31, 1987, p. 37. To take another example, the *Newsweek* photographs accompanying Nordland, "Africa in the Plague Years," have been widely reprinted. One (p. 44) shows an emaciated woman framed in the doorway of her home, holding a small thin baby in her lap. The *Newsweek* print is captioned "Two victims: Uganda barmaid and son," and is credited to

Ed Hooper—Picture Search. Appearing on the cover of the May 24, 1988, issue of the *Washington Post*'s weekly journal *Health* (vol. 4, no. 21) is a photograph of the identical woman shot at a slightly different angle; accompanying Philip J. Hilts's featured story "Out of Africa" (pp. 12–17), the photograph is now captioned as follows: "In the Ugandan village of Kinyiga, Florence Masaka, 22, and her 2-month-old daughter have both tested positive for the AIDS virus." The byline accompanying the story incorrectly credits the photos to "Al Hooper." Hilts's article and the photographs were reprinted in *Africa Report,* November–December 1988, pp. 26–31, to accompany "Dispelling Myths about AIDS in Africa"; the photos were captioned only with text from the story. The Hooper photographs also accompanied Catharine Watson's "Africa's AIDS Time Bomb: Region Scrambles to Fight Epidemic," *The Guardian,* June 17, 1987, pp. 10–11; and the *Weekly Review* (Nairobi), June 24, 1988, p. 18, reprinted the mother and child photograph with the caption "Ugandan AIDS victims" and no picture credit. Most recently it appears in Hooper's book *Slim: A Reporter's Own Story of AIDS in East Africa* (London: The Bodley Head, 1990), where the caption reads: "Florence and Ssengabi, sitting outside their hut in Gwanda. Florence died one month after this picture was taken; her baby, Ssengabi, died four months later." (Picture follows p. 170.)

14. Sabatier quotes a Nigerian prostitute named Juliet as follows: "Although white clients generally pay better than their African counterparts, I will never go to bed with a white man unless he wears a condom. As far as I am concerned, AIDS is a white man's disease" (René Sabatier, *Blaming Others: Prejudice, Race, and Worldwide AIDS* [Washington, D.C.: Panos Institute; Philadelphia: New Society Publishers, 1988], p. 96). Similarly, a letter to the editor of the *Weekly Review* in Nairobi even inverted the Western argument for gender-neutral transmission to argue that AIDS in Africa could not really be affecting men and women equally because why should a disease that is homosexual in one country be heterosexual in another?

15. Ann S. Anagnost, "Magical Practice, Birth Policy, and Women's Health in PostMao China," paper presented at the Unit for Criticism and Interpretive Theory Colloquium, University of Illinois at Urbana, December 7, 1988.

16. Edward Said, "In the Shadow of the West," *Wedge* 7–8 (Winter–Spring 1985): 4–11, at p. 5.

17. Jean William Pape, a leading AIDS researcher in Haiti and one of the physicians Selzer consulted, expresses disenchantment with the Western press for consistently ignoring "the efforts of the Haitian people to fight, with almost no resources, the most devastating disease of this century." He told the Panos Institute: "I have given over 60 interviews to American and other reporters about AIDS in Haiti. It is very time-consuming and exhausting, and takes energy I would like to put into my work. Of all those interviews there are only one or two that recorded what I said, and the context in which I said it, accurately. The others often painted a picture of AIDS in Haiti that was unrecognizable to me" (quoted in Sabatier, *Blaming Others,* p. 90). (Selzer also consulted Pape, but I have no evidence that Pape found his report objectionable.) But negative reactions to Western media reports do not necessarily disrupt the cycle of representation. Some African governments, for example, angry at what they

believed to be inflations of their statistics or simply wishing to deflect focus on the AIDS problem, prohibited AIDS researchers and physicians from giving interviews to the Western press. "One result of such attempts at control," said James Brooke, West Africa correspondent for the *New York Times,* in an interview with the Panos Institute in November 1987, "has been to force foreign reports to rely more heavily on foreign researchers working in those countries, making it more difficult than before to convey an authentically African point of view" (quoted in Sabatier, *Blaming Others,* p. 95). See also James Kinsella, *Covering the Plague: AIDS and the American Media* (New Brunswick, N.J.: Rutgers University Press, 1989). A series in the *New York Times* entitled "A Continent's Agony" ran from September 16 to 19, 1990 (see note 30 for a listing of lead articles). I discuss this series in "AIDS, Africa, and Cultural Theory," in *Transition* 51 (1991): 86–103.

18. "Regime of truth" is Michael Foucault's term. See "The Political Function of the Intellectual," *Radical Philosophy,* no. 17 (1977): 13–14. See also Treichler, "AIDS, Homophobia, and Biomedical Discourse."

19. René Dubos, *Mirage of Health: Utopias, Progress, and Biological Change* (New Brunswick, N.J.: Rutgers University Press, 1987), pp. 218, 219. Originally published 1959.

20. John Tagg, using Foucault to analyze the function of photographs in representing "the true," in *The Burden of Representation* (Amherst: University of Massachusetts Press, 1988), p. 94.

21. Ronald Reagan, press conference after returning from a Latin American trip, December 15, 1987.

22. Raymond Williams, *Keywords: A Vocabulary of Culture and Society,* rev. ed. (New York: Oxford University Press, 1985); in discussing the word *experience* in *Keywords,* pp. 126–29, Williams refers to his earlier analysis in *The Country and the City* of experience and statistical analysis as different ways of producing knowledge (London: Chatto and Windus, 1973), especially pp. 215–32.

23. See, for example, the testimony of Bradshaw Langmaid, Bureau of Science and Technology, USAID, on funding criteria for AIDS aid to African countries, in *AIDS and the Third World: The Impact on Development,* Hearing before the Select Committee on Hunger, U.S. House of Representatives, 100th Cong., 2d sess., June 30, 1988, Serial No. 100–29 (Washington, D.C.: U.S. Government Printing Office, 1988), pp. 33–34.

24. Most studies depend on some degree of cooperation between the First and the Third World and are thus influenced by the scientific and political commitments of given agencies and their ability to find common grounds of inquiry as well as resources. Scarce resources have created wide variation in scientific research in Africa; yet much more research goes on than stereotypes about Africa would suggest. Needless to say, views on cooperation with Western scientists are also highly variable, reflecting in some respects the ideological commitments of the state as a whole. See Sabatier, *Blaming Others,* pp. 108–9, on the distinction between the many long-term collaborative projects that predate AIDS and what African commentators call "parachute research" or "tourist research," in which foreign researchers drop in "to collect blood samples, data or

clinical observations, and just quickly [take] off again, to write up their findings for a (Western) scientific journal."

25 Jonathan M. Mann et al., "The International Epidemiology of AIDS," *Scientific American*, October 1988, pp. 82–89, at p. 82. See also Peter Piot et al., "AIDS: An International Perspective," *Science* 239 (1988): 573–79. Monthly statistical updates are available from the Pan-American Health Organization in Washington, D.C., WHO's regional health office for the Americas. Though the worldwide estimate of HIV infection is often given in the press as five to ten million, official estimates are somewhat lower: six to eight million was the estimate given at the Sixth International Conference on AIDS in San Francisco by Dr. Michael Merson, Mann's replacement as head of WHO's Global AIDS Program (Roland De Wolk, "Parley Opens with a Bleak Prognosis," *Oakland Tribune*, June 21, 1990, pp. A1, A4).

26. Mann et al., "International Epidemiology of AIDS," p. 84; Piot et al., "AIDS: An International Perspective," p. 576.

27. Mann et al., "International Epidemiology of AIDS," p. 84. The Soviet Union did not report its first official "indigenous" death from AIDS until September 1988—a pregnant Leningrad prostitute named Olga Gaeevskaya; "Epidemiologists were incensed that the woman's doctors failed to diagnose AIDS before she died" (*Edmonton Journal*, October 11, 1988, p. A2). Another "outbreak" of HIV infection (the headline says "AIDS") occurred among twenty-seven babies and five of their mothers in a hospital in Elista, capital of a region along the Caspian Sea. Some authorities blame unsterilized needles for the babies' infection and suggest that the mothers' infection was contracted while they were breast-feeding the infected babies (John F. Burns, "Outbreak of AIDS Triples Testing in a Soviet City," *New York Times*, February 5, 1989, p. 29).

28. For assessments of the impact of AIDS on the Third World, see testimony in *AIDS and the Third World: The Impact on Development; AIDS Prevention and Control: Invited Presentations and Papers from the World Summit of Ministers of Health on Programs for AIDS Prevention* (Geneva: World Health Organization; Oxford: Pergamon Press, 1988) [Jointly organized UK government and WHO; held at Queen Elizabeth II Conference Centre, Westminster, London, on January 26–28, 1988]; Panos Institute, *AIDS and the Third World* (London: Panos, in assoc. with Norwegian Red Cross, 1989; Philadelphia: New Society Publishers, 1989 [trade edition of nontrade dossier published 1986, 1987]; Sabatier, *Blaming Others*; Cindy Patton, *Sex and Germs: The Politics of AIDS* (Boston: South End Press, 1985); Norman Miller and Richard C. Rockwell, eds., *AIDS in Africa: The Social and Policy Impact* (Lewiston, N.Y.: Edwin Mellen Press, 1988); R. M. Anderson, R. M. May, and A. R. McLean, "Possible Demographic Consequences of AIDS in Developing Countries," *Nature* 332 (1988): 228–34; Robert J. Biggar, "Overview: Africa, AIDS, and Epidemiology," in *AIDS in Africa*, ed. Miller and Rockwell, pp. 1–8; Raymond W. Copson, *AIDS in Africa: Background/Issues for U.S. Policy* (Washington, D.C.: Congressional Research Service, Library of Congress, 1987 [17 pp.]); Christine Hawkins, "AIDS Expected to Slow Population Growth," *New Africa* 251 (August 1988): 25; Charles Hunt, "Africa and AIDS," *Monthly Review* 39, no. 9 (February 1988): 10–22; Institute of Medicine and National Academy of Sci-

ences, *Confronting AIDS: Update 1988* (Washington, D.C.: National Academy Press, 1988); Nancy Krieger, "The Epidemiology of AIDS in Africa," *Science for the People,* January–February 1987, pp. 18–21; M. Over et al., "The Direct and Indirect Costs of HIV Infection in Developing Countries: The Cases of Zaire and Tanzania," paper presented at the International Conference on the Global Impact of AIDS, London, March 8–10, 1988; Kenneth Prewitt, "AIDS in Africa: The Triple Disaster," in *AIDS in Africa,* ed. Miller and Rockwell, pp. ix–xv; Jane Perlez, "Africans Weigh Threat of AIDS to Economies," *New York Times,* September 22, 1988, p. 16; Al J. Venter, "AIDS: Its Strategic Consequences in Black Africa," *International Defense Review* 21 (April 1988): 357–59; Gloria Waite, "The Politics of Disease: The AIDS Virus and Africa," in *AIDS in Africa,* ed. Miller and Rockwell, pp. 145–64; Catharine Watson, "Africa's AIDS Time Bomb: Region Scrambles to Fight Epidemic," *The Guardian,* June 17, 1987, pp. 10–11.

29. Miller and Rockwell, "Introduction," in *AIDS in Africa,* pp. xxiv–xiv.

30. Quoted in Marilyn Chase, "Rich Nations Urged to Help Poor Lands Fight AIDS by Backing WHO Program," *Wall Street Journal,* June 17, 1988, p. 4. On the evolution of the epidemic in Third World countries, see Lawrence K. Altman, "New Support from Africa as WHO Plans Effort on AIDS," *New York Times,* December 22, 1985, p. 11; Erik Eckholm, "AIDS, an Unknown Disease before 1981, Grows into a Worldwide Scourge," *New York Times,* March 16, 1987, p. 11; Thomas W. Netter, "AIDS Spurs Countries to Act as Cases Rise around World," *New York Times,* March 22, 1987, p. 18; Steven V. Roberts, "Politicians Awaken to the Threat of a Global Epidemic," *New York Times,* June 7, 1987, sec. 4, p. 1; "AIDS Now Is a Global Public Health Crisis, Harvard MD Stresses," *American Medical News,* June 12, 1987, p. 19. On international cooperation see Simon Watney, "Our Rights and Our Dignity," *Gay Times,* March 1988, pp. 32–34; Sabatier, *Blaming Others;* Amadou Traore, "Meeting Point: Dr. Gottlieb Monekosso, WHO Regional Director for Africa," *The Courier* [Africa-Caribbean-Pacific-European Community] 105 (September–October 1987): 2–5. A cooperative international policy is outlined in the document *Concerning a Common European Public Health Policy to Fight the Acquired Immunodeficiency Syndrome (AIDS),* Council of Europe Committee of Ministers Recommendation No. R (87) 25; adopted at the 81st session, November 26, 1987. Jonathan Mann, former director of the Global AIDS Program, advocates aggressive, activist strategies to achieve global cooperation; in an "AIDS Monitor" column on the January 1988 global summit (*New Scientist,* February 4, 1988, p. 32), Mann states that the international declaration reached at the summit represents "an extraordinary consensus." The impact of the epidemic at decade's end is assessed in a four-part series in the *New York Times* which ran from September 16 to 19, 1990: Erik Eckholm with John Tierney, "AIDS in Africa: A Killer Rages On," September 16, pp. A1, A11; John Tierney, "AIDS Tears Lives of the African Family," September 17, pp. A1, A6; John Tierney, "With 'Social Marketing,' Condoms Combat AIDS," September 18, pp. A1, A6; Erik Eckholm, "Confronting the Cruel Reality of Africa's AIDS Epidemic," September 19, pp. A1, A14.

31. (1) Mann et al., "International Epidemiology of AIDS," p. 84; (2) Cop-

son, *AIDS in Africa*, p. 9; (3) Mann et al., "International Epidemiology of AIDS," p. 84; (4) Watson, "Africa's AIDS Time Bomb," p. 10; (5) Hilts, "Out of Africa," p. 12; (6) Mary Harper, "AIDS in Africa—Plague or Propaganda?" *West Africa*, November 7–13, 1988, pp. 2072–73, at p. 2072.

32. For an overview of problems associated with diagnosis and testing, see Albert E. Gunn et al., *AIDS in Africa* (Washington, D.C.: Foundation for America's Future, 1988); R. Sher, "Seroepidemiology of HIV in Africa from 1970–1974," *New England Journal of Medicine* 317, no. 7 (August 13, 1987): 450–51; I. Wendler, "Seroepidemiology of HIV in Africa," *British Journal of Medicine* 293 (September 27, 1986): 782–85; World Health Organization and Centers for Disease Control, "HIV Not Related to Monkeys," *WHO-CDC AIDS Weekly Report*, July 25, 1988, p. 8. See also Dieter Koch-Weser and Hannelove Vanderschmidt, eds., *The Heterosexual Transmission of AIDS in Africa* (Cambridge, Mass.: Abt Books, 1988), especially Felix I. D. Konotey-Ahulu, "AIDS in Africa: Misinformation and Disinformation," pp. 24–25.

33. Sander I. Gilman, *Disease and Representation: Images of Illness from Madness to AIDS* (Ithaca, N.Y.: Cornell University Press, 1988). An influential anthropological source for rumors about exotic behaviors has been Daniel B. Hrdy, "Cultural Practices Contributing to the Transmission of HIV in Africa," *Reviews of Infectious Diseases* 9, no. 6 (November–December 1987): 1109–19. The rumors preserve bits and pieces of such anthropological research without its larger cultural context. The first major study of prostitutes is Joan K. Kreiss et al., "AIDS Virus Infection in Nairobi Prostitutes: Spread of the Epidemic to East Africa," *New England Journal of Medicine* 314, no. 7 (February 13, 1986): 414–18. A detailed critique of many studies can be found in Richard C. Chirimuuta and Roaslind J. Chirimuuta, *AIDS, Africa, and Racism* (London: Free Association Books, 1989), who also suggest that "underreporting" is no more a problem than "overdiagnosing." See also Cynthia Haq, "Data on AIDS in Africa: An Assessment," and Barbara Boyle Torrey, Peter O.Way, and Patricia Rowe, "Epidemiology of HIV and AIDS in Africa: Emerging Issues and Social Implications," both in *AIDS in Africa*, ed. Miller and Rockwell, pp. 9–19 and 31–54. A general critique of studies on AIDS in Africa is provided by Margaret Cerullo and Evelynn Hammonds, "AIDS in Africa: The Western Imagination and the Dark Continent," *Radical America* 21, nos. 2–3 (March–April 1987): 17–23, and Krieger, "Epidemiology of AIDS in Africa." An attempt to place AIDS statistics within a broader political and economic perspective is presented in Carol Barker and Meredeth Turshen, "Briefings: AIDS in Africa," *Review of African Political Economy* 27, no 105 (January–March 1986): 51–54. An elaborate web of speculation about Haiti can be found in Alexander Moore and Ronald LeBaron, "The Case for a Haitian Origin of the AIDS Epidemic," in *The Social Dimensions of AIDS*, ed. Douglas Feldman and Thomas Johnson (New York: Praeger, 1986), pp. 77–93. The historical debate over "the Haitian origin of syphilis," of course, goes back centuries, a debate noted in his critique of Moore and LeBaron by Paul Farmer, "The Exotic and the Mundane: Human Immunodeficiency Virus in Haiti," *Human Nature* 1, no 4 (1990): 415–45.

34. Nathan Clumeck, "AIDS in Africa," in *AIDS: Pathogenesis and Treat-*

ment, ed. Jay A. Levy (New York: Marcel Dekker, 1989), pp. 37–63. Existing studies are summarized by Clumeck; by Hilts, in "Out of Africa"; and by Torrey et al., in "Epidemiology of HIV and AIDS in Africa." On the clinical manifestations of AIDS in Haiti, see Warren D. Johnson, Jr., and Jean W. Pape, "AIDS In Haiti," in *AIDS: Pathogenesis and Treatment,* ed. Levy, pp. 65–78; interactions of AIDS with tuberculosis are discussed on pp. 72–77.

35. See, for example, Caputo, "Uganda: Land beyond Sorrow"; Lloyd Timberlake, *Africa in Crisis: The Causes, the Cures of Environmental Bankruptcy,* ed. Jon Tinker (Philadelphia: New Society Publishers, 1986); and ongoing coverage in the Nairobi *Weekly Review.*

36. Jamie Feldman, "Identity, Illness, and the Process of Giving Meaning: French Medical Discourse on AIDS," unpublished manuscript, University of Illinois at Urbana-Champaign, July 1988. See also Michael Pollack, *Les homosexuels et le SIDA: Sociologie d'une épidémie* (Paris: Éditions A. M. Metailie, 1988).

37. Richard Parker, "Acquired Immunodeficiency Syndrome in Brazil," *Medical Anthropology Quarterly* 1, no. 2 (1987): 155–75, at pp. 158, 159.

38. David Seftel, "AIDS and Apartheid: Double Trouble," *Africa Report* (November–December 1988): 17–22, at p. 21.

39. See Elizabeth Fee, "Sex Education in Cuba: An Interview with Dr. Celestino Alvarez Lajonchere," *International Journal of Health Services* 18, no. 2 (1988): 343–56; Nicholas Wade, "Cuba's Quarantine for AIDS: A Police State's Health Experiment," *New York Times* editorial, February 6, 1989, p. A14; Richard Goldstein, "AIDS Arrest: The Cuban Solution," *Village Voice,* February 14, 1989, p. 18.

40. Though these dichotomies are primarily social, the differentiation among types of AIDS and strains of HIV is also a scientific and clinical question. See, for example, Clumeck, "AIDS in Africa."

41. Hilts (in "Out of Africa," p. 12) notes the incredulity that greeted the appearance of AIDS in Africa. He quotes a pulmonary specialist in Uganda who first saw AIDS there in 1983: "It looked like the new American disease. But none of us could believe it." But before too long, AIDS began to be blamed on the loose morals of African people—always those in other countries, classes, or ethnic groups. Thus, an editorial in the *Kenya Times* (Nairobi), May 26, 1987, blamed Uganda for lax sexual behavior, noting that "nature has its own law of retribution." See discussion in Sabatier, *Blaming Others,* p. 105. In contrast, see Frank Browning, "AIDS: The Mythology of Plague," *Tikkun* 3, no. 2 (March–April 1988): 69–71. Browning says that most descriptions of U.S. subcultures involved in AIDS make them sound "as strange as those of Bantu twig gatherers" (p. 70).

42. Clyde Haberman, "Japan Plans to Deny Visas over AIDS," *New York Times,* April 1, 1987, p. A18. According to a report in the *Independent* (London), February 14, 1987, when the death of a Japanese prostitute in Kobe was attributed to AIDS, the immediate conclusion was that she had been infected by sexual contact with a foreigner; as one Japanese newspaper put it, "Her death was the result of an infatuation with Europe." Sabatier (in *Blaming Others,* p. 114) notes that "in the red light district of Tokyo warning signs suddenly

appeared: '*Gaijin* [foreigners] off limits.' " For a more extended discussion, see James W. Dearing, "Foreign Blood and Domestic Politics: The Issue of AIDS in Japan," in this volume.

43. Parker, "Acquired Immunodeficiency Syndrome in Brazil," p. 157; and Alan Riding, "AIDS in Brazil: Taboo of Silence Ends," *New York Times,* October 28, 1987, p. 8.

44. Sabatier, *Blaming Others,* pp. 106–7. See also Robert Pear, "U.S. Seeks to Bar Aliens with AIDS," *New York Times,* March 27, 1987, p. A18; and Serge Schmemann, "Calls of 'Hi Sailor' Get the Heave-Ho," *New York Times,* May 14, 1988, p. 4.

45. Dubos, *Mirage of Health,* p. 218; many researchers characterize AIDS as a "disease of development," among them Marc H. Dawson, "AIDS in Africa: Historical Roots," in *AIDS in Africa,* ed. Miller and Rockwell, pp. 58–69. Virchow is cited in Paul Epstein and Randall Packard, "Ecology and Immunology," *Science for the People* (January–February 1987): 10–17, who also discuss AIDS and development.

46. Brooke Grundfest Schoepf et al., "AIDS and Society in Central Africa: A View from Zaire," in *AIDS in Africa,* ed. Miller and Rockwell, pp. 211–35, at p. 218.

47. Ibid., p. 228; the authors observed (as USAID, apparently, did not) that condoms "which hurt their wearer or break during normal use may limit the effectiveness of AIDS prevention efforts." See also Hooper, *Slim.*

48. Gill Gordon and Tony Klouda, *Preventing a Crisis* (London: International Planned Parenthood Federation, 1988). Reviewed by Harper, "AIDS in Africa—Plague or Propaganda?"

49. Schoepf et al., p. 219. Few alternatives to the condom exist. At the Fifth International Conference on AIDS in Montreal, there was for the first time discussion of a female condom and of the use of spermicides without the use of condoms; but at the Sixth International Conference in San Francisco, some data suggested that for some women the use of spermicides might *increase* the risk of HIV transmission by causing inflammation and breakdown of the vaginal mucosa.

50. Parker, "Acquired Immunodeficiency Syndrome in Brazil," p. 161.

51. Ibid., pp. 160–63. I have greatly oversimplified Parker's intricate representation of Brazilian sexuality, which, as he emphasizes, is not the mere overlay of a Western ethnographer but permeates language, slang, informal discussion, and ongoing open debate about sexuality as an essential aspect of cultural identity and "Brazilianness." But the penetrator/recipient and other distinctions that construct masculinity/femininity between same-sex partners occur elsewhere, including the United States. See Charles F. Turner, Heather G. Miller, and Lincoln E. Moses, eds., *AIDS: Sexual Behavior and Intravenous Drug Use* (Washington, D.C.: National Academy Press, 1989), pp. 73–185, for an illuminating review of recent research on "same-gender sexual behaviors" in several cultural settings. See also Ralph Bolton, "A Selected Bibliography on AIDS and Anthropology" (forthcoming in *Journal of Sex Research*). For an analysis of sexuality from a different perspective, but one potentially helpful in articulating women's concerns, see the conclusions and recommendations "adopted by the group of

experts" at a UNESCO conference in Madrid, March 12–21, 1986 ("UNESCO: On Prostitution and Strategies against Promiscuity and Sexual Exploitation of Women," *Echo* [Newsletter of the Association of African Women for Research and Development] 1, nos. 2–3 (1986): 16–17).

52. Sabatier, *Blaming Others*, p. 134.

53. Timberlake, *Africa in Crisis*, p. 8.

54. Sabatier, *Blaming Others*, p. 4.

55. Williams, *The Country and the City*, p. 284.

56. *Emerging AIDS Markets: A Worldwide Study of Drugs, Vaccines, and Diagnostics* (New Haven, Conn.: Technology Management Group, August 1986). See also Vicki Glaser, "AIDS Crisis Spurs Hunt for New Tests,"*High Technology Business* 8, no. 1 (January 1988); and Manny Ratafia and Frederick I. Scott, Jr., "AIDS: A Glimpse of Its Impact," *American Clinical Products Review* (May 1987): 26–29; this article also makes clear the size and diversity of the "AIDS market" for the development of clinical products.

57. See Gina Kolata, "Africa Is Favored for AIDS Testing," *New York Times*, February 19, 1988, p. 7; the "AIDS Monitor" column in the *New Scientist*, February 18, 1988, p. 36; and Jane Perlez, "Scientists from Western Countries Pressing for AIDS Studies in Africa," *New York Times*, September 18, 1988, p. B5. Perlez, reporting vaccine discussions at a conference in Tanzania on AIDS and Africa, writes: "In Africa, unlike the United States, the virus is most commonly spread through heterosexual contact. Officials believe that, despite warnings to use condoms and avoid multiple partners, further spread of the virus is inevitable. . . . Because of behavioral changes brought about by extensive education about AIDS, the spread of the infection among gay men in the United States has slowed. Thus, there would be few new infections in a study group, whether or not its members took the vaccine, the scientists said. The scientists said they regarded intravenous drug users, a group that continues to have a high incidence of AIDS in the United States, as unreliable for the necessary follow-up that is needed for a study group." A WHO committee developing ethical guidelines for vaccine testing said the decision to go ahead should be made by three groups: scientists developing the vaccine, scientists knowledgeable about vaccine development but with no academic or commercial stakes in it, and "government officials and their scientific advisers from the population where the vaccine is to be tried." No representatives of the population to be tested are mentioned.

58. V. Y. Mudimbe, *The Invention of Africa: Gnosis, Philosophy, and the Order of Knowledge* (Bloomington: Indiana University Press, 1988), p. 195.

59. Pratt, "Fieldwork in Common Places."

60. Nairobi *Standard*, January 15 and 18, 1985. For the development of research on AIDS in Africa, see Ruth Kulstad, ed., *AIDS: Papers from Science, 1982–1985* (Washington, D.C.: American Association for the Advancement of Science, 1986); and Koch-Weser and Vanderschmidt, *The Heterosexual Transmission of AIDS in Africa*.

61. Lawrence K. Altman, "Linking AIDS to Africa Provokes Bitter Debate," *New York Times*, November 21, 1985, p. 1.

62. Altman, "Linking AIDS," p. 1. On the "international furor" see espe-

cially Chirimuuta and Chirimuuta, *AIDS, Africa, and Racism;* and Richard C. Chirimuuta, Rosalind Harrison, and Davis Gazi, "AIDS: The Spread of Racism," *West Africa,* February 9, 1987, pp. 261–62.

63. In the Western media AIDS in the Third World is used to draw conclusions about the West. Thus, Selzer's view that Haiti is "devastated" is intended to serve as a cautionary lesson about gay excess. Stories about Africa may likewise serve to warn Western readers about themselves. "FUTURE SHOCK," proclaimed the cover of *Newsweek* in December 1986, citing new worrisome projections of AIDS increases in the United States; a related cover headline was titled "AFRICA: THE FUTURE IS NOW." On AIDS and the media in general, see James Dearing and Everett M. Rogers, "The Agenda-Setting Process for the Issue of AIDS," paper presented at the International Communication Association, May 28–June 2, 1988; and Kinsella, *Covering the Plague.*

64. Quoted in Sabatier, *Blaming Others,* p. 97.

65. Alfred J. Fortin, "The Politics of AIDS in Kenya," *Third World Quarterly* 9, no. 3 (July 1987): 906–19, at p. 907. See also Alfred J. Fortin, "AIDS and the Third World: the Politics of International Discourse," paper prepared for the 14th World Congress of the International Political Science Association, Washington, D.C., August 28–September 1, 1988.

66. Hilary Ng'weno, "The Politics of AIDS in Kenya," *Weekly Review,* September 4, 1987, pp. 11–13.

67. Mudimbe, *The Invention of Africa.*

68. The naming of AIDS internationally is addressed by Sabatier, *Blaming Others;* Hooper, *Slim;* and Farmer, "The Exotic and the Mundane."

69. Miller and Rockwell, *AIDS in Africa,* p. xxiii.

70. Ibid., p. xxiii.

71. Nancy Schmidt, "African Press Reports on the Social Impact of AIDS on Women and Children in Africa," paper presented at conference on the Impact of AIDS on Maternal-Child Health Care Delivery in Africa, University of Illinois, Urbana-Champaign, May 6, 1990.

Notes on Contributors

Ronald Bayer is associate professor at the School of Public Health, Columbia University. He spent ten years at The Hastings Center, a research institute devoted to the study of ethical questions in medicine, and has authored or edited many books and articles on ethical and political controversies in medicine, including his most recent book, *Private Acts, Social Consequences: AIDS and the Politics of Public Health* (1991).

Virginia Berridge is senior lecturer and deputy director of the AIDS Social History Programme at the London School of Hygiene and Tropical Medicine. Her previous publications include *Opium and the People: Opiate Use in Nineteenth-Century England* (1987) and "Health and Medicine, 1750–1950" in the *Cambridge Social History of England* (1990).

Stephen L. Boswell is director of HIV Clinical Services at Massachusetts General Hospital and a researcher in the Harvard/Boston City Hospital AIDS Clinical Trials Unit. He is a Kaiser Scholar in health policy and management at the Massachusetts Institute of Technology, and his research interests include the organization and operation of the U.S. blood industry.

David C. Colby is principal policy analyst at the Physician Payment Commission, and has previously been a Robert Wood Johnson Faculty Fellow in health care finance. He has published

articles on health cost containment, physician payment methodologies, Medicaid policies, and AIDS issues.

Timothy E. Cook is associate professor and chair of the Department of Political Science at Williams College, Williamstown,
Massachusetts. An American Political Science Congressional Fellow in 1984–85, he is the author of *Making Laws and Making
News: Media Strategies in the U.S. House of Representatives*
(1989). In addition to his continuing work on television news
and the politics of AIDS, he is currently writing a book on the
national news media as a political institution.

James W. Dearing is assistant professor in the Department of
Communication at Michigan State University, East Lansing. He
has lived for two years in Tokyo, investigating mass media and
scientific communications in Japan.

Don C. Des Jarlais is director of research for the Chemical Dependency Institute at Beth Israel Medical Center, deputy director
for AIDS research with Narcotic and Drug Research, Inc., and
professor of community medicine at Mount Sinai's Department
of Community Medicine, all in New York City. A leader in the
field of AIDS and intravenous drug use, he is a member of the
U.S. National Commission on Acquired Immune Deficiency Syndrome.

Harold Edgar is Julius Silver Professor of Law at Columbia University School of Law. His fields of expertise include food and
drug law, and he is a founding fellow of The Hastings Center, a
research institute for the study of ethical questions in medicine.

Paul Epstein is medical director of the Cambridge Hospital Mul-
tidisciplinary AIDS program, instructor of medicine at Harvard
School of Medicine, and of the Cambridge City AIDS Task Force,
which focuses on multicultural education, public and school policy, and care for HIV infected persons. He has worked as a physician in Mozambique and has visited Kenya, Uganda, Zambia,
Zimbabwe, South Africa, and Mozambique investigating AIDS
programs.

Elizabeth Fee is associate professor of history and health policy
at the Johns Hopkins School of Hygiene and Public Health and
member of the Johns Hopkins Institute of the History of Medi-

cine. Her books include *Disease and Discovery* (1987), *AIDS: The Burdens of History* (with Daniel M. Fox, 1988), and *A History of Education in Public Health: Health That Mocks the Doctors' Rules* (with Roy M. Acheson, 1991).

Daniel M. Fox is president of the Milbank Memorial Fund in New York City. He has written, coauthored, or edited fifteen books and published many articles about health and social policy, the history of economic and social thought, and the history of medicine. His previous work on AIDS includes *AIDS: The Burdens of History* (with Elizabeth Fee, 1988).

Samuel R. Friedman is senior principal investigator for Narcotic and Drug Research, Inc. and has been engaged in research into AIDS epidemiology and prevention since 1983. He is author of over one hundred publications in this field.

Larry Gostin is executive director of the American Society of Law and Medicine, adjunct associate professor of health law at Harvard School of Public Health, lecturer on law at Harvard Law School, and associate director of the World Health Organization/ Harvard University International Collaborating Center on Health Legislation. In 1983 he received the distinguished Rosmary Delbridge Memorial Award for the person in Great Britain "who has most influenced Parliament and government to act for the welfare of society."

Ann Meredith has chronicled women's culture since 1970. Through oral histories and photographic portraits, she has documented the issues of women and aging, women in nontraditional work, alternative life-styles, international concerns, cowgirls of the West, incest, rape and abuse, and women living with AIDS.

Stephen S. Morse is assistant professor of virology at Rockefeller University, New York. He was chair of the Conference on Emerging Viruses (National Institutes of Health, 1989), is editor of the forthcoming *Emerging Viruses* and *Evolutionary Biology of Viruses,* and serves on the Committee on Microbial Threats to Health at the Institute of Medicine–National Academy of Sciences.

Gerald M. Oppenheimer is associate professor of health sciences and nutrition at Brooklyn College and staff associate in the G. H.

Sergievsky Center, Faculty of Medicine, Columbia University. He has published papers on AIDS and health insurance, epidemiology, and the history of medicine.

Randall M. Packard is professor of history, chair of the History Department at Tufts University, and chair of the Joint Committee on African Studies of the Social Science Research Council. A former research fellow of the Harvard School of Public Health, he has done extensive research on the social history of health and disease in southern Africa. His recent publications include *White Plague, Black Labor: Tuberculosis and the Political Economy of Health and Disease in South Africa* (1989).

Robert A. Padgug was trained as a classical historian and is currently employed at a large insurance company, where he deals with health policy. His publications on the AIDS crisis include articles on cost and utilization issues and the role of the lesbian/gay community in the epidemic.

David J. Rothman is Bernard Schoenberg Professor of Social Medicine, professor of history, and director of the Center for the Study of Society and Medicine at Columbia University. His most recent book is *Strangers at the Bedside: A History of How Law and Bioethics Transformed Medical Decision Making* (1991).

Harvey M. Sapolsky is professor of public policy and organization in the Political Science Department at the Massachusetts Institute of Technology. He is a specialist in public policy issues involving large science and technology components, including particularly those in the health, communications, and defense fields.

Jo L. Sotheran is project director of Narcotic and Drug Research, Inc., and has worked as a sociologist in the AIDS field since 1984. Her current research is on the relation of social contexts, especially household and domestic factors, to risk behavior and services utilization among drug users.

Philip Strong, a microsociologist and ethnographer, is director of the AIDS Social History Programme at the London School of Hygiene and Tropical Medicine. His previous work includes *The Ceremonial Order of the Clinic* (1979); the eight-volume series *Health and Disease* (1985); and *The NHS: Under New Management* (1990).

Paula A. Treichler teaches at the University of Illinois at Urbana-Champaign in the College of Medicine, the Institute of Communications Research, and the Department of Women's Studies. Her books include *A Feminist Dictionary* (with C. Kramarge, 1986) and *Language, Gender, and Professional Writing* (with F. Frank, 1989). Her work on AIDS has appeared in *October, ArtForum, Transition,* and *Science.*

Index

Compositor: Maple-Vail Book Manufacturing Group
Text: 10/13 Sabon
Display: Sabon
Printer: Maple-Vail Book Manufacturing Group
Binder: Maple-Vail Book Manufacturing Group

JAN